To Dan, Mom, Dad, and my sisters and brothers:
Joanne, Joe, Alan, and Amy

Paulette Rollant

To David and my family

Joyce Hamlin

To my parents, Edward and Lottie, my nephew, Matthew, and my
nieces, Elizabeth and Sara

Karen Piotrowski

Preface

HOW TO USE *MOSBY'S RAPID REVIEW SERIES*

Mosby's Rapid Review Series is designed to help you get the most from your prep, study and review time for nursing exams. These books can be used to review essential concepts, theory, and content prior to nursing courses and challenge, certification, or licensing examinations. The rapid review series can also be used to prepare for clinical experiences and as a quick reference while in the clinical setting. *Mosby's Rapid Review Series* consists of three books:

Maternal-Child Nursing
Medical-Surgical Nursing
Nursing Pharmacology

The series is designed to highlight and prioritize important information about the specific content as indicated in each title. It is not meant to provide comprehensive, in-depth coverage of the selected area of nursing.

In the revised editions, the new features, "Fast Facts," "Warning," "Essential Odds and Ends" chapter, "WEB Resources," the updated bibliography, the glossary, and the revised questions, answers, and test tips give you the added advantage for test prep. The CD-ROM disk of 265 new higher level questions, which include management and home care content, provides an opportunity to practice for the real test.

Keep in mind that this series, in combination with other texts, should be consulted when a more comprehensive discussion of a particular topic is desired. Use these books to jog your memory, to reinforce what you know, to guide you to identify what you don't know, and to lead you to appropriate sources for more details. If you are in a formal education setting, these books are not intended as a substitute for class attendance or the completion of any required reading assignments.

Used consistently and correctly, *Mosby's Rapid Review Series* can help you to:

1. Enhance your skills to prioritize in clinical situations, especially management and home care situations, by applying the nursing process.
2. Increase your ability to easily remember essential content.

3. Increase the productivity of your review and study time to leave time for you and your family.
4. Apply new behaviors for the improvement of your test-taking skills.
5. Evaluate your strengths and weaknesses for specific content areas or testing situations.

WHAT IS UNIQUE ABOUT *MOSBY'S RAPID REVIEW SERIES?*

1. The 265-question test on an accompanying CD-ROM
2. Comprehensive rationales for each answer option
3. Test-taking tips to eliminate test-taking errors
4. Chapter format of the nursing process with prioritized content
5. Web sites and traditional bibliography for further exploration of content areas
6. Odds and Ends chapter for the unfamiliar
7. Glossary of key terms

Test questions on CD-ROM

Each book in the series is accompanied by a comprehensive exam of 265 questions. The comprehensive exam questions, like the end-of-chapter questions, include the answers, comprehensive rationales, and test-taking tips. The disk has a tutorial and a test mode. Both allow you to repeat the test as many times as you wish. The level of the questions varies from knowledge, recall, application, and analysis. In many of the questions, all the options are correct; the task of the test taker is to select the highest priority.

Comprehensive rationales

The rationales include the answers and the rationales for each option. In questions where all options are correct but they must be prioritized, rationales state why or how each option is correct and why only one option is the best answer.

Test-taking tips

These tips build your decision-making skills to set nursing priorities and for managing and delivering home care wisely. The tips help to further develop your logical thinking skills to narrow the options to two and then select the correct answer based on what you know. After working with the questions in these books or on the CD-ROM, you will more often select the correct answer on those harder questions. You will have increased confidence from new learning methods and actions to think "how can I answer this question" rather than "if I only knew. . . ." You will learn how to get the correct answer on those questions about content you don't know.

Chapter format

Each chapter contains an easy-to-follow format divided into five sections:

1. "Fast Facts" are placed at the beginning of each chapter. These items are the "must know" information in that chapter.

2. "Content Review" is organized and structured by the nursing process to help you identify what is most important. Within each chapter the highlights include:
   • Prioritized information within each heading
   • Prioritized nursing diagnoses
   • Client-centered goals
   • The "Warning" feature is used throughout and focuses on critical and life-threatening issues
   • Client education is focused for the settings of hospital, clinics, and home
   • Management and home care content are included where applicable
   • You are alerted to issues regarding older adults where applicable
   • Evaluation criteria include decision-making tools about which actions to take when the client's clinical status shows improvement or deterioration
   • Tables, charts, and figures contrast, cluster, and simplify information for ease of grasp, recall, and review
3. "Review Questions" are stand-alone, four-option multiple choice questions. The test questions are of all difficulty levels and include management and home care situations for decision-making. The stems vary from being brief to lengthy to provide a realistic drill that mimics the NCLEX exam.
4. "Answers, Rationales, and Test-Taking Tips" focus on:
   • Comprehensive rationales, which are given for each option to explain why or how it is correct or incorrect. Additional information is given for less common facts or entities in the options. Other pertinent advice is also included to help you recall or review unfamiliar content or issues.
   • Test-taking tips, which give actions and strategies to use. For the more difficult questions, such as when options are narrowed to two; when you have no idea of a correct answer; when the content or issue is unfamiliar; or when all of the options are correct answers, specific approaches are given for each type of situation. The explanations include ways to prevent test-taking errors and ways to change your reading of the stem and options to get results—more correct answers. Specific prescriptions are given to raise your test scores.

"WEB resources" and bibliography

Web site resources for a particular condition, disorder, or topic are found throughout each book. A bibliography, including some books used in the development of the series, suggests areas for further study if more in-depth facts are needed.

Glossary

This list of key terms is provided to save you time in looking up unfamiliar terms or words.

WHAT'S IN *MOSBY'S RAPID REVIEW SERIES: MATERNAL-CHILD NURSING?*

This book is divided into two parts. It begins with coverage of the pregnant woman and her support system during the periods of the antepartal, labor process, and fetal birth. The needs of the postpartal woman and her support system during the fourth trimester are then emphasized. The processes of recovery and adaptation, with the resolution of problems during the puerperium are included. The remaining chapters in the maternal section focus on the needs of the newborn. The physiologic adaptations to extrauterine life, alterations in the newborn's health status, and the application of the nursing process to the needs of the newborn are presented.

Part two of the book is devoted to child nursing with the focus on the more common pathological entities in children. The initial chapters take a head-to-toe systems approach, with the neurologic, cardiovascular, hematologic, immunologic, and respiratory systems detailed. The rest of the chapters have a more global and safety approach, with the areas of elimination, mobility, endocrine disorders, and the special needs of children covered.

This sequence of content will enhance your ability to recall content, especially if you have developed a study or review plan that is similar. This type of sequence is also typically used to complete a normal nursing assessment during pregnancy and afterwards.

Each chapter is a synthesis of the many essentials needed by nurses in practice. The content is prioritized in the major and minor lists. The most common elements are written to include what is essential for study, review, and to reference items in an expedient manner. The most common normal and abnormal events are included in each chapter. Acute and home care is part of each discussion.

ABOUT THE AUTHORS

The original idea, the design, and the development of the *Rapid Review Series* were by Dr. Rollant. The original co-authors were the content experts for their respective books. They provided their expertise and hard work to develop the specific content and the questions. In the first edition, Dr. Rollant expanded the rationales for the question answers and then added the test-taking tips for each question.

In this revised second edition, each book has an author who is expert in the field, and Dr. Rollant is the series editor. Content experts Joyce Hamlin, author of the pediatric section, and Karen Piotrowski, author of the maternity section, have united their efforts in this combined Maternal-Child Nursing review book to create the most effective study tool available. Dr. Rollant has directed, coordinated, and managed the consistency of the revision as well as provided additional test questions, rationales, and test-taking tips. Dr. Rollant, with the expertise of test-taking skills development, expanded the discussion in the rationales for the correct answer and the discussion of each option for the questions written by the authors.

As a team, the series editor and the authors have worked diligently to provide the best test preparation and review format available to nursing students and graduates. We wish you the best in your nursing career. We encourage you to let us know what you have found the most or least helpful and what other needs you may have for test preparation. You can contact us through Mosby, Inc. Nursing Editorial Department, 11830 Westline Industrial Drive, St. Louis, MO 63146, or e-mail Dr. Rollant at rollant@bellsouth.net.

ACKNOWLEDGMENTS

I express my heartfelt gratitude to those who have endured with me throughout this publication opportunity of a nursing review series: an adventure from idea to reality.

I especially want to thank the following people who were involved in the first edition of the review series:

Beverly Copland, who thought that I had the potential to complete this project and who eagerly gave me tons of strong support in the initial and ongoing book development phases.

Laurie Muench, who picked up the ball in the middle of manuscript preparation and persisted with me through the process to completion of book publication. The response "OK . . . when can I expect it?" provided silent encouragement and sometimes comic relief when my mental and physical energies ran quite low. Laurie's thoughtfulness and guidance to help me set priorities were invaluable! I am very grateful and fortunate to have worked with Laurie.

Suzi Epstein, who was full of enthusiasm and total support from the birth of the idea to the final publication of the books. Suzi's creativity and suggestions provided essential building blocks in the overall development of the series.

My *coauthors*, for their enormous efforts to produce manuscript in a short time. Their nursing expertise was helpful for the development of the unique aspects of each book.

I also want to thank the following people who were involved in this second edition of the series:

Brian Dennison, who headed up the meeting of the authors for the revisions, coordinated the manuscript schedule and provided guidance up to the production of the changes. Brian's creativity, framed with his organizational skills, allowed for the process to be quite enjoyable. Brian's patience and steadiness were of great strength to me.

Nancy O'Brien, who entered at the production phase and carried the task to completion; however, not without a lot of bumps along the way. Nancy left no stone unturned as she strongly supported my colleagues and me. I appreciate her talent, skills, and patience to enter a project midway and complete it with ease and detail.

My wonderful husband, *Dan*, for his patience, humor, support, and love. His faith in my abilities has sustained my energies and maintained my sense of self. He has been my sounding board throughout both editions of the review series and through the publication of the *Soar to Success: Do Your Best on Nursing Tests* book.

My parents, *Joseph* (deceased March 7, 2000) and *Mildred Demaske*, for their love, encouragement, and prayers.

Paulette Demaske Rollant

I wish to acknowledge *Paulette Rollant, Loren Wilson, Brian Dennison,* and *Karen Piotrowski* for their support and dedication to the Rapid Review Series. Special thanks to my husband, *David,* and to my mother, *Helen Kosco,* for their encouragement and support.

Joyce Hamlin

I wish to acknowledge with special thanks:

My parents, *Edward* and *Lottie Piotrowski,* for their unwavering support and encouragement.

Irene M. Bobak, Beverly Copland, and *Debra Roberts,* for providing me with the opportunity to begin writing for Mosby.

Paulette Rollant, Laurie Muench, and *Brian Dennison,* for their invaluable guidance during the preparation of both the first and second editions of this text.

My coauthor, *Joyce Hamlin,* for her support and for her commitment to working together to create a text that combines the specialty areas in nursing that we both love.

And finally, *my colleagues* in the Department of Nursing at D'Youville college, for their inspiration and encouragement.

Karen Piotrowski

Contents

PART TWO
Pediatric Nursing
by Joyce Hamlin

INTRODUCTION
How to Use This Book
for Rapid Review &
Study

This book is designed to work for you at your convenience to save you time and energy. Read the following guidelines first. They will help save you additional time and energy for test preparation. These guidelines are divided into three areas of concern: the NCLEX–RN test plan structure, rapid study steps, and rapid review tips.

The chapters in this book are designed for short, quick intervals of review. Carry this book with you to catch the those times when you are stuck and have nothing to do for that 5 to 15 minutes, and talk yourself into a brief rapid review and study period.

The directions for rapid review and study will give you the edge to:

- Maximize your individual performance on test prep and test questions
- Identify your personal priorities for test prep
- Sharpen your thinking and discrimination skills on multiple choice tests*

NCLEX–RN test plan structure

The framework of *client needs* is the universal structure used on the NCLEX-RN. This framework of client needs defines the nursing actions and expected competencies across all settings for all clients. An integration of concepts and processes with nursing practice will be tested on the NCLEX-RN throughout the following four major categories of *client needs*. These categories, their subcategories, and related content, which includes but is not limited to this list, are:

1. Safe, effective care environment
   - Management of care: advanced directives, advocacy, case management, client rights, concepts of management, confidentiality, continuity of care,

delegation, ethical practice, continuous quality improvement,
incident/irregular occurrence/variance reports, informed consent, legal
responsibilities, organ donation, consultation and referrals, resource
management, supervision
- Safety and infection control: accident prevention, disaster planning, error
prevention, handling hazardous and infectious materials, medical and
surgical asepsis, standard (universal) precautions, use of restraints
2. Health promotion and maintenance
- Growth and development through the life span: the aging process,
ante/intra/postpartum and newborn stages, developmental stages and
transitions, expected body image changes, family planning, family systems,
human sexuality
- Prevention and early detection of disease: disease prevention, health and
wellness, health promotion programs, health screening, immunizations,
lifestyle choices, techniques of physical assessment
3. Psychosocial integrity
- Coping and adaptation: coping mechanisms, counseling techniques, grief
and loss, mental health concepts, religious and spiritual influences on health,
sensory/perceptual alterations, situational role changes, stress management,
support systems, unexpected body image changes
- Psychosocial adaptation: behavioral interventions, chemical dependency,
child abuse/neglect, crisis intervention, domestic violence, elder
abuse/neglect, psychopathology, sexual abuse, and therapeutic milieu
4. Physiological integrity
- Basic care and comfort: assistive devices, elimination, mobility/immobility,
non-pharmacologic comfort interventions, nutrition and oral hygiene,
personal hygiene, rest and sleep
- Pharmacological and parenteral therapies: administration of blood and blood
products, central venous access devices, chemotherapy, expected effects,
intravenous therapy, medication administration, parenteral fluids,
pharmacologic actions and agents, side effects, total parenteral nutrition,
untoward effects
- Reduction, risk potential: alterations in body systems, diagnostic tests,
laboratory values, pathophysiology, therapeutic procedures, potential
complications after tests, procedures, surgery, and health alterations
- Physiological adaptation: alterations in body systems, fluid and electrolyte
imbalances, hemodynamics, infectious diseases, medical emergencies,
pathophysiology, radiation therapy, respiratory care, unexpected response to
therapies

Website: http://www.ncsbn.org/dxp.html
Other helpful sites:
National Student Nurses Association
http://www.NSNA.org/index.htm
American Nurses Association
http://www.ANA.org/index.htm

Rapid study steps

Step 1. Identify a study routine—What can be changed for efficiency and effectiveness?

a. What are your best days to study? First, list or think about all weekly activities that are set, such as work time, your children's school obligations, or attendance at church.

b. Write these activities on the days of your personal calendar and the calendar at home – yes, the big one that everyone uses to coordinate family activities; it is usually in the kitchen on the refrigerator. Be sure to include the time needed for each activity, including travel time to and from the activity.

c. Oh! You don't use one. Maybe it is time to get one and get writing! This communicates the weekly needs to your family or support systems. It highlights the time you will be available or unavailable to them.

d. Now write in your study times. What are the best times to study? Just look at "the time left" on each day. Decide if you desire to schedule in study, relaxation, or catch-up activities at these times. Then stick to it.

e. To have designated study time written on a readily accessible calendar is a nice reminder every day to yourself that study is important to you. Be sure to cross off completed tasks! You will feel great as you cross off the completed daily or weekly study times. These actions give you a sense of accomplishment.

   1) Does the designated study time have to be blocked for at least a few hours? No. Set aside your designated study time in 15- to 30-minute increments. These times might be set when you know that others in the family will be involved in their own activities.

   2) Remember the nursing process: assessment of the immediate situation is the first step in any given client situation. Get started with the application of the nursing process to your own life. The more you use these steps in your daily life, the more skilled you become in answering those test questions based on the nursing process. Weekly, assess what time you have and what content is weak and needs attention.

Step 2. Launch a rapid textbook study routine for each given class

a. Scan the table of contents in your textbook, noting assigned required reading

   1) Put a check mark in front of the content for 10 items with which you are comfortably strong.

   2) Circle 10 content areas with which you are shaky or which you dislike.

   3) Prioritize the shaky content, then the comfortable content.

     i. Put numbers from 1 to 10 in front of your shaky content, and then in front of the comfortable content.

     ii. Number 1 should be the weakest content area and number 10 should be the strongest area within each category of shaky or comfortable content.

b. When you are feeling a high-energy day, go to the number 1 chapter of the shaky content area and read.

c. When you are having a low-energy day, go to the number 1 chapter of the comfort content area and read.

d. Continue to work your way through all 10 areas of each category. Once you have completed all areas, start again with this process for the remainder of the content.

Step 3. Resort to rapid chapter reading

a. Read the summary at the end of the chapter or the introduction if no summary is provided.
b. Read the major and minor headings in the chapter in an attempt to put together a picture of the importance and the sequence of the content.
   1) If you are at this point and it is before class, make a brief list of what you don't understand. Use this list as the basis of the questions that you ask during class.
   2) If you are doing this after you have attended the class, more in-depth reading of the selected subject matter may be needed.
c. Next, read each chapter. Start by first reading the sections of the unfamiliar subject matter. Use this process to read the paragraphs: Read the first and the last sentence of each paragraph. Then, if you need to read the entire paragraph, do so. Recall from English class that paragraphs are formed with the key sentences at the first and last position. Apply this "process of writing" to your "process of reading."
d. Continue to use this process for assigned readings, such as journal articles, as well as for your enjoyment in reading books, newspapers or magazines.

Step 4. Achieve actions for accurate and retentive rapid study

a. Develop a system of study that meets the needs of your schedule.
   1) Select time when you are least tired or stressed, both mentally and physically.
   2) Limit your study time to a maximum of 90 minutes. This time frame results in the most effective, efficient retention of content.
b. If possible, relax and take a nap after the study period to cement the information into your long-term memory. Some research reveals that sleeping for 2 to 3 hours after studying results in a 70% to 80% retention rate of content in long-term memory. In contrast only a 30% to 40% retention rate is achieved when you are active after the study session.
c. Breathe deeply and slowly three times at the onset and at the end of your study time. S-L-O-W, deep breathing with concentration on the air going in and out is one of the best ways to get relaxed, both physically and mentally.
d. Use one other relaxation technique at the halfway mark of your study session.
e. If your time is limited, use 10- to 15-minute intervals to study small pieces of the content. For example, you may want to review the different aspects of hypertension in one study session.

Step 5. Select a theme for the day

a. When you plan at the beginning of the semester, use the approach of selecting a theme or topic for the day. For example, if there is enough time between your test and when you begin to study, review something every Monday on sodium from the book. Then, at work, find clients with sodium imbalances, review their charts, and discuss their situations with colleagues or with the clients' physicians. Continue with themes for each day such as:

1) Tuesdays: potassium.
2) Wednesdays: calcium.
3) Thursdays: magnesium.
4) Fridays: acidosis situations.
5) Saturdays: alkalosis situations.
6) Sundays: fun days. Don't forget to keep one day to relax and have fun. This allows your mind to work; your mind will automatically reorganize the retained content for better recall.

b. Weekly themes also might be of help. Do one system per week, such as pulmonary, endocrine, and so forth. Think of a way to associate the theme with meaning. For example, during the first week, study the pulmonary system since this is the first system with basic cardiac life support (BCLS). Then during the second week, study the cardiovascular system.

Step 6. Set up a study place

a. Designate a place to sit and study. Have all of your schoolbooks, references, computer, and so forth, at this location for ease of access.
b. A designated study place eliminates the "set up" time if all of your stuff is centralized and not scattered throughout the house. You can get more done in less time.
c. On days you aren't motivated to study, simply sit at this location for a minimum of 5 minutes. Within that time frame, tell yourself you might "flip through" a book. Before you know it, you will be into a productive study session.

Rapid review tips

1. Are there a few basic essential actions I can use for recall? Yes! Yes! Yes!
   a. Use yellow or lime green notebook paper or index cards. These colors enhance recall in long-term memory.
   b. Underline single words instead of phrases. The mind becomes more alert and attentive.
   c. Use a lime green or yellow highlighter.
   d. PRINT with CAPS when you make notes. Recall is enhanced. Avoid cursive writing of notes.
   e. Talk out loud to whomever will listen—even talk to your pets—cat, dog or fish.
   f. Review for 15 to 30 minutes before you go to sleep.
   g. Repeat items at least 3 times.
2. How can I use this review book for a rapid review before my class?
   a. Complete the review questions at the end of each chapter for a specified content area.
   b. Review the answers, rationales, and test-taking tips.

c. Review content for the missed areas.

d. Refer to your textbook, which has more details, if you still do not understand the information.

3. How should I use my notes from class?

   a. Read over your notes from class—every day! Yes, every day! Three repetitions enhance recall: You hear the instructor. You take notes. You reread your notes.

   b. Every day before going to sleep, take 10 minutes for a quick read-over of your class notes.

   c. Read over the notes for each class in the same sequence as the classes were attended that day.

4. What is an easy way to know key terms or content?

   a. Card them.

   b. Use a 3- x 5-inch index card to write the terms or condition on one side and the definitions of the key terms or the content information on the opposite side.

   c. Use the nursing process format to outline critical content.

   d. Look at the term and state your definition out loud.

   e. Uncover the definition and read the given definition out loud.

   f. Speaking the content as well as seeing the content will enhance your retention. If you have a few related terms that you can't remember, make a story out of the terms.

   g. Carry the card with you for a few days to review this content again. Suggestion: put these cards on your sunvisor in the car and review them at the stoplight or if stopped in traffic.

5. How can I prepare for the end of the semester comprehensive exam?

   a. Complete the comprehensive exam on the CD-ROM. Use it in the test mode.

   b. Review which questions were missed. Be sure to read the rationales and test-taking tips.

   c. Note if the test item was missed because of a lack of content knowledge or because you simply misread the question or some of the options.

   d. If a content problem is identified, list the specific content missed. Then cluster these under umbrellas of similar content. Use index cards for this activity.

      1) Prioritize these clusters, with number 1 being the least familiar content.

      2) Review additional content as indicated by the questions that you missed.

      3) Review the most familiar content last, or on low-energy days. Review the weakest content first, or on high-energy days.

   e. If your problem was identified as misreading, make a list of where the misreading occurred—in the question? In an option? If in an option, which one? Is there a pattern to the misread options? Was the misread option a series of items or a two-part option? Did you misread the second part of the option? Identify the pattern of errors you made in reading. Most test takers have 3 to 5 consistent errors that they repeat over and over again.

Think of actions that you can take to eliminate or minimize these types of testing errors.

6. Should I repeat the same practice test questions?
   a. Yes. However, do practice questions at different times of the day than when the comprehensive test was initially done. Repeat the comprehensive exam on the CD-ROM in the test mode, and then in the tutorial mode, and then again in the test mode.
   b. Note whether the test item was missed because of a lack of content knowledge or because of simply misreading the question or some of the options.
   c. Note that even though the questions are repeated, you should evaluate how your reading of the questions and options differed.
   d. Do you have a pattern in perception and consistent ability to identify key words, terms, age, and developmental needs?
   e. Did the fatigue factor or tenseness influence your thinking skills? And what did you do or could you have done to minimize these factors to improve your abilities?
   f. Did anticipatory thinking of the correct answer enhance or hinder your selection of the correct answer?
   g. Doing the same test questions over can be helpful to reinforce content, fine tune test skills, and establish better reading habits.
7. How do I evaluate my performance for testing?
   a. For any practice test questions, read all of the rationales and test-taking tips. Do this for the questions you got correct and those that you missed. The rationales and test-taking tips often contain pearls of wisdom on how to remember or get a better understanding of the content.
   b. Remember to do a relaxation exercise before you begin your questions, during the examination, and as you review the results. Do at least one mental and one physical relaxation exercise at least every 30 minutes or every 30 questions.
   c. When you miss a question ask yourself:
      1) Did I not know the content?
      2) Did I misread the question or options?
   d. If you miss questions because of a knowledge deficit.
      1) Make a list on a 3- x 5-inch card for 3 to 4 days.
      2) Group or cluster the content according to the steps in the nursing process, the content area, or a system.
      3) Look up that content.
      4) Do not look up content after every practice test. A better approach is to cluster the content and look it all up every 3 to 4 days. With this approach you will have better retention in long-term memory and the best recall at a later time.
   e. If you misread the question or the option(s):
      1) Try to identify new ways to approach reading questions and their options.
      2) Try to identify what key words, time frames, ages, and developmental stages that you may have overlooked.

8. How can I improve my test scores?
   a. Practice, practice, and practice doing questions.
   b. Practice, practice, and practice doing relaxation before you begin the practice exam, after every 10 to 20 questions, and then at the end of the examination to refresh your thinking and diminish your tenseness or tiredness.
   c. Look for a pattern or cluster of wrong answers.
      1) Where did you miss questions?
      2) Are there clusters of missed questions? If so, did this happen after what type of question? One related to the nursing process? One that had a priority and where all of the options are correct? One that asks in terms of "all but the following"? One that asked for the most or the least important item? One that had information you had never seen?
      3) Did you miss clusters of questions at the beginning of the test?
         1. If so, you have a tension or anxiety problem at the start of the test
         2. Simply do at least one mental and physical relaxation exercise before the test and at question 25 to control your thinking.
      4) Did you miss clusters of questions at the middle or the end of the test?
         i. Then you have a fatigue or tiredness problem.
         ii. First be alert to the event of "feeling tired" or fatigued.
         iii. When you feel this way, get up and leave the room for 2 to 4 minutes. While you are out of the room, MOVE and be active. Touch your toes 10 times. Swing your arms from side to side. Mentally tell yourself: "I know something. I'll figure it out."
         iv. Return to the test in a more sharp, attentive state.
9. What is most essential to preparation for the NCLEX? What are the most essential actions to prepare for "the big test"?
   a. Be sure to do a practice exam with the exact number of questions as the NCLEX or your "big test."
   b. Write down on a note card when you were the most tired, anxious, or nervous during this examination. List the question number you were at when you were feeling this way.
   c. Do a relaxation exercise at these tense or fatigued times during the exam. Note which actions helped the most.
   d. Avoid the thought, "I am tired and just want to get done with the test."
   e. Your success is directly correlated to your degree of effort to review content as well as to deal with tension and fatigue during the review and exam processes.

Summary

We would be pleased if you use this book as a major tool to supplement your textbooks, clinical, and classroom activities. We hope that after you have used this book you will have learned to take actions to:

- Maximize your individual performance in study, review, and testing situations.
- Identify personal actions to help you set priorities for test preparation.
- Sharpen your thinking and reading skills during tests.

We hope that this book makes it easy, enjoyable, and effective to study and review at convenient times. The short, condensed, and prioritized chapter content may spark new ways to develop your skills in critical thinking and recall of content.

It is feedback from students, graduates, and practitioners in nursing that prompted the development and publication of this rapid review series. We welcome your comments. Please contact Dr. Rollant@bellsouth.net or 22 Village Lane, Newnan, GA 30265. We wish you a successful career in the nursing profession and hope that *Mosby's Rapid Review Series* has made that success a little easier to obtain!

The material on rapid study steps and rapid review tips was taken from Rollant PD: Soar to Success: Do Your Best on Nursing Tests, St. Louis, 1999, Mosby.

1

Human Genetics, Conception, and Fetal Development

FAST FACTS

1. The genetic material carried in the nucleus of each cell of the body determines the physical characteristics of a human being.
2. Abnormalities in the genes and chromosomes adversely affect fetal and newborn growth and development.
3. Defective genes can be transmitted to the offspring of gene carriers regardless of whether the carriers have the disorder.
4. **Teratogens** are environmental substances or exposures known to be harmful to humans that adversely affect fetal and newborn growth and development.
5. **Congenital disorders** are present at birth from an interference in the process of fetal growth and development; these disorders can result from a single or a combination of abnormal chromosomes or genes and environmental factors, including teratogens.
6. **Conception** that results in a pregnancy requires the following: (1) maturation of **gametes,** that is, sperm and ova; (2) a menstrual cycle that results in both ovulation and preparation of the uterine endometrium for implantation; (3) an intact female and male reproductive system that allows passage of both sperm and ovum so that fertilization can occur; (4) fertilization of an ovum with a sperm; and (5) implantation of the fertilized ovum in the secretory endometrium where further development takes place.

CONTENT REVIEW

I. Basic principles of human genetics

A. Genetic material

1. Definition for chromosomes and genes which are found in nucleus of human cells
2. **Chromosome**—threadlike strands composed of the hereditary material known as deoxyribonucleic acid (DNA)
3. **Gene**—a small segment of DNA; each chromosome is comprised of many genes, and each gene occupies a specific location on the chromosome
4. Somatic cells—contain 46 chromosomes
   a. There are 23 pairs, one pair from each parent
      (1) Autosomes—22 pairs that control most body traits
      (2) Sex chromosomes—1 pair that determines the gender and other selected traits
         (a) Male, XY
         (b) Female, XX
   b. Each of the 23 pairs of chromosomes is *homologous* (matched) in terms of composition and traits regulated
5. Traits—each person has two genes for every trait, one maternal and one paternal
   a. *Alleles* refer to the different variations of a trait, for example, eye and hair color
      (1) If both alleles for a trait are the same they are *homozygous* for that trait; for example, when the two gene alleles for eye color are blue, the person will have blue eyes
      (2) If both alleles for a trait are different they are *heterozygous* for that trait; for example, a person may have one gene for brown hair and one for blond hair
   b. Genes are dominant or recessive for a trait
      (1) The dominant gene in a pair is expressed even if the other gene is different. For example, the gene for brown eyes is dominant, the gene for blue eyes is recessive; when a person has one of each, he or she will have brown eyes.
      (2) The recessive gene for a trait is only expressed if the other gene in the pair is recessive. For example, two genes for blue eyes are required for a person to have blue eyes.
6. *Genotype*—an individual's entire genetic makeup created when an ovum and sperm unite at fertilization
7. *Phenotype*—an individual's physical appearance that results from expression of genotype
8. *Karyotype*—a photograph of an individual's chromosomes arranged in pairs in terms of order, form, and size; used to detect chromosomal abnormalities

B. **Chromosomal abnormalities—Two predisposing factors for their occurrence are advanced maternal age (over 35 years) and exposure to teratogens. Two types of abnormalities that can occur during cellular division and replication include the following:**
  1. Abnormal number of chromosomes—more than or less than the required 46 chromosomes
      a. Down syndrome (trisomy 21)—three of chromosome 21
      b. Turner's syndrome (monosomy of the X chromosome as XO instead of XX)—one X chromosome is missing, resulting in the abnormal development of the female reproductive system and secondary sexual characteristics and infertility
      c. Klinefelter's syndrome (trisomy of the sex chromosomes as XXY instead of XY)—results in abnormal development of the male reproductive system and secondary sexual characteristics and infertility
  2. Abnormality in chromosomal structure as a result of breakage leads to translocation, addition, or deletion of genetic material. An example is *cri du chat syndrome* in which a deletion of the short arm of chromosome 5 occurs that results in the infant being born with microcephaly, severe mental retardation, and abnormal facial characteristics. The infant also has a catlike cry.
C. **Transmission of abnormal genes**
  1. **Unifactorial (single gene) inheritance—**a particular trait, health problem, or defect is controlled by one gene as a result of a variety of transmission patterns
      a. *Autosomal dominant inheritance—*an abnormal gene is dominant; a disorder is expressed when the gene is present even if the other gene in the pair is normal
          (1) Examples are polydactyly, Huntington's chorea, and achondroplasia
          (2) Transmission probability for each pregnancy when one parent is affected and one parent is normal: a 50% chance offspring will be affected, and a 50% chance offspring will be unaffected
      b. *Autosomal recessive inheritance—*an abnormal gene is recessive; a disorder is expressed only when both genes in the pair are the same recessive gene
          (1) If the second gene in the pair is normal, the disorder is not expressed but the person is a carrier of the abnormal gene and can transmit it to offspring
          (2) Examples are phenylketonuria (PKU), Tay-Sachs disease, sickle cell anemia, and cystic fibrosis
          (3) Transmission probability for each pregnancy when both parents are carriers of the recessive gene: a 25% chance offspring will be unaffected, a 25% chance offspring will be affected, and a 50% chance offspring will be unaffected but will be a carrier

    c. *X-linked recessive inheritance*—a defective recessive gene is carried on the X chromosome
       (1) Females are predominately carriers
       (2) Males predominately express the disorder when they receive the recessive gene from their mothers because there is no corresponding gene on their Y chromosome. Males can transmit the defective gene only to their female offspring.
       (3) Females can only express the disorder if they receive a recessive gene from their mother and a recessive gene from their affected father
       (4) Examples are hemophilia, color blindness, and Duchenne muscular dystrophy

    d. *X-linked dominant inheritance*—a defective dominant gene is carried on the X chromosome; it is expressed in both male and female offspring who inherit the defective gene
       (1) Females are less severely affected than are males because females also carry a normal gene on their second X chromosome
       (2) An example is vitamin D-resistant rickets

    e. *Inborn errors of metabolism*—absence of or defect in enzymes responsible for the metabolism of proteins, fats, or carbohydrates leads to an accumulation of harmful substances (e.g., phenylalanine), causing health problems
       (1) An autosomal recessive pattern of inheritance is followed
       (2) Physical growth and mental development are adversely affected as the harmful substance accumulates with age; death can occur
       (3) Examples are phenylketonuria (PKU), Tay Sachs disease, and cystic fibrosis

  2. **Multifactorial inheritance**—a pattern of inheritance reflecting the interaction of several genetic and environmental factors that create mild to severe defects, depending on the number of factors present
    a. Expression of the health problem occurs when either
       (1) The required number of defective genes are transmitted, or
       (2) Less than the required defective genes are transmitted but the required environmental factors also are present
    b. Family history of the disorder often is present
    c. Examples include cleft lip and palate, neural tube defects, pyloric stenosis, congenital heart disease, and club foot

D. Genetic counseling
  1. Counseling should be provided when parents give birth to a child with an inheritable disorder or there is a family history of genetic problems

2. Counselors use therapeutic communication techniques to develop a trusting relationship and provide education, guidance, and support
3. Counseling consists of
   a. Determination of the transmission probability for each pregnancy
   b. Discussion of the implications for health problems created
      (1) Affect on fetal and neonatal growth and development
      (2) Availability of treatment
      (3) Impact on family processes. Provide an opportunity to talk with other parents who have children with the same disorder.
   c. Description of the advantages, risks, and costs of diagnostic interventions used to determine if the fetus is affected; examples of diagnostic interventions include chorionic villi sampling, **amniocentesis,** and sonography
   d. Assistance with decision-making using an unbiased, nonjudgmental approach that maintains confidentiality and privacy
      (1) Determine influencing factors such as personal resources and religious and cultural beliefs
      (2) Determine if the parents want to take the risks associated with the pregnancy or seek alternatives to biologic children
      (3) Determine if the parents want to continue with the pregnancy, seek an abortion, or allow the child to be adopted
   e. Support for parents in their decision. Provide emotional support, encourage open communication, and make referrals to support groups
   f. Facilitation of the grieving process as parents cope with loss of a "perfect" child or loss of the ability to have biologic children

II. *Conception*—fertilization of the ovum creates a *zygote* (first cell of a new human being); interrelated steps comprise conception and the beginning of pregnancy

A. *Gametogenesis*—maturation of gametes (sperm and ovum) using meiosis to create haploid cells with 23 single chromosomes. Gametes unite during fertilization to create a diploid cell with 46 chromosomes. *Spermatogenesis* is the maturation of spermatocyte to sperm; *oogenesis* is the maturation of oocyte to ovum.

B. *Menstrual cycle*—recurring hormone-regulated process of follicle maturation and endometrial development, resulting in ovulation and preparation of the uterus for implantation of a fertilized ovum
   1. Gonadotrophin releasing hormone (GnRH) is secreted by the hypothalamus when estrogen and progesterone levels decrease at end of the menstrual cycle; the pituitary is stimulated to secrete FSH and LH
   2. Follicle-stimulating hormone (FSH) develops the graafian follicle

3. Luteinizing hormone (LH) completes follicle development, stimulates ovulation (release of the maturing ovum from the ruptured follicle), develops the corpus luteum
4. Estrogen is secreted by a maturing follicle and corpus luteum, and stimulates
   a. Proliferation of endometrium; thicker, more vascular
   b. Motility of fallopian tubes, which facilitates the capture of an ovum and propels it through the tube to the ampulla for fertilization
   c. Motility of the uterus (along with prostaglandin) to facilitate forward movement of sperm through the uterus to the tube for fertilization
   d. Production of copious thin, elastic, alkaline cervical mucous that is receptive to sperm to facilitate their passage
5. Progesterone is secreted by the corpus luteum formed at the site of the ruptured follicle
   a. Continues endometrial development into the secretory layer; provides an implantation site capable of nourishing the blastocyst
   b. Raises body temperature, which is one of the objective signs of ovulation
   c. Reduces uterine motility to facilitate implantation
6. Fertilization occurs
   a. The corpus luteum continues to function as a result of human chorionic gonadotrophin (HCG) secreted by the implanted blastocyst

⚠ Warning!

HCG, which is found in maternal urine and serum, is the basis for a positive pregnancy test.

   b. The corpus luteum maintains pregnancy by the secretion of estrogen and progesterone until the placenta can take over at 6 to 10 weeks
7. If fertilization does not occur
   a. The corpus luteum degenerates
   b. Estrogen and progesterone levels decrease
   c. Menstruation occurs (day one of cycle) as a result of endometrial breakdown
   d. The cycle begins again with secretion of FSH
C. **Sexual intercourse during a fertile period**
1. Ovum capable of fertilization 24 hours after ovulation; optimum time is 2 hours
2. Sperm is viable for about 48 hours after ejaculation into the uterus and is capable of fertilization for about 24 hours. About 4 to 6 hours are required for the sperm to reach the ampulla; ideally, the sperm should be in the tube at ovulation.

D. Fertilization—a union of one ovum and one sperm to create a zygote
1. Once fertilized, the cell membrane of ovum becomes impenetrable to other sperm
2. The zygote continues to grow and develop using mitosis to replicate cells with the same genetic composition (46 chromosomes) as the parent cell
3. The progression is as follows: zygote to morula (16 cells), to blastocyst, to embryo, to fetus
4. During development the zygote travels through the tube to the uterus to be implanted as a blastocyst

E. Implantation *(nidation)*—the blastocyst reaches the uterus in 3 to 4 days where it burrows into the endometrium, usually in the upper uterine segment, within 7 to 10 days of conception

⚠ Warning!

Slight bleeding may be noted at time of implantation and may be mistaken for a menstrual period. This contributes to the inaccuracy of Nägele's rule for determination of the estimated date of birth.

III. Fetal growth and development
A. Three periods or stages have been identified
1. Pre-embryonic or ovum
   a. The period from conception until day 14
   b. The zygote develops into the blastocyst that implants into the endometrium
2. Embryonic
   a. The period from day 15 until 8 weeks' gestation
   b. **Embryo** is the term now used to refer to the fertilized ovum
   c. This is the critical stage for organ and external feature development. The embryo is especially vulnerable to teratogen exposure
3. Fetal
   a. The period from 9 weeks' gestation until pregnancy ends
   b. Characterized by refinement of structure and function developed during the previous stages
   c. **Fetus** is the term now used to describe the embryo
   d. The fetus is less vulnerable to teratogens, except for those that can interfere with the development of the brain and central nervous system (CNS)

B. The progress of fetal development is illustrated in Figure 1-1. These illustrations can be an effective prenatal teaching tool when working with pregnant women and their families, especially during the second trimester.

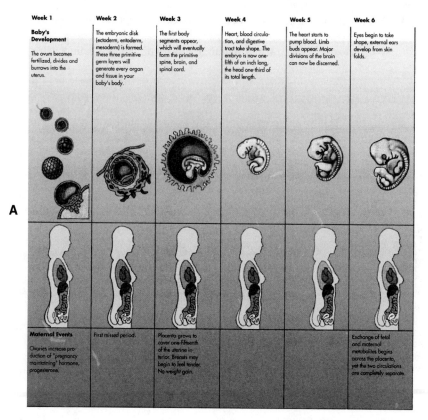

Week 1	Week 2	Week 3	Week 4	Week 5	Week 6
Baby's Development The ovum becomes fertilized, divides and burrows into the uterus.	The embryonic disk (ectoderm, entoderm, mesoderm) is formed. These three primitive germ layers will generate every organ and tissue in your baby's body.	The first body segments appear, which will eventually form the primitive spine, brain, and spinal cord.	Heart, blood circulation, and digestive tract take shape. The embryo is now one-fifth of an inch long, the head one-third of its total length.	The heart starts to pump blood. Limb buds appear. Major divisions of the brain can now be discerned.	Eyes begin to take shape, external ears develop from skin folds.
Maternal Events Ovaries increase production of "pregnancy maintaining" hormone, progesterone.	First missed period.	Placenta grows to cover one-fifteenth of the uterine interior. Breasts may begin to feel tender. No weight gain.			Exchange of fetal and maternal metabolites begins across the placenta, yet the two circulations are completely separate.

Figure 1-1   Summary of fetal development and maternal events. **A,** Weeks 1 to 6.

IV. Structures essential to fetal growth and development

A. *Amniotic membranes*
1. Amnion (inner) and chorion (outer) membranes enclose the fetus in the amniotic fluid
2. Provide protection from infectious organisms that can be transmitted vertically from the maternal vagina

B. *Amniotic fluid*
1. Definition—clear, slightly yellow, alkaline fluid (approximately 1 L at term) that surrounds the fetus
2. Derived from maternal plasma, the cells of the amnion, and fetal fluids from the lung, skin, and urine
3. Essential functions
   a. Cushions fetus from trauma
   b. Facilitates fetal movement to enhance the development of the musculoskeletal system
   c. Facilitates symmetrical growth, prevents fetal entanglement in membranes, and allows for unrestricted positioning
   d. Regulates intrauterine temperature

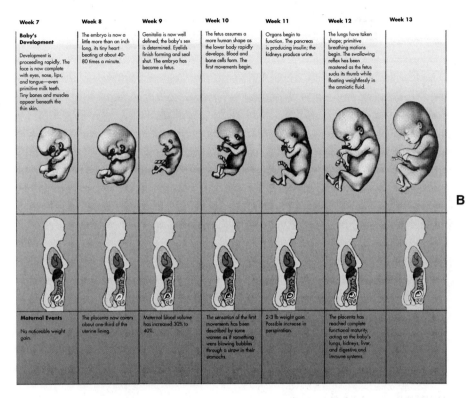

	Week 7	Week 8	Week 9	Week 10	Week 11	Week 12	Week 13
Baby's Development	Development is proceeding rapidly. The face is now complete with eyes, nose, lips, and tongue—even primitive milk teeth. Tiny bones and muscles appear beneath the thin skin.	The embryo is now a little more than an inch long, its tiny heart beating at about 40-80 times a minute.	Genitalia is now well defined; the baby's sex is determined. Eyelids finish forming and seal shut. The embryo has become a fetus.	The fetus assumes a more human shape as the lower body rapidly develops. Blood and bone cells form. The first movements begin.	Organs begin to function. The pancreas is producing insulin; the kidneys produce urine.	The lungs have taken shape; primitive breathing motions begin. The swallowing reflex has been mastered as the fetus sucks its thumb while floating weightlessly in the amniotic fluid.	
Maternal Events	No noticeable weight gain.	The placenta now covers about one-third of the uterine lining.	Maternal blood volume has increased 30% to 40%.	The sensation of the first movements has been described by some women as if something were blowing bubbles through a straw in their stomachs.	2-3 lb weight gain. Possible increase in perspiration.	The placenta has reached complete functional maturity, acting as the baby's lungs, kidneys, liver, and digestive and immune systems.	

B

Figure 1-1, cont'd Summary of fetal development and maternal events. **B,** Weeks 7 to 13.   *Continued*

e. Provides a source of oral fluid
f. Cushions the umbilical cord to prevent its compression
g. Serves as a receptacle for fetal substances: fluid can be analyzed to determine fetal health status by way of **amniocentesis**

C. *Placenta*
1. Definition—organ specific to pregnancy that is formed as the *chorionic villi* (projections from the chorion) are imbedded into the decidua
2. Fully functional by week 12; continues to grow and develop until aging process begins at about 36 weeks' gestation
3. Maternal factors inhibit uteroplacental circulation (e.g., diabetes, hypertension, cardiac disease, and smoking), adversely affecting placental development. Placenta will be smaller and age sooner, which compromises fetal growth and development.
4. It has essential functions
   a. Respiration—transports oxygen and removes carbon dioxide
   b. Nutrition—stores and transports nutrients, fluid, vitamins, and minerals from the mother to support fetal growth and development
   c. Waste removal—removes by-products of fetal metabolism
   d. Protection—prevents exposure to some but not all harmful substances; allows for the passage of maternal antibodies

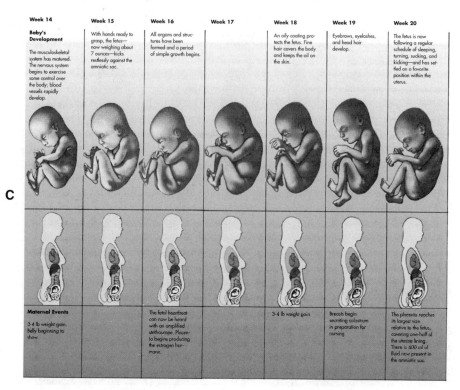

Week 14	Week 15	Week 16	Week 17	Week 18	Week 19	Week 20
Baby's Development The musculoskeletal system has matured. The nervous system begins to exercise some control over the body; blood vessels rapidly develop.	With hands ready to grasp, the fetus—now weighing about 7 ounces—kicks restlessly against the amniotic sac.	All organs and structures have been formed and a period of simple growth begins.		An oily coating protects the fetus. Fine hair covers the body and keeps the oil on the skin.	Eyebrows, eyelashes, and head hair develop.	The fetus is now following a regular schedule of sleeping, turning, sucking, and kicking—and has settled on a favorite position within the uterus.
Maternal Events 3-4 lb weight gain. Belly beginning to show.		The fetal heartbeat can now be heard with an amplified stethoscope. Placenta begins producing the estrogen hormone.		3-4 lb weight gain	Breasts begin secreting colostrum in preparation for nursing	The placenta reaches its largest size relative to the fetus, covering one-half of the uterine lining. There is 400 ml of fluid now present in the amniotic sac.

Figure 1-1, cont'd   Summary of fetal development and maternal events. **C,** Weeks 14 to 20.

  e. Endocrine—secretes estrogen, progesterone, HCG, and human placental lactogen (HPL), which are essential to maintain pregnancy

 D. *Umbilical cord*
  1. Connects the fetus to the placenta
  2. It is composed of one vein that carries oxygenated blood and nutrients to the fetus; two arteries that carry deoxygenated blood and waste to the placenta; Wharton's jelly, which supports and separates the vessels; and amnion, the membrane cover

V. Factors influencing fetal growth and development
 A. Exposure to teratogens can adversely affect fetal and newborn health, well-being, and survival
  1. The nature of the harmful effect is influenced by
   a. Toxicity of teratogens
   b. Amount and length of exposure compared with the amount required for damage to occur
   c. Degree of embryo and fetal susceptibility
   d. Timing of exposure
    (1) Pre-embryonic period—spontaneous abortion

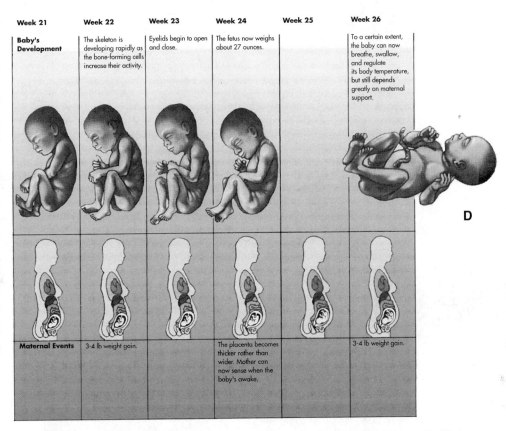

Week 21	Week 22	Week 23	Week 24	Week 25	Week 26
Baby's Development	The skeleton is developing rapidly as the bone-forming cells increase their activity.	Eyelids begin to open and close.	The fetus now weighs about 27 ounces.		To a certain extent, the baby can now breathe, swallow, and regulate its body temperature, but still depends greatly on maternal support.
Maternal Events	3-4 lb weight gain.		The placenta becomes thicker rather than wider. Mother can now sense when the baby's awake.		3-4 lb weight gain.

D

Figure 1-1, cont'd   Summary of fetal development and maternal events. **D,** Weeks 21 to 26.   *Continued*

  (2) Embryonic period—structural and anatomic abnormalities as well as spontaneous abortion

  (3) Fetal period—behavioral abnormalities, intrauterine growth retardation, and fetal demise

 e. Single or combination exposure, for example, cigarette smoking alone or the abuse of tobacco, alcohol, caffeine, and marijuana

 2. Teratogens include

  a. Drugs and chemicals—nicotine, alcohol, certain hormones, medications, cocaine, heroin, and marijuana

  b. Environmental pollutants—lead, chemicals in soil, water, air, and radiation

  c. Infectious agents—rubella, syphilis, toxoplasmosis, cytomegalovirus, herpes simplex virus, and human immunodeficiency virus (HIV)

B. Maternal health habits and lifestyle may expose the fetus to teratogens or limit the amount of substances required for optimal growth and development. Preconception care helps women adopt

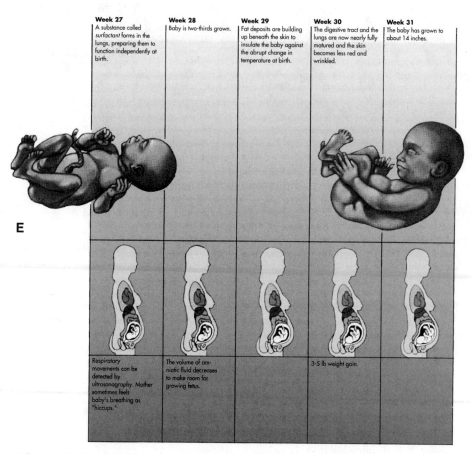

Week 27	Week 28	Week 29	Week 30	Week 31
A substance called *surfactant* forms in the lungs, preparing them to function independently at birth.	Baby is two-thirds grown.	Fat deposits are building up beneath the skin to insulate the baby against the abrupt change in temperature at birth.	The digestive tract and the lungs are now nearly fully matured and the skin becomes less red and wrinkled.	The baby has grown to about 14 inches.

E

| Respiratory movements can be detected by ultrasonography. Mother sometimes feels baby's breathing as "hiccups." | The volume of amniotic fluid decreases to make room for growing fetus. | | 3-5 lb weight gain. | |

Figure 1-1, cont'd   Summary of fetal development and maternal events. **E,** Weeks 27 to 31.

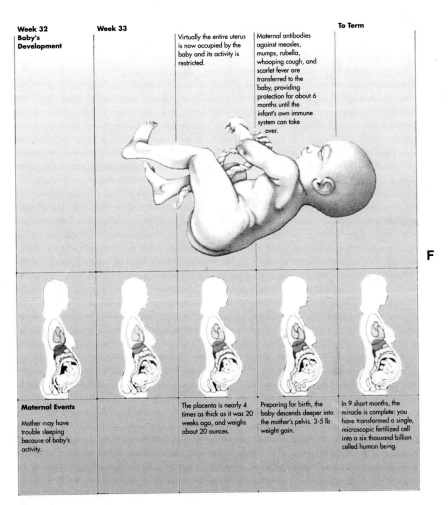

**Week 32
Baby's
Development**

Week 33

To Term

Virtually the entire uterus is now occupied by the baby and its activity is restricted.

Maternal antibodies against measles, mumps, rubella, whooping cough, and scarlet fever are transferred to the baby, providing protection for about 6 months until the infant's own immune system can take over.

F

Maternal Events

Mother may have trouble sleeping because of baby's activity.

The placenta is nearly 4 times as thick as it was 20 weeks ago, and weighs about 20 ounces.

Preparing for birth, the baby descends deeper into the mother's pelvis. 3-5 lb weight gain.

In 9 short months, the miracle is complete: you have transformed a single, microscopic fertilized cell into a six thousand billion celled human being.

Figure 1-1, cont'd Summary of fetal development and maternal events. **F,** Weeks 32 to term.

Box 1-1
Effects of Alcohol, Tobacco, and Cocaine on Fetal Growth and Development

Alcohol

The effects of alcohol are related to the amount and timing of exposure as well as concurrent abuse of other substances.

Fetal alcohol syndrome is common among women considered to be alcoholics and is characterized in children by retardation, poor fine motor skills, behavioral problems, growth restriction, structural abnormalities of the face and limbs, and cardiac and circulatory problems.

Fetal alcohol effect occurs among women who are light-to-moderate drinkers and is characterized in children by emotional problems, insomnia, and hyperactivity. These children also have difficulties with learning, speech, decision-making, and coping with school and employment. Binge drinking exposes the fetus to large amounts of alcohol at one time.

The effects of alcohol on a fetus are influenced by the timing of alcohol consumption. For example, during the fetal stage of development, the major effect is on the development of the brain and CNS.

Intrauterine growth restriction (IUGR) and low birth weight (LBW) occur as a result of a smaller placenta and maternal nutritional intake being less than body requirements as a result of alcohol abuse.

Women who drink have a higher rate of stillbirth.

Stopping or reducing the intake of alcohol during pregnancy appears to improve outcome.

Alcohol enters breast milk during lactation.

Research has not identified a safe level of or safe time for alcohol consumption during pregnancy. Women should abstain from alcohol use during pregnancy and lactation.

Tobacco

The effects of tobacco use in the form of cigarette smoking are related to the degree to which the mother smokes during pregnancy and her age and health status. For example, pregnant women over the age of 35 years, who are already at risk for cardiovascular problems (e.g., heart disease, hypertension, and pregnancy-induced hypertension), experience more harmful effects.

The circulatory effects of tobacco use are placental damage with smaller vessels and increased incidences of miscarriage, preterm birth, stillbirth, and low birth weight.

healthy lifestyles before pregnancy. Habits and lifestyle that adversely affect fetal and newborn development are
1. Poor nutrition
2. Stressful lifestyle
3. Inadequate hygiene or unsafe sex practices
4. Environmental pollutants at home and in the workplace
5. Use of tobacco, alcohol, or cocaine (Box 1-1)

C. **Paternal health habits and exposure to environmental influences increasingly are the subject of research**
1. Fertility, in terms of sperm and penile erection, and the quality of genetic material transmitted have already been shown to be

Box 1-1
Effects of Alcohol, Tobacco, and Cocaine on Fetal Growth and Development—cont'd

Tobacco—cont'd

The nutritional effect of tobacco use is interference with nutrient intake and absorption to result in lower maternal weight gain.

The carcinogenic effect of tobacco by-products has been found, in some studies, to increase the risk for brain cancer and leukemia among children exposed to these by-products while in utero.

The potential long-term effects of intrauterine and second-hand exposure to tobacco are slower rate of growth with less adipose tissue; language and learning deficits; lower IQ; developmental delays; behavioral problems, including hyperactivity, anxiety, depression, and disobedience; increased incidence of serious infections, including respiratory and ear infections; and increased incidence of asthma and sudden infant death syndrome (SIDS).

Stopping or reducing the smoking of cigarettes during pregnancy will favorably affect the outcome.

Cocaine

Cocaine has a major effect on pregnancy. Vasoconstriction increases the risk of spontaneous abortion, preterm labor and birth, abruptio placentae, and low birth weight.

Women may use cocaine to induce labor and control the time of birth. For example, an adolescent may have difficulty coping with a pregnancy that lasts 40 weeks.

Fetal and neonatal effects: congenital anomalies including microencephaly; defects in the development of the skull, limbs, CNS, kidneys, urinary tract, heart, and abdomen; and intracranial hemorrhage and seizures from fetal hypertension. These infants are hyperactive, irritable, and hard to console, with muscular rigidity. They are poor feeders and may have diarrhea. They have the following: irregular sleep patterns; limited ability to interact and make eye contact; hypersensitivity to environmental stimuli, with limited ability for *habituation* (shutting out of stimuli); and the possibility of long-term behavioral and learning problems.

Because the breathing patterns of these infants may be affected especially during sleep, they are at increased risk for SIDS.

Coping with a newborn affected by cocaine is especially difficult for a mother who still abuses drugs or is recovering from drug abuse herself.

adversely affected by the same health habits and lifestyle practices identified for women

2. Prospective fathers should receive preconception care to help them adopt healthy lifestyles before pregnancy

WEB Resources

http://www.modimes.org
March of Dimes

http://www.pregnancycalendar.com/first9months
A multimedia journey through the first 9 months of an unborn child's life using illustrations, sonographic pictures, and sound

REVIEW QUESTIONS

1. A pregnant woman has been told that her fetus will be born with Down syndrome. Down syndrome is an example of which of these problems?
   1. Unifactorial inheritance
   2. X-linked recessive inheritance
   3. Trisomy of chromosome 21
   4. Chromosomal translocation

2. Based on genetic testing of a newborn, a diagnosis of dwarfism has been made. The parents ask the nurse if this could happen to future children. Because this is an example of autosomal dominant inheritance, the nurse would tell the parents:
   1. For each pregnancy, there is a 50-50 chance the child will be affected by dwarfism
   2. This will not happen again because the harmful genetic effects of the infection you had during pregnancy caused the dwarfism
   3. For each pregnancy there is a 25% chance the child will be a carrier of the defective gene but will be unaffected by the disorder
   4. Because you already have had an affected child there is a decreased chance for this to happen in future pregnancies

3. If a woman experiences a deficiency in the secretion of lutenizing hormone (LH) from her pituitary gland, the result will be an interference with which process?
   1. Initial development of the graafian follicle
   2. Proliferation of the endometrium after menstruation
   3. Release of the ovum from a ruptured follicle—ovulation
   4. Formation of copious, thin, elastic cervical mucous

4. A woman who is trying to get pregnant asks the nurse why her level of estrogen is so important for pregnancy. The nurse should tell her that estrogen has which of these actions?
   1. Increases movement in the fallopian tubes so the ovum can be captured into the tube where it will be fertilized
   2. Creates a secretory lining in her uterus to nourish the fertilized ovum until the placenta is formed
   3. Quiets the uterus so the fertilized ovum will not be expelled
   4. Stimulates the development of the follicle that contains the ovum until ovulation occurs

5. A woman who uses cocaine during pregnancy is at increased risk for giving birth to a newborn that exhibits which of these findings?
   1. Postmaturity syndrome
   2. Limited ability to interact with parents, make eye contact, or respond to stimuli
   3. Clinical findings of withdrawal from cocaine
   4. Depression of the CNS, sleepiness, and lethargy

ANSWERS, RATIONALES, AND TEST-TAKING TIPS

Rationale	Test-Taking Tips

1. Correct answer: 3

Down syndrome is a chromosomal disorder related to an extra chromosome, three instead of two of chromosome 21. Unifactorial and X-linked recessive inheritance refer to genetic disorders. Translocation relates to structural abnormality of chromosomes associated with breakage.

Associate that the number 21 is important for the legal "D"rinking age in most states and that chromosome 21 is associated with "D"own syndrome.

2. Correct answer: 1

Autosomal dominant inheritance is unrelated to exposure to teratogens. Each pregnancy has the same potential for expression of the disorder. There is no reduction if one child is already affected. If the gene is inherited, the disorder is always expressed.

Eliminate option 3 with the vague words "a decreased chance." Eliminate option 2 with the introduction of new information. If you have no idea between options 1 and 3, select option 1 with the 50-50 chance, the same chance you have of a correct answer when you narrow the options to two.

3. Correct answer: 3

Follicle-stimulating hormone (FSH) is responsible for the initial development of the graafian follicle. Estrogen is responsible for endometrial proliferation and increased production of cervical mucous.

Associate "L"H with "L"etting go or the release of the ovum from a ruptured follicle, which is ovulation; "F"SH with the "F"irst in the development of the "F"ollicle; and "E"strogen with "E"ndometrial function and the site of the "E"xit for mucus.

4. Correct answer: 1

Options 2 and 3 are the result of progesterone secretion. Option 4 is the result of FSH and LH.

Associate that "E"strogen is "E"ssential for "E"nsuring the getting pregnant. Once a woman is pregnant, "P"rogesterone keeps her "P"regnant. Associate "L"H with "L"etting go or the release of the ovum from a ruptured follicle, which is ovulation.

Rationales	Test-Taking Tips

5. Correct answer: 2

Newborns of mothers who use cocaine are more likely to be preterm. While newborns do not experience manifestations of withdrawal from cocaine, they do experience neurotoxic effect including CNS irritability that can interfere with their ability to interact effectively with parents, caregivers, and stimuli in the environment.

Associate "C"ocaine abuse with "C"ommunication difficulties whether the client is an adult or a newborn. Also associate "C"ocaine and "C"igarette use increases the "C"hances of early births.

2

Anatomic, Physiologic, and Psychological Adaptations to Pregnancy

FAST FACTS

1. The **antepartal (prenatal, gestation) period** of pregnancy begins with conception and ends with the onset of labor.
2. Pregnancy duration is about 40 weeks, or 280 days from last menstrual period: (1) **term** birth occurs after 37 weeks' and before 42 weeks' gestation, (2) **preterm** birth occurs before 38 weeks' gestation but after viability is reached at about 20 to 24 weeks' gestation; and (3) **post-term** birth occurs after 42 weeks' gestation.
3. There are three **trimesters,** which are segments of the prenatal period, each lasting approximately 12 weeks or 3 months.
4. The estimated date of birth (EDB) can be determined three ways: (1) By *Nägele's rule*—first day of the last menstrual period (LMP) minus 3 months, plus 7 days, and in most cases, add 1 year; for example,

	Months	Days	Year
LMP began on	7	14	1999
Nägele's rule	−3	+7	+1
EDB	4	21	2000

(2) by **ultrasonography,** which measures the gestational sac and fetus for comparison with measurements expected for a particular gestational age; and (3) by the date of occurrence of significant events, such as auscultation of fetal heart beat with Doppler ultrasonography or ultrasound stethoscope

(weeks 10 to 12) or a fetoscope (weeks 18 to 20); or such as by the date of *quickening,* which is the maternal perception of fetal movement at 16 to 20 weeks' gestation.

> ⚠ **WARNING!**
>
> Nägele's rule has limited value if dates are forgotten, menstrual cycles are irregular, or intermittent spotting (vaginal bleeding) occurs during pregnancy. Using a combination of all methods enhances the accuracy of the EDB.

5. Family is defined as an open living system composed of two or more persons who support each other physically, economically, and emotionally. The degree of support may vary among family members and may be influenced by age, need, and other factors.
6. A nuclear family is composed of parents and their children and is less common as a family form in the United States. A binuclear family is a family after divorce; children are members of both the maternal and paternal households.
7. A single parent family is composed of one parent and children and is more common as a family form in the United States from separation, divorce, death, or never being married.
8. An extended family is expansion of a nuclear or single-parent family to include other family members such as grandparents, siblings, aunts, uncles, and cousins.
9. A blended, reconstituted, or combined family is composed of parent and stepparent, and children and stepchildren.
10. A homosexual (gay or lesbian) family is composed of two parents of the same gender. Note that these parents and children often experience negative attitudes and discrimination from society, including the health care system and health care providers.
11. The three major tasks of childbearing and childrearing families are (1) altering careers and lifestyles to meet the needs of children for physical care, emotional support, nurturing, and developmental guidance; (2) incorporating children into the family system by assigning developmentally appropriate roles and responsibilities, developing communication patterns, providing morals and values, and preserving cultural and religious beliefs and traditions; and (3) preparing children to enter society *(socialization)*.
12. The nurse needs to determine for each pregnant woman: (1) her meaning and definition of family; (2) the composition of her family and degree of support received from each member; the person in her family most important to her; and (3) the nature of her relationship with the father and the amount of responsibility he is willing to assume with regard to supporting her and parenting the child.
13. A *support system* is defined as a group of individuals deemed by a person to be important to their well-being. Examples include family members and friends, health care providers, clergy, social workers, counselors, teachers, supervisors, colleagues, and others.

14. The nurse needs to determine the composition of each pregnant woman's support system as well as the degree and type of support offered by each individual.
15. Pregnancy and birth affect the woman, her family, and her family-support system by (1) their reaction to physical and emotional changes of pregnancy; (2) alteration of the family dynamics in terms of roles, responsibilities, and relationships; and (3) accomplishment of the developmental tasks during transition to role of mother or father.

CONTENT REVIEW

I. **Pregnancy—healthy state of maternal adaptation to support fetal growth and development. Adaptations:**
   A. Are ongoing throughout the *antepartal* period as a result of mechanical and hormonal factors
   B. Affect nearly every system to some degree (Table 2-1)
   C. Increase a woman's vulnerability to health problems, especially for women at high risk
   D. Help to diagnose pregnancy: presumptive, probable, and positive changes (Box 2-1)
   E. Are the bases for pregnancy-related discomforts
   F. Require careful assessment to determine if changes
      1. Fall within the expected range for pregnancy
      2. Reflect a warning sign of a pathophysiologic process that represents ineffective adaptation (e.g., physiologic anemia versus pathologic anemia)

II. **Pregnancy creates the potential for a *maturational crisis*, which is associated with an expected change resulting from growth and development, or a *situational crisis*, which is associated with a change in circumstances, or both**
   A. Examples of change in circumstances include family finances, stability of relationships, health status of a family member, complication of pregnancy, and preterm birth
   B. Risk for crisis is influenced by three factors:
      1. Perception of the event
         a. Realistic—pregnancy is viewed as a growth experience; the need for adjustments and the increase in responsibilities are acknowledged
         b. Unrealistic—pregnancy is viewed with fear and as a stressful time; the newborn is seen as someone to love them or as someone who can strengthen a shaky relationship, and it is anticipated that life will go on as usual after childbirth

Text continued on p. 33

TABLE 2-1	Anatomic and Physiologic Adaptations Associated with Pregnancy		
Anatomic and Physiologic Adaptations	**Expected Assessment Findings**	**Warning Signs of Ineffective Adaptation**	

Breasts

Bilateral changes, stimulated by estrogen, progesterone, human placental lactogen (HPL):

Glandular and duct tissue develops; alveoli hypertrophy

Fluid is produced

Precolostrum (thin, clear) at 6 wk

Colostrum (thick, yellowish, precursor to milk) during the third trimester

Vascularity increases

Appearance:

Full, heavy, enlarged, *striae gravidarum*

Increased pigmentation of nipples and areola

Montgomery's tubercles (sebaceous glands) of areola enlarge

Nipples larger, more erect

Leakage of precolostrum, colostrum

Sensitive and tender

Nodular on palpation

Breast self-examination (BSE) distinguishes expected change from pathology; assess for the following:

Masses: fixed, firm, unilateral

Skin changes: dimpling, erythema, rashes, ulcerations, edema

Nipple retraction

Painful breasts

Note: Pathologic changes usually are unilateral, not bilateral

Reproductive System (Uterus, Vagina, Perineum)

Changes stimulated by effects of estrogen, progesterone, and fetal growth:

Uterus enlarges into a thin, soft-walled organ

Uterus softens progressively from lower segment to cervix

Endometrium thickens, becomes velvety and more vascular to support implantation; now termed *decidua*

Increase in fundal height (Fig. 2-1)

Above symphysis pubis by 12-14 wk

At umbilicus by 20 wk

At zyphoid process by 36 wk

Decrease in fundal height with lightening (movement of fetus into pelvic inlet)

Primigravida: 2-4 wk before onset of labor

Multipara: just before labor onset

Softened lower uterine segment (Hegar's sign)

Vaginal bleeding to any degree must be evaluated to determine cause

Risk for reproductive tract infections increase as evidenced by:

Lesions, pruritus, erythema

Vaginal discharge changes: color, amount, odor, consistency

Signs of preterm labor:

Pelvic pressure; sensation of something falling out

Vascularity increases:

Deepening color of cervix and vagina

Softening from lower uterine segment to perineum and vulva

Increasing stretching of cervix, vagina, and perineum

Increasing friability (fragility)

Increasing pelvic congestion results in greater sexual arousal and orgasms in second trimester

Increased pelvic pressure related to enlarged uterus inhibits venous return

Increased activity of cervical and vaginal glands produce more mucous; mucous plug (*operculum*) fills cervical canal to create a barrier to infection

Cessation of menstrual cycle and menses related to suppression of follicle-stimulating hormone (FSH) and luteinizing hormone (LH) by elevated levels of estrogen and progesterone

Softened cervix (Goodell's sign)

Reddish-purple color of vagina and cervix (Chadwick's sign)

WARNING! Spotting can occur after vaginal examination and intercourse from the increased vascularity and increasing friability (fragility) of the cervix.

Enlarged vulva and labia majora

Varicosities are noted on vulva, perineum, around anus (hemorrhoids)

Increased vaginal discharge (*leukorrhea*) whitish-gray, less acidic, faint musty odor

WARNING! Increased risk for vaginal infections especially yeast (candidiasis)

Braxton Hicks contractions—irregular, painless tightening of uterus as it enlarges most noticeable by 28 weeks' gestation; often confused with true labor

Amenorrhea

Low backache; menstrual-like or intestinal cramps with or without diarrhea

Uterine contractions every 10 min or less (six or more per hour)

Change in vaginal discharge

Diagnosis confirmed by cervical changes: effacement (80%) or cervical dilation (more than 1 cm), or both

Continued

TABLE 2-1 Anatomic and Physiologic Adaptations Associated with Pregnancy—cont'd

Anatomic and Physiologic Adaptations	Expected Assessment Findings	Warning Signs of Ineffective Adaptation
Oxygenation Diaphragm pushed upward by enlarging uterus Ribs flare, chest expands Increased oxygen demand related to increased maternal basal metabolic rate (BMR), development of reproductive structures, and fetal growth and development Increased vascularity of upper airway and respiratory system	Respirations: Slight increase in baseline respiratory rate (2 breaths per min) Volume deeper (hyperventilation of pregnancy) Thoracic breathing pattern Some shortness of breath and slight dyspnea even at rest; diminishes after lightening Chest circumference expands by 2-3 in (5-7 cm) Nasal mucosa is swollen, moist, reddened Nasal and sinus stuffiness, with clear, watery discharge Increased inflammatory response to upper respiratory infections (colds) Episodes of epistaxis (nosebleeds) Sense of fullness in ears, slight impairment of hearing, earaches Voice deepens Slight respiratory alkalosis, compensated by mild metabolic acidosis	Signs and symptoms indicative of cardiac decompensation and pulmonary edema especially in high-risk women with cardiac, hypertensive, or renal health problems: Anxiety; fatigue Rapid, weak, irregular pulse Moderate to severe dyspnea with tightness in chest Orthopnea Crackles; productive cough with frothy sputum

Circulation

Increase in blood volume peaks at about 20-26 weeks' gestation

Increase of 30-50% or 1500 ml (singleton pregnancy)

Increase of 2000 ml or more (multiple gestation)

Dilation of vascular network accommodates volume

Purpose of volume increase is to:

Fill expanded vascular network: placenta, enlarged uterus

Protect maternal-fetal unit from hypotension related to impaired venous return

Protect from hemorrhagic shock related to blood loss during childbirth

Hemodilution (peaks in second trimester)

Initially plasma increases faster than red blood cells (RBCs)

RBC production catches up by third trimester as plasma volume expansion levels off

Cardiac output (CO) increases by 30-50% peaking at 32 wk, then declines

Cardiac workload increases

Heart enlarges slightly

Heart is moved upward and to the left

Blood pressure:

Decreases 5-10 mm Hg systolic and diastolic during first and second trimester

Returns to prepregnant baseline during third trimester

Supine hypotension: blood pressure decreases as a result of uterine compression of vena cava and aorta when in supine position (see Fig. 2-2) (not found in 1st trimester)

Postural hypotension: decrease in blood pressure with sudden change from supine to upright position

Hypotension results in: dizziness, lightheadedness, pallor, diaphoresis, anxiety

Heart rate and pattern:

Point of maximal intensity (PMI) shifts upward to left

Rate increases 10-15 beats per minute by 14-20 wk persisting until term

Transitory systolic murmurs, benign dysrhythmias, palpitations

Dependent edema of lower extremities

Varicosities in lower extremities, vulva, and perineum and around anus

Physiologic anemia related to hemodilution

Hematocrit 33% or higher and hemoglobin 11 g/dl or higher (1st and 3rd trimester)

Signs of pregnancy induced hypertension (PIH)

Hypertension: 140/90 mm Hg or higher after 20 weeks' gestation, two measurements 4-6 hr apart

Pathologic edema: upper body edema: face, hands, fingers, abdomen; unresponsive to bed rest

Sudden increase in weight over 2 kg in 1 wk

Headaches, visual disturbances (double vision, spots before eyes, blurring)

Epigastric pain

CNS irritability, brisk deep tendon reflexes, ankle clonus

Proteinuria: 2+ or more, in two specimens 6 hr apart

Signs of pathologic anemia:

Hematocrit and hemoglobin levels decrease below accepted minimums

Often related to iron deficiency

Signs of thrombophlebitis commonly unilateral in lower extremity (calf):

Discomfort, feeling of heaviness in leg

Heat, erythema, over-inflamed vein (especially if superficial vein is affected)

Edema, increase in calf size

Continued

| TABLE 2-1 Anatomic and Physiologic Adaptations Associated with Pregnancy—cont'd |||
Anatomic and Physiologic Adaptations	Expected Assessment Findings	Warning Signs of Ineffective Adaptation
Circulation—cont'd Inferior vena cava, abdominal aorta, and pelvic blood vessels are compressed by enlarging uterus and maternal position (supine, upright) to result in: Impaired venous return Decreased CO Diminished perfusion of placenta, kidneys Increased venous pressure in the lower extremities Circulation and CO enhanced in lateral position which remove uterine compression effect on blood vessels Hypercoagulability of blood Protects against hemorrhage Hypercoagulability with sluggish circulation in lower extremities increases risk for thrombus formation	Hematocrit at least 32% and hemoglobin at least 10.5 g/dl (2nd trimester) Stabilizes by midpregnancy with gradual return to prepregnant range	Positive Homans sign: sharp pain in calf on dorsiflexion of the foot **WARNING!** Once a positive Homans' sign is established, do not recheck since clots may be dislodged.

Nutrition and Fluid-Electrolytes

BMR increases by approximately 20%

Increased activity of thyroid gland; slight enlargement; elevated thyroid hormone levels

Nutrient needs increase and metabolism is altered to meet demands of increased BMR, maternal adaptations, and fetal growth and development:

Increased nitrogen (protein) retention

Moderate increase in iron absorption

Increased calcium absorption

More complete fat absorption with deposition in subcutaneous tissue in preparation for lactation

Glucose level regulated by a changing production of insulin (diabetogenic effect of pregnancy) to preserve glucose for fetal use; placenta produces insulin antagonists in second and third trimesters

Weight increases related to: fetal growth, placenta and amniotic fluid, expansion of maternal blood and fluid volume, maternal fat deposition, breast and uterine development

Weight gain recommendations for pregnancy are based on the woman's body mass index (BMI)

First trimester weight gain: 3.5-5 lb (1.6-2.3 kg) for all BMI classifications

Normal weight (BMI 19.8-26):

Total gain: 25-35 lb (11.5-16 kg)

0.8 lb/wk (0.4 kg) 2nd, 3rd trimesters

Underweight (BMI <19.8):

Total gain: 28-40 lb (12.5-18 kg)

1.1 lb/wk (0.5 kg) 2nd and 3rd trimesters

Overweight (BMI 26-29):

Total gain: 15-25 lb (7-11 kg)

0.6 lb/wk (0.3 kg) 2nd and 3rd trimesters

Obese (BMI >29):

Total gain of at least 15 lb (7 kg)

Less than 0.6 lb/wk (0.3 kg) 2nd and 3rd trimesters

Morning sickness—nausea or vomiting or both

Occurs at any time of day

Subsides by second trimester

Nutritional and fluid deficits do not occur

Increased appetite; cravings for or aversion to certain foods

Weight gain pattern that does not follow expected norms:

Weight loss

Gain of too much or too little related to excessive or inadequate nutrient intake

Sudden, sharp increase related to fluid retention of pregnancy-induced hypertension

Hyperemesis gravidarum—severe vomiting leads to weight loss over 5%, fluid-electrolyte and acid-base imbalance

Pica—ingestion of nonnutritive substances (clay, laundry starch, dirt, chalk) or food stuffs low in nutritional value (ice, freezer frost, baking powder, cornstarch) which can lead to anemia and malnutrition

Signs of cholecystitis or cholelithiasis

Pathologic anemia related to low iron intake

Continued

TABLE 2-1	Anatomic and Physiologic Adaptations Associated with Pregnancy—cont'd	
Anatomic and Physiologic Adaptations	**Expected Assessment Findings**	**Warning Signs of Ineffective Adaptation**
Nutrition and Fluid-Electrolytes— cont'd		
Motility of upper gastrointestinal tract decreases (progesterone effect)	Pyrosis	
Relaxation of cardiac sphincter with reflux of gastric contents into esophagus leads to pyrosis (heartburn)	Oral cavity	
Maximum nutrient absorption	Softened, tender, vascular gums bleed more easily	
Slower emptying time of gallbladder increases risk for cholelithiasis	*Epulis*—localized vascular lesion on gums	
Nausea and vomiting from slower emptying time of stomach, elevated level of human chorionic gonadotrophin (HCG), fetal demand for glucose, emotions (stress, anxiety, ambivalence)	Laboratory values:	
Vascularity of oral cavity increases from higher estrogen level	Lower fasting blood sugar (FSB): 65 mg/dl	
	Higher cholesterol levels: 243-305 mg/dl	
Bowel Elimination		
Intestinal displacement	Diminished bowel sounds	Abdominal cramping and pain could indicate ruptured ectopic pregnancy, appendicitis, separation of placenta, miscarriage
Increased pressure on anal blood vessels from enlarging uterus	Flatulence	Assess: location, frequency, onset, character of pain and accompanying signs and symptoms
Decreased peristalsis (progesterone effect)	Constipation	
Increased fluid absorption from feces related to slower movement through intestine	Hemorrhoids related to pelvic pressure and straining to pass constipated stool; aggravated after lightening occurs	

Urinary Elimination

Increased metabolic wastes to excrete

Increased renal blood flow and glomerular filtration rate

Maternal position (supine, upright) reduces renal blood flow as a result of uterine pressure; leads to fluid retention and edema

Lateral position enhances renal blood flow

Decreased bladder capacity related to displacement and compression by enlarging uterus (1st trimester and after lightening)

Decreased renal tone and peristalsis in pelvis, ureters, bladder and peristalsis (progesterone effect) leads to stasis and back flow of urine

Urinary frequency, urgency, stress incontinence, especially during the 1st trimester and after lightening

Increased urine production when in lateral position

Decrease in edema

Nocturia

Alteration in urine characteristics:
Glycosuria (trace, +1)
Proteinuria (trace, +1, especially if urine is concentrated)
Higher nutrient content

Positive pregnancy test indicates the presence of HCG

Diarrhea could indicate presence of intestinal tract infection, influenza; assess frequency, onset, duration, and accompanying signs and symptoms

Risk for urinary tract infection (UTI) increased

Asymptomatic bacteriuria; positive urine culture with no clinical signs of UTI; associated with pregnancy and fetal complications

Signs of pyelonephritis or UTI:
Flank pain; positive costovertebral angle (CVA) tenderness
Fever
Frequency, urgency accompanied by dysuria
Change in characteristics of urine (cloudy, hematuria, odor)
Presence of casts, blood cells, microorganisms in urine

Physical Activity and Rest

Decreased abdominal muscle tone; stretches from enlarging uterus

Pressure on nerves and postural changes from the enlarged, heavier breasts and enlarged uterus

Increased joint and ligament mobility (relaxin)

Alteration in appearance:
Lordosis (accentuated lumbar curve)
Waddling gait, awkward movement

Discomfort:
Neck and shoulder strain, numbness and tingling of hands
Low back pain
Muscle cramps in lower extremities

Signs of carpal tunnel syndrome—sustained tenderness and weakness of thumb muscles that radiates to the elbow

Signs from pregnancy-induced hypertension
Severe persistent headache
Irritability, restlessness, insomnia
Brisk deep tendon reflexes (DTR), ankle clonus

Continued

TABLE 2-1	Anatomic and Physiologic Adaptations Associated with Pregnancy—cont'd	
Anatomic and Physiologic Adaptations	**Expected Assessment Findings**	**Warning Signs of Ineffective Adaptation**
Physical Activity and Rest—cont'd Hypocalcemia from an increased fetal demand and low intake Changes in blood pressure and cardiac output occur with changes in maternal position (i.e., upright to supine, supine to lateral) Stressors from pregnancy may interfere with rest and sleep	Faintness, dizziness Fatigue, decreased energy level especially in the first and third trimester *Diastasis recti abdominis*—separation of recti muscles of abdomen Tension headache	
Integument Deepened body pigmentation from increased melanin Increased activity of sweat and sebaceous glands (estrogen) Increased fragility and elasticity of connective tissue (adrenocortical activity)	Pigmentary changes: *Melasma* (*chloasma*, mask of pregnancy)— blotchy brownish discoloration of face usually over cheeks, forehead, nose *Linea nigra*—darkening of vertical line along abdominal midline lengthens as fundal height increases	Signs of physical abuse Common sites: head, neck, chest, breasts, abdomen, upper extremities; during pregnancy: breasts, abdomen, genitalia Types of injuries: burns, bruises, abrasions, fractures, and other traumatic injuries Take note of pattern: hand print, belt buckle, strap

Integument—cont'd

Increase in basal body temperature from an increased BMR and progesterone effect; heat dissipation through sweat gland activity and peripheral vasodilation

Darkening of nipples, areola, vulva, moles, freckles and birth marks

Increased sensitivity to sunlight; sunburn occurs more easily

Diaphoresis, acne, oily skin

Striae gravidarum—reddish-purple stretch marks on breasts, abdomen, buttocks, thighs

Changes from peripheral vasodilation:

Hair is lustrous, fuller; hirsutism

Fingernails are thinner, softer, fragile

Palmar erythema

Vascular spiders (spider angiomas, telangiectasis)—tiny red circular elevations with several thin branching arms; found on neck, thorax, arms of fair-skinned women

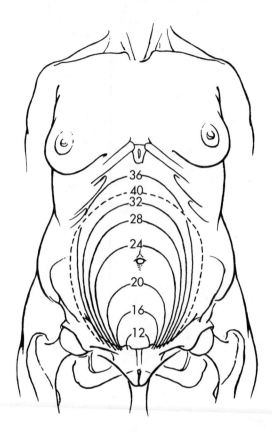

Figure 2-1   Approximate levels of the uterine fundus at various gestational points. Numbers indicate weeks of gestation. The dotted line indicates height after lightening. (From Barkauskas V, Baumann LC, Stoltenberg-Allen K, Darling-Fisher C: *Health and physical assessment,* ed 2, St. Louis, 1998, Mosby.)

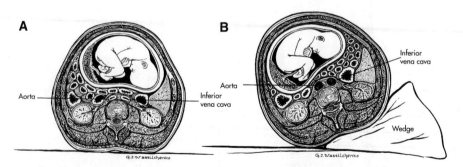

Figure 2-2   Supine hypotension. **A,** Compression of aorta and inferior vena cava with woman in supine position. **B,** Compression of these vessels is relieved by placement of a wedge pillow under the woman's right or left hip. (From Lowdermilk DL, Perry SE, Bobak IM: *Maternity and women's health care,* ed 7, St. Louis, 2000, Mosby.)

Box 2-1
Presumptive, Probable, Positive Changes of Pregnancy

Presumptive changes are subjective findings felt by the woman. They are suggestive of but not diagnostic of pregnancy. These changes include breast tenderness, tingling, and heaviness; nausea and vomiting; fatigue; quickening; amenorrhea; and urinary frequency.

Probable changes are objective findings noted by the examiner that are more suggestive of but not yet diagnostic of pregnancy. These changes include the pigmentary changes of the integument, *striae gravidarum,* uterine enlargement, uterine souffle, Braxton Hicks contractions on palpation, Hegar's sign, Goodell's sign, Chadwick's sign, ballottement, and a positive pregnancy test.

Positive changes are objective findings that are diagnostic of pregnancy and that cannot be attributed to any other cause but pregnancy. These changes include fetal heart beat, fetal outline on ultrasonography, and fetal movements seen or by palpated by the examiner.

2. Coping mechanisms
   a. Usual methods of coping with stress and responding to change often are used during pregnancy
   b. Constructive—healthy lifestyle changes are made; participation in parenting groups, childbirth classes, and prenatal care occurs
   c. Ineffective—delay in confirming pregnancy or seeking prenatal care; attempt to conceal pregnancy by limiting weight gain or wearing baggy clothing
3. Situational supports
   a. Availability and degree of support offered by the family-support system
      (1) Emotional support, especially from partner or the father of the baby
      (2) Physical support in terms of household tasks, transportation, and child care
      (3) Role models and sources of information and expertise related to pregnancy and parenting
   b. Willingness of the pregnant woman to accept support
   c. Availability of health care and community support agencies to meet the needs of a pregnant woman and her family-support system; consider eligibility, quality of services, and convenience of location and appointment times

III. Maternal psychosocial adaptations to pregnancy and impending parenthood
A. **Maternal role and responsibilities**
   1. Activities acceptable and required during pregnancy. Examples include self-care interventions, nutrition, activity and rest patterns, and prenatal care.
   2. Prohibited activities

3. Birthing practices
4. Parenting activities

B. Factors influencing maternal role and responsibilities
1. Family experiences, especially relationship with own mother
2. Cultural norms and expectations about a woman's behavior when pregnant and as a mother
3. Previous experiences with pregnancy and as a mother or caretaker of children
4. Attitude toward the pregnancy—desired and planned, or unplanned and unwanted
5. Society's views about women and motherhood
   (1) Combining career or work role with the role of a parent
   (2) Involving father and other family members to assist the mother in meeting her parenting responsibilities
   (3) Choosing single parenthood
   (4) Postponing childbearing until the woman is ready

C. Developmental tasks in the preparation for the maternal role
1. First trimester—acceptance of pregnancy; woman states "I am pregnant."
   a. Seeks confirmation of pregnancy
   b. Reacts to confirmation of pregnancy influenced by readiness for and desire to be pregnant. Most women experience *ambivalence,* that is, wanting to be pregnant and not wanting to be pregnant at the same time.
   c. Adjusts to physical changes and sensations. Examples include morning sickness, fatigue, breast tenderness, and frequent urination.
   d. Exhibits *egocentricity,* that is, the woman's concerns center on self and physical changes
   e. Exhibits *emotional lability* (moods swings) from hormonal changes and anxiety about her ability to cope successfully with pregnancy
   f. Has diminished sex drive from physical changes, fear of harming fetus, and mood swings
2. Second trimester—acceptance of the fetus as distinct from herself; woman states "I am going to have a baby."
   a. Fetus becomes a reality; attachment to the fetus is stimulated by hearing the heart beat and feeling movement *(quickening)*
   b. The woman becomes introspective and focuses on the fetus and motherhood
      (1) Fantasizes about the baby and herself as a mother
      (2) Reviews relationship with own mother
      (3) Observes mothering activities of other women
      (4) Decreases focus on family members
   c. Discomforts of first trimester diminish
   d. Sexual drive increases; pelvic congestion enhances orgasm
   e. Body contours change; pregnancy "shows"

3. Third trimester—acceptance of impending birth and the reality of parenthood; woman states "I am going to be a parent."
  a. Concerns center on
    (1) Securing safe passage of fetus
    (2) Separating self from fetus
    (3) Obtaining acceptance of newborn by others
  b. Discomforts increase, which enhance readiness for labor
    (1) Fetal activity interferes with rest
    (2) Enlarging uterus changes the woman's center of gravity; she is more awkward and clumsy; she finds it more difficult to ambulate, move, find a comfortable position, and generally accomplish the tasks of living
    (3) Altered body contour increases her sensitivity to the reaction of others
    (4) Decreased sex drive from discomforts, body image, dyspareunia, and concerns about fetal injury and stimulation of preterm labor
  c. Lightening leads to urinary frequency; varicosities of legs, vulva, rectum and anus; and edema of legs, ankles, and feet
  d. Impending birth motivates woman to
    (1) Participate in childbirth and parenting classes
    (2) Prepare a birth plan with her partner and primary health care provider; the plan should be a realistic, mutually acceptable birth guide

D. Difficulty in accomplishing the tasks of pregnancy in adolescent women
1. Pregnancy is often unexpected; fear of discovery and possible rejection by family and support system results in
  a. Denial; delay in the acceptance of pregnancy
  b. Avoidance of prenatal care
  c. Attempt to conceal pregnancy
2. Immaturity in terms of her own development
  a. Limits motivation to seek and follow through with prenatal care, healthy lifestyle, or childbirth preparation classes
  b. Leads to an unrealistic, idealized view of babies and the impact of parenting
3. Successful physical and psychosocial adaptation to pregnancy depends on support and acceptance provided by the family-support system, including peers

E. Warning signs of ineffective maternal psychosocial adaptation to pregnancy
1. Intense denial of pregnancy results in
  a. Avoidance of confirmation of pregnancy and participation in prenatal care and expectant parents' classes
  b. Attempts to conceal pregnancy by limiting weight gain, refusing to wear maternity clothes

      c. Lack of preparation for newborn in terms of name, living space, and supplies

  2. Unrealistic expectations about birth and parenting

  3. Low tolerance for pregnancy's physical changes, which interfere with the woman's ability to participate in daily activities of living

  4. Refusal to alter lifestyle to ensure a healthy outcome of the pregnancy and optimal fetal growth and development

IV. Paternal psychosocial adaptation to pregnancy and impending parenthood

A. Perception of the paternal role is influenced by six factors:

  1. Family experiences; relationship with own father

  2. Views of partner about paternal role responsibilities; paternal responsibilities should be mutually negotiated to avoid conflict

  3. Cultural beliefs and expectations about paternal behaviors during pregnancy, birth, and parenting

  4. Previous experiences with fatherhood or as a caregiver to children

  5. Attitude toward his partner and the pregnancy

  6. Societal norm: equitable sharing of parenting responsibilities

B. Developmental tasks to prepare for the paternal role

  1. Accepts reality that partner is pregnant; man states "I am going to be a father."

    a. Views pregnancy as a confirmation of virility

    b. Experiences doubt about his ability to support partner, especially during childbirth, and ability to be a father

    c. Experiences concern about impact on finances, lifestyle, and sexuality

    d. Is influenced by **couvade,** that is, the culturally determined pattern of expected paternal behaviors during pregnancy and birthing

      (1) Identifies with partner's pregnancy-related discomforts. Examples include experiencing nausea and vomiting, weight gain, and fatigue.

      (2) Identifies the responsibilities during childbirth and the nature of participation

    e. Reviews relationship with own father

    f. Becomes introspective, fantasizing about the baby and himself as a father; develops attachment to fetus

  2. Copes in a positive manner with partner's changing body and emotions

    a. Views physical and emotional changes of pregnancy as natural and beautiful

    b. Alters sexual relationship in tune with partner's changing sex drive, body contours, and needs

    c. Openly communicates concern while working with partner to find mutually satisfying ways to express love and affection

3. Participates in the process of pregnancy and birth
   a. Increases "creative" activities such as self-improvement, enhancement of living space, and job advancement
   b. Negotiates his role during childbirth with his partner; participates in the development of a birth plan
   c. Copes effectively with fears about the safety of the mother and fetus and his effectiveness as a labor participant
C. **Paternal feelings and behaviors have an influence on the success and ease of the mother's adaptation to pregnancy and parenting**
D. **Warning signs of ineffective paternal psychosocial adaptation to pregnancy**
   1. Is unwilling or unable to meet the physical and emotional needs of his partner or to participate in preparation activities
   2. Refuses to discuss the fetus or newborn; views or fantasizes about the baby as an older child
   3. Expresses anger about changes in lifestyle, sexuality, and financial situation; may lead to abuse of partner, infidelity, or abandonment
   4. Expresses displeasure with the changes in his partner's appearance
   5. Experiences difficulty about the sexual relationship with partner, which may lead to infidelity or impotence

⚠ Warning!

The incidence of physical or psychological abuse, or both, of a woman by her partner can begin or intensify during pregnancy.

V. Sibling responses to pregnancy and the newborn

A. **Pregnancy and addition of a new family member has a major impact on siblings**
   1. May be the child's first crisis
   2. Feels anxiety about changes in the familiar daily patterns of living and relationships
   3. Perceives a loss of position and status in family and this results in feelings of jealousy
   4. Feels stress resulting from separation from the mother during her hospitalization
B. **Sibling reactions depend on age, developmental level, and life experiences**
   1. Toddlers—are aware of the mother's changing appearance; difficulty with separation from the mother; may exhibit regression
   2. Preschoolers and school-aged children—ask detailed questions about the pregnancy; are eager to participate in the care of the newborn
   3. Adolescents—may be embarrassed about the evidence of parental sexual activity and change in the mother's appearance; may be very sensitive to the mother's needs
C. **Parental views and practices about sibling preparation are critical to successful sibling adjustment (Box 2-2)**

Box 2-2
Sibling Preparation for a New Baby

Begin preparations and use methods consistent with the developmental level of each child involved, for example:
- Toddlers and preschoolers should be told about the pregnancy when changes in the mother become noticeable.
- Children of school age and adolescents should be told about the pregnancy as soon as the parents know.

Include children in preparations made for the new baby:
- Discuss anticipated changes in the roles and responsibilities of each family member and the impact the baby will have on family life.
- Have children help with choosing a name, getting the baby's room ready, and picking out toys and clothing.

Make plans in advance for the care of children during the time of birth:
- Seek input from the children involved, for example, who they would want to stay with and where they would want to go, and honor their input as much as possible.
- Arrange for introductions and sleepovers to help very young children become familiar with temporary caregivers and to prepare for the separation.

Make changes, especially those concerning very young children, early in pregnancy:
- Make environmental changes such as advancing from a crib to a bed.
- Make developmental changes, for example, toilet training and enrollment in day care.
- Preserve rituals, for example, at mealtime and bedtime, of young children as much as possible.

Use developmentally appropriate books, videos, and classes to educate children about the following:
- Sexuality
- Pregnancy and birth
- The characteristics, needs, and care of a newborn
- Children's roles when the newborn comes home

Enhance the development of a realistic view of newborns:
- Provide opportunities for children to interact with families who have newborns.
- Allow older children to accompany the mother to a prenatal care visit to hear the fetal heart beat and learn the importance of health care during pregnancy.
- Encourage children to feel the movements of the fetus and to talk to the fetus.
- View family photo albums, showing the children what they looked like as babies.
- Enroll children in sibling preparation classes.

VI. Grandparents' response to their child's pregnancy and parenting
   A. **Reactions to the event that their child is having a child**
      1. Realizations that they are old enough to be grandparents and their child is an adult
      2. Their views may conflict with current pregnancy, birthing, and parenting practices
      3. Opportunity to do things with grandchildren they did not have the time nor resources to do with their own children
   B. **Grandparents serve as family historians; role models; teachers; and sources of support, strength, and nurturing**

C. **Nature of grandparents' role and degree of involvement are influenced by**
1. Their experiences with their own parents in the role of grandparents
2. Their view of grandparents' role contrasted with society's view
3. The view of grandparents' role held by the expectant parents
4. Nature of the relationship between the grandparents and the expectant couple
    a. Ability to develop with their children mutually agreed-on role responsibilities and involvement
    b. Failure to develop responsibilities may increase the risk for family conflict and crisis

WEB Resources

http://www.pregnancy.about.com
This site fully covers all aspects of pregnancy, birth, and postpartum periods. It is part of the about.com network of sites led by expert guides.

http://www.abcbirth.com
Online textbook about pregnancy, childbirth, and early parenting.

http://www.awhonn.org
Association of Women's Health, Obstetric, and Neonatal Nurses.

http://www.pampers.com
Pampers Parenting Institute provides expert advice, information, and support for parents from pregnancy through the toddler period.

http://www.newdads.com
Boot Camp for New Fathers provides information and programs for first-time fathers beginning in pregnancy and continuing through the care and nurturing of the infant and new mother.

REVIEW QUESTIONS

1. The first day of a woman's LMP was September 7, 1999, and it ended on September 12. Use Nägele's rule to determine this woman's estimated date of birth (EDB), which would be which of these specific dates?
   1. January 10, 2000
   2. June 14, 2000
   3. June 19, 2000
   4. November 30, 2000

2. Which of these findings, if exhibited by a pregnant woman, represents a probable change of pregnancy?
   1. Morning sickness
   2. Quickening
   3. Positive pregnancy test
   4. A fetal heart beat auscultated with a Doppler or fetoscope

3. On examination of a pregnant woman at 10 weeks' gestation the nurse notes that her vagina and cervix are a deep reddish-purple color. The nurse would record this as which of these documentation notes?
   1. Chadwick's sign
   2. Hegar's sign
   3. Goodell's sign
   4. Hyperpigmentation of the genitalia

4. While her fundal height is being measured, a pregnant woman at 20 weeks' gestation begins to complain of dizziness and lightheadedness. The nurse notes that the woman's skin has become pale and diaphoretic. The nurse recognizes that this woman is most likely experiencing which of these findings?
   1. Supine hypotension
   2. Anxiety reaction to the examination
   3. Postural hypotension
   4. Circulatory collapse

5. A pregnant woman's prepregnant weight is 125 pounds and her body mass index (BMI) is 24. By the end of her pregnancy, her weight should fall between which range of pounds?
   1. 140-150
   2. 150-160
   3. 153-165
   4. 160-180

6. Which of these behaviors will reduce a family's risk for maturational crisis during pregnancy?
   1. A mother plans to surprise her pregnant daughter by moving in with her after birth and show her daughter the right way to take care of a baby

2. A woman, pregnant for 7 months, expresses pride that by limiting her weight gain, she can still wear her regular clothes
3. A pregnant woman has started to modify her work schedule in anticipation of the added responsibilities of parenting after her baby is born
4. A 19-year-old single woman, pregnant for the first time, decides not to participate in parenting classes because she has experience as a babysitter and therefore knows how to take care of babies

7. During the second trimester, the nurse would expect a pregnant woman to exhibit which one of these behaviors?
1. Excitement when quickening occurs
2. Egocentricity
3. Interest in childbirth techniques
4. Diminished sex drive from fatigue, nausea, and breast tenderness

8. A Chinese–American expectant father tells the nurse he does not view his role during childbirth to be that of a coach. The nurse recognizes that this behavior is most likely a reflection of which perception?
1. Limited interest in the well-being of his wife
2. Embarrassment
3. Couvade
4. Ambivalence about the pregnancy

9. Which of these findings, if exhibited by an expectant father, would be a warning sign of ineffective adaptation to his partner's first pregnancy?
1. Views pregnancy with pride as a confirmation of his virility
2. Consistently changes the subject when the topic of the fetus or newborn is raised
3. Expresses concern that he might faint at the birth of his baby
4. Experiences nausea and fatigue, along with his partner, during the first trimester

10. Expectant parents, in the first trimester of pregnancy, ask the nurse how they can prepare their 3-year-old preschool daughter for the new baby. Which of these actions would be least effective to facilitate adjustment?
1. Tell the child about the pregnancy as soon as mom begins to "show"
2. Arrange for a few "sleepovers" with the person who will care for their child at the time of the birth
3. Wait to transfer their child to her new room and bed just before the expected birth of the baby
4. Enroll their child in a sibling preparation class for young children

ANSWERS, RATIONALES, AND TEST-TAKING TIPS

Rationale	Test-Taking Tips

1. Correct answer: 2

Nägele's rule: subtract 3 months and add 7 days and 1 year to the first day of *the last menstrual period:*

```
   9    7   1999
  -3   +7    +1
   6   14   2000
```

Avoid confusion when the first and last day of the menstrual cycle is given. Remember that the first day is most important. Most nurses can recall counting back 3 months, which narrows your answers to options 2 and 3. To recall how many days to add, simply remember the number of days in a week—7. Add 7 days to the first day of the cycle.

2. Correct answer: 3

Options 1 and 2 are presumptive changes. Option 3 is a probable change. Option 4 is a positive change.

Associate PREsumptive changes with the PREgnant mother's findings that are suggestive of but not diagnostic of pregnancy. Associate PROBable changes with the PRactitioner of OB findings that are more suggestive but not diagnostic of pregnancy. Then associate that the pOsitive changes are Only Objective findings by the Obstetric practitioner: fetal heart beat is heard, fetus is outlined with ultrasonography, and fetal movement is detected by the examiner. In summary, the mother finds the first changes, presumptive, suggestive of pregnancy. Then the practitioner finds probable changes. Lastly, the practitioner ultimately makes *the* diagnosis of pregnancy. The sequence is typically as follows: the presumptive, probable, and positive changes of pregnancy. Avoid a common error. Make a note of this—a positive pregnancy test falls under the *probable* category of changes, not the positive change category.

3. Correct answer: 1

The color change exhibited is related to the increased vascularity of genitalia, not an increased pigmentation. Hegar's sign is softening of the lower uterine segment. Goodell's sign is softening of the cervix.

Think alphabetically for these signs with the anatomic inspection from external to internal:
Chadwick's = vagina with color changes;
Goodell's = cervix with a softening of it;
Hegar's = uterus with a softening of the lower segment.

4. Correct answer: 1

The signs exhibited relate to a decrease in blood pressure from uterine compression of the vena cava. It is an expected finding and unrelated to circulatory problems or maternal anxiety. Postural hypotension, a systolic decrease of at least 20 mm Hg, occurs when rising from a supine to an upright position. The most common cause of this finding is a decrease in the circulating volume—*hypovolemia*—from dehydration, blood loss, or excessive diuresis.

Eliminate options 2 and 4 because there is not enough information in the stem to support their selection. Reread the stem to note that with fundal measurement the client would be flat on her back or in a supine position. Simply match the position in the question with the position in the option, option 1. Eliminate option 3 because posture was not changed from a supine to an upright, dangling, or standing position in this situation.

5. Correct answer: 2

A BMI of 24 indicates a normal weight. Therefore, the recommended weight gain would be 25 to 35 pounds. BMI is the body mass index, which is calculated using height and weight measurements. Standardized tables are available. This index guides the weight gain recommendations for the entire pregnancy and the weekly pattern of weight gain during the second and third trimesters.

If you have no idea of a correct answer, use the "eliminate the extremes" approach. Eliminate options 1 and 4, which are the highest and lowest ranges for pounds gained. Reread the question. Then go with what you know: the recommendation of weight gained on the average is between 25 and 35 lb. Add the minimum of this—25 lb—to the prepregnancy weight of 125 lb for a minimum total of 150 lb. Select option 2. Another approach is to subtract 125 lb from the 150 and 160 lb of option 2 to get 25 to 35 lb. Then subtract 125 lb from the 153 and 165 lb of option 3 to get 28 to 40 lb.

Rationales	Test-Taking Tips

6. Correct answer: 3

Option 3 represents a realistic perception of the impact of parenthood and constructive coping mechanisms. Option 1 represents a situational support problem. Option 2 represents ineffective coping to deal with changes in body image. Option 4 represents an unrealistic perception of full-time parenting and ineffective coping mechanisms.

The clues in the stem are the direction of the action "reduce the family's risk. . . for crisis" and the timeframe "during pregnancy." Option 1 focuses on after the pregnancy and also would increase the risk of crisis from the surprise. Weight gain restriction is a threat to the well-being of the mother and fetus, which may lead to a physiologic crisis. Option 4 reflects an immature perception of the needs during pregnancy.

7. Correct answer: 1

Egocentricity is typical of the first trimester. Diminished sex drive typically occurs during the first and third trimesters. Interest in childbirth is prominent in the third trimester as the onset of labor approaches.

Associate the behaviors exhibited by the mother during the trimesters with the letter "E." Behaviors "E"xhibited by the mother are the three Es. Ego "for me go" the first trimester with no entertainment of sexual activity. Excitement—the baby is really there during the second trimester. Exit plans and preparation during the third trimester take up all the interest, with none left for sexual activity.

8. Correct answer: 3

Couvade refers to culturally determined paternal behaviors during pregnancy and birth. The fact that the father's ethnic background is specifically cited in the stem of the question should lead you to choose an option that is culturally based. The given situation lacks information to support your selection of option 1, 2, or 4.

Read carefully to note the limited information given in the stem. Even if you have no idea of what the word couvade means, you could have eliminated the other options because no data in the stem supported them. This is an example of a time to select what you do not know. Based on the knowledge you have, the other three options do not fit the given situation and information. Avoid reading information into the stem.

9. Correct answer: 2

Options 1, 3, and 4 are normal behaviors of an expectant father, especially during a first pregnancy. Persistent refusal to talk about the fetus or newborn may be a sign of a problem and should be assessed further.

Careful reading leads to the correct selection of the option. The clues are "warning sign" and "ineffective adaptation." Options 1, 3, and 4 can be clustered or grouped as positive and reflect some type of interaction with the mother. Option 2 is of a negative tone, different than the other options, the odd option, and most likely is the best choice if you are guessing.

10. Correct answer: 3

Options 1, 2, and 4 are all effective measures. Whereas changes may need to be made in the living space to accommodate the new baby, all major changes that involve the child should be initiated early in the pregnancy, not just before the birth.

Read carefully and methodically. With questions that ask for the "least," reverse the order in which you read the options from 1, 2, 3, 4 to the sequence 4, 3, 2, 1. This forces your mind to be more alert to select the last item as you prioritize the options. Be alert and prepare as you read with these types of question that all of the options are usually correct actions. Your goal is to prioritize them. Then reread the question one last time before you make a final selection.

3

Nursing Process Application and Fetal Health Assessment in Antepartal Care

FAST FACTS

1. The prospective father of the baby should also be included in preconception care.
2. Prenatal care reduces the incidence of low birth weight (LBW) and preterm birth and increases the likelihood of a positive pregnancy outcome.
3. Recommended prenatal care schedule based on the woman's risk status: first 28 weeks, once a month; weeks 28 to 36, every 2 weeks; week 36 until birth, weekly; post-term, twice a week.
4. Test findings during pregnancy should be evaluated based on the expected ranges for a pregnant woman because in some situations these ranges differ from those for a nonpregnant woman.
5. As pregnancy progresses observe for signs of supine hypotension as the physical assessment is completed during the clinic visits.
6. Good nutrition is a major factor in preventing LBW.
7. Pregnant women should not ingest mineral oil because it adversely affects absorption of fat-soluble vitamins.
8. Pregnant women must avoid saunas and hot tubs because they can elevate body temperature, which leads to fetal damage.
9. Inadequate protein intake has been associated with onset of pregnancy-induced hypertension (PIH).
10. Current research is demonstrating an association between adequate calcium intake and the prevention of PIH.

11. Iron deficiency anemia is the most common nutritional disorder of pregnancy. Iron from food sources is more readily absorbed when served with foods high in vitamin C.

12. Assessment methods used to determine fetal health status vary according to the risk status of the pregnancy: (1) In a *low-risk pregnancy,* the mother exhibits good health status at the start of pregnancy, the maternal-fetal unit adapts to the changes of pregnancy and parturition in an effective manner, and risk factors known to jeopardize the maternal-fetal unit are absent; (2) In a *high-risk pregnancy,* the risk factors that place the maternal-fetal unit in jeopardy are present before pregnancy or develop as the maternal-fetal unit adapts to the changes of pregnancy and parturition.

13. The mother and her family must be prepared for diagnostic testing with an explanation of each test and results obtained.

14. The best site to detect the point of maximum intensity of the fetal heart rate (FHR) is to locate the fetal back.

15. When a low FHR (under 100 beats per minute) is obtained, count the maternal pulse because the uterine souffle may have been counted. The expected FHR is 110 to 160, regular, and strong.

16. Be alert for findings of supine hypotension during ultrasound testing and postural hypotension when the woman arises at the end of the test.

CONTENT REVIEW

I. Preconception and prenatal care

A. *Preconception care*—**health assessment and guidance within the year before becoming pregnant to ensure the optimal physical and psychosocial condition for pregnancy**

B. Prenatal care—**early, comprehensive, ongoing health care during pregnancy. Factors interfering with participation in prenatal care:**

1. Demographic—age (under 20 and over 40 years), education level (under 12 years), unmarried, and minority status
2. Financial—unemployed, poor, and inadequate or lack of health care insurance
3. Health care system—limited capacity or access (hours open, location), culturally insensitive, and an unwelcoming approach to care
4. Mother
   a. Personal or cultural views with regard to health care during pregnancy
   b. Knowledge deficit about the importance of prenatal care
   c. Concurrent stressful life experiences affecting priority for prenatal care
   d. Fear and embarrassment; attitude toward the pregnancy
5. Prenatal health care provider: ongoing assessment of health and risk status health guidance; prompt intervention when signs of problems occur (Box 3-1)

Box 3-1
Recommended Content of Prenatal Visits

First Visit
Assessment—determine baseline health status:
  Health history
  Psychosocial status
Physical examination:
  Vital signs
  General assessment of body systems with emphasis on changes associated with pregnancy
  Height and weight with determination of body mass index (BMI)
  Reproductive assessment of breasts, external and internal pelvic examination, and determination of pelvic adequacy now or near term
  Laboratory testing (see Table 3-3, p. 61)
Health guidance:
  Emphasize importance of regular prenatal health care to promote and maintain the health of the mother and her baby.
  Discuss the components of prenatal care: the schedule of visits, what to expect and why.
  Begin health teaching about pregnancy, self-assessment about expected findings and warning signs, self-care measures and healthy lifestyle.
  Make an appointment for the next visit.

Subsequent Visits
Assessment—monitor changes from the baseline data and progress of adaptations to the pregnancy:
  Update health history
  Psychosocial status
Physical examination:
  Vital signs
  Physical adaptations to pregnancy: expected assessment findings, presence of warning signs
  Weight
  Reproductive assessment of breasts, fundal height, and external genitalia. Repeat internal examination near term to determine cervical changes or as required, that is, with signs of preterm labor or reproductive tract infection
  Fetal status: FHR, fetal movements (FMs), presentation
  Laboratory testing (see Table 3-3, p. 61)
Health guidance:
  Discuss areas of concern such as discomforts of pregnancy, health and lifestyle habits
  Provide health teaching consistent with developmental tasks of pregnancy
  Facilitate preparation of birth plan

C. **Care management follows a nursing process framework**
    1. Assessment
        a. Consider woman's health history and that of her family, especially female relatives; involve the pregnant woman and her family in the assessment process; teach them to recognize the expected changes and warning signs
        b. Determine reaction to pregnancy

c. Observe progress in physical and psychosocial adaptation to pregnancy noting expected assessment findings and warning signs (Tables 2-1 and 3-1 on pp. 22 and 51, Box 3-2 on p. 55)

d. Address discomforts of pregnancy because they may represent a developing health problem, increase anxiety, or interfere with the adjustment to pregnancy (Table 3-2, p. 57)

e. Use consistent assessment protocol to allow comparison of findings over time. Examples include blood pressure (BP) technique, weight, and fundal height measurement.

f. Monitor laboratory testing—a variety of tests are performed according to trimester of pregnancy and health status of the maternal-fetal unit; tests are used to monitor adaptations to pregnancy and to detect health problems early (Table 3-3, p. 61)

2. Nursing diagnoses associated with pregnancy relate to

a. Ineffective anatomic and physiologic adaptation to pregnancy

b. Difficulty coping with the required alterations in lifestyle behaviors to promote health of maternal-fetal unit

c. Discomforts that accompany the adaptations to pregnancy (see Table 3-2, p. 57)

d. Knowledge deficits in terms of pregnancy, childbirth, nutritional requirements, and parenting (Tables 3-2 on p. 57, 3-4 on p. 64, 3-5 on p. 67)

e. Anxiety from pregnancy and parenting

f. Deficits in family and support system

3. Plans of care and the expected outcomes for the common nursing diagnoses are described in Table 3-5, p. 67

II. Methods to determine fetal health status in a low-risk pregnancy

A. **Assess FHR—fetal heart sounds are detected by 10 to 12 weeks' gestation with Doppler ultrasonography and by 18 to 20 weeks' gestation with a fetoscope**

1. Doppler or ultrasound stethoscope used most often

a. Sound waves detect blood flow and produce an audible sound that can be counted

b. Conduction gel is used to enhance sound transmission

2. Fetoscope: stethoscope designed to auscultate FHR; less sensitive than Doppler ultrasonography

B. **Assessment methods**

1. Use Leopold's maneuvers to determine location of fetal back, which is the best site to detect the point of maximum intensity of the fetal heart beat

2. Identify sounds

a. Fetal heart beat

b. *Uterine souffle*—beatlike sound of blood flowing through enlarged uterine blood vessels; rate corresponds to the mother's heart beat

TABLE 3-1	Prenatal Assessment of Physical Status

History	Physical Assessment

Reproductive System and Breasts

Gynecologic history:
  Menstrual pattern
  Reproductive problems such as infections, neoplasms, infertility, surgeries
  Birth control and sexuality practices
Obstetrical history:
  Gravida—total number of pregnancies
    Nulligravida—never pregnant
    Primigravida—first pregnancy
    Multigravida—two or more pregnancies
  Para—number of pregnancies reaching viability (approximately 20 to 24 weeks' gestation); fetus is born alive or is stillborn
    Nullipara—no pregnancy completed to viability
    Primipara—completion of one pregnancy to viability
    Multipara—completion of two or more pregnancies to viability
  Five-digit system to describe pregnancies and outcomes:
    "G"—gravida
    "T"—number of term birth(s)
    "P"—number of preterm birth(s)
    "A"—number of **abortion**(s)—termination of pregnancy before age of viability; can be spontaneous or induced
    "L"—number of living children
  Past obstetrical outcomes from pregnancy, birth, or postpartum events and fetus-newborn status
  Current pregnancy experiences
    Adaptations made
    Progress noted and warning signs observed
    FM patterns experienced

Breasts:
  Observe appearance, leakage
  Palpate consistency, tenderness
  Review breast self-examination technique
Fundal height measurement
  Use pliable, nonstretchable tape
  Assist woman into supine position with head and shoulders elevated with small pillow for comfort
  Measure along midline of abdomen from notch of symphysis pubis to top of fundus
  As pregnancy progresses observe for signs of supine hypotension
Uterus: palpate
  Braxton Hicks contractions
  Fetal movement
  Fetal presentation and position using systematic abdominal palpation (Leopold maneuvers)
Lower uterine segment, cervix, vagina:
  Palpate softening of lower uterine segment (Hegar's sign)
  Palpate softening of cervix (Goodell's sign)
  Observe change in color of cervix and vagina to deep reddish-purple from increased vascularity (Chadwick's sign)
  Perform pelvic examination at first visit and again near term; obtain specimens for testing as indicated
Observe and palpate external genitalia and vaginal discharge for evidence of reproductive tract infection
Observe vulva and perineum for varicosities, lesions, rashes

Continued

TABLE 3-1	Prenatal Assessment of Physical Status—cont'd

History	Physical Assessment

Oxygenation and Circulation

History	Physical Assessment

History of health problems
  Asthma, respiratory infections
  Cardiac disorders
  Hypertension
  Thrombophlebitis
Harmful lifestyle practices and situations
  Tobacco, drug abuse, alcohol use
  Exposure to environmental pollutants
Changes with this pregnancy
  Nasal stuffiness, epistaxis, altered
    hearing, discharge
  Dyspnea, shortness of breath (SOB),
    orthopnea
  Cough, sputum production
  Palpitations
  Varicosities
Signs from cardiac decompensation, pulmonary edema, pregnancy induced hypertension (PIH)
Dizziness, faintness, fatigue, difficulty performing activities of daily living
	Measure BP using standard protocol:
	  Same position (upright position), same
	    arm (right)
	  Allow woman to rest for at least 5
	    minutes before measuring
	  Use appropriately sized cuff
	Determine temperature, pulse (apical, radial), respiratory rate and effort
	Auscultate breath sounds
	Assess FHR
	Observe and palpate extremities:
	  Circulatory status—color, temperature,
	    peripheral pulses, capillary refill
	  Edema—generalized, dependent, pitting
	  Signs of thrombophlebitis—positive
	    Homans' sign, erythema, pain, edema

Nutritional, Fluid and Electrolyte Adaptation

History	Physical Assessment

Useful tools: nutritional self-assessments, nutrition diaries for 3 days or 24-hour nutritional recalls; facilitate individualized approach to nutrition counseling and teaching
Nutritional habits and resources
  Typical food and fluid intake; food
    preferences
  Food preparation methods
  Facilities for food preparation and
    storage
  Availability of and ability to obtain
    food
  Knowledge of nutritional requirements
    for pregnancy
  Cultural and religious influences, vegetarianism
History of nutritional problems
  Inappropriate intake leading to dietary
    imbalance
	Measure weight:
	  Prepregnant weight, height, BMI
	  Pattern of weight gain
	  Protocol for weight measurement
	    Reduce stress involved in the "weigh
	    in"
	    Use same scale; balance before use
	    Have woman wear same amount of
	      clothing: examination gown, no
	      shoes
	    Teach woman how to measure her
	      own weight at home; compare
	      findings
	Evaluate hydration status for turgor, diaphoresis, edema, concentration and amount of urine
	Observe condition of oral cavity for integrity of gums and teeth, vascular lesions, bleeding
	Palpate thyroid gland

TABLE 3-1	**Prenatal Assessment of Physical Status—cont'd**

History	Physical Assessment

Nutritional, Fluid and Electrolyte Adaptation—cont'd

Underweight, overweight, obese
Bulimia, anorexia
Cholecystitis, cholelithiasis, ulcers
Food allergies
History of endocrine problems
  Pregestational or gestational diabetes mellitus
  Hyper-, hypothyroidism
  Adrenal insufficiency; steroid use with health problems such as lupus erythematosus, arthritis
Changes with this pregnancy:
  Appetite
  Pyrosis
  Cravings, pica; altered food tolerances (e.g., pain after fatty meals, aversions)
Nausea, vomiting: onset, duration, pattern, severity, precipitating factors

Elimination

History	Physical Assessment
History of elimination problems (e.g., urinary tract infections (UTIs), pyelonephritis, colitis)	Auscultate bowel sounds
Usual pattern of bowel and bladder elimination	Observe urethral meatus for redness and edema
Any recent changes such as pain, decreased or increased frequency	Observe anus for hemorrhoids and vulva for dilated veins
Usual characteristics of feces and urine	
Any recent changes noted in consistency, color, odor, clarity, amount	
Interventions used to facilitate bowel elimination such as specific foods, fluids, medications	

Physical Activity and Rest

History	Physical Assessment
Usual activity patterns and types of activities	Muscle tone: overall; abdominal muscles; check for diastasis recti abdominus
Usual energy level and any recent change in energy levels	Range of motion
Participation in exercise programs	Ambulation, gait, balance
Any changes in activity patterns or tolerance since pregnant	Posture
	Signs of fatigue
	Appropriateness of dress in terms of nonrestrictive clothing, low-heeled shoes

Continued

TABLE 3-1	Prenatal Assessment of Physical Status—cont'd
History	**Physical Assessment**

Physical Activity and Rest—cont'd
Usual rest and sleep patterns
  Changes in usual rest and sleep patterns
  Sufficiency of rest and sleep for feeling
   of well-being
  Interference in rest and sleep since
   pregnant
Interventions used to facilitate rest and
  sleep
Knowledge of safety interventions and
  body mechanics from changing body
  contours and center of gravity
Use of appropriate safety interventions
  when in a car or traveling	

Integument
History of integument problems such as
  rashes, birth marks, acne
Hygiene and grooming practices, products
  used for care
Changes noted in skin, mucous mem-
  branes, hair, nails since pregnancy
	Appearance in terms of hygiene and
	  grooming
	Condition of skin and mucous membranes
	  Color
	  Integrity, texture, moisture
	Signs indicative of physical abuse
	Condition of hair and nails: integrity, growth
	Expected pregnancy changes
	  Pigmentary
	  Acne, oily skin
	  Striae gravidarum
	  Palmar erythema, spider nevi

c. *Funic souffle*—beatlike sound of blood flowing through umbilical cord; rate corresponds to fetal heart beat

3. Count fetal heart beat for one full minute
4. Expected rate is 110 to 160 beats per minute, regular, and strong

 Warning!

When a low FHR (less than 100 beats per minute) is obtained, count the maternal pulse because the uterine souffle may have been counted.

5. Allow the mother and family to hear the fetal heart beat; reassures and facilitates attachment

C. **Fundal height measurement: enlargement of uterus indirectly implies fetal growth**

Box 3-2
Assessment of Psychosocial Adaptations to Pregnancy

Assessment of Self-Concept

Perceptions of physical self:
- Description of current health status
- Feelings expressed about a changing body image and sensations
- Interventions taken to enhance health during pregnancy, including views about health guidance during pregnancy (prenatal care)

Perceptions of personal self:
- Reaction to and feelings about pregnancy
- Perception of pregnancy and parenting: realistic, unrealistic
- Coping mechanisms used to respond to stress; interventions used to cope with the demands of pregnancy and parenting: effective or ineffective
- Cultural beliefs and practices about pregnancy and parenting
- Progress in meeting the developmental tasks of pregnancy and age-related developmental tasks
- Moral, ethical, and spiritual values; beliefs; and standards of behavior

Experience of abuse. Ask direct questions of all women:
- Have you ever been abused (emotionally or physically) by your partner or someone else close to you?
- Within the past year have you been hit, slapped, kicked, or otherwise physically harmed by someone?
- Within the past year, have you ever been forced to have sex?
- Are you afraid of your partner or a person close to you?

Level of knowledge about the pregnancy:
- Adaptations
- Self-assessment and self-care interventions

Father: consider assessment in all areas of Perceptions of Physical Self, Personal Self, and Knowledge listed above

Assessment of Role Function

Description of the following:
- Current roles
- Role responsibilities and expectations as defined by self, family, and support system
- Role performance as determined by self, family, and support system
- Presence of role conflicts

Awareness of potential for role conflicts and preparations made

Perceptions about the role of the mother

Present knowledge and skill level in the role of mother and interventions taken to prepare for the role of mother

Assess father and the paternal role

Continued

D. *Leopold maneuvers*—systematic palpation of the abdomen to determine fetal presentation and position, degree of fetal descent into pelvis, and uterine contours

E. **Daily Fetal Movement Count (DFMC):**
   1. Assessment of fetal movement (FM) by the mother is the DFMC
      a. Vigorous fetal activity is associated with fetal well-being
      b. Alteration in pattern of FM may indicate fetal compromise from

Box 3-2

Assessment of Psychosocial Adaptations to Pregnancy—cont'd

Assessment of Interdependence

Family and support system:
- Identity (partners, siblings, grandparents, friends, co-workers)
- Capability of providing support
- Degree of support offered during pregnancy and after the baby is born

Relationship of expectant mother and father with each other and with family and support system:
- Willingness to accept support
- Strength to appropriately refuse or limit support

Responses of family and support system to pregnancy
Preparation interventions for siblings of expected baby
Stability and safety of the home and work environment
Financial security
Community agency availability
   Acceptance or rejection of required community agency support

---

hypoxia. Examples of alteration in movement include decreased frequency, weakening, and cessation.

2. Assessment performed at home, results recorded, and reviewed at prenatal visits

3. Maternal attachment to fetus may be enhanced as she recognizes the unique responses of her fetus to environmental stimuli. Examples include voices, music, emotions, and foods.

4. Protocol to follow for DFMC
   a. Begin at the 27th week when 90% of FMs can be perceived
   b. Count when fetus is likely to be awake; for example after the mother eats
   c. Assume a lateral position to enhance uteroplacental perfusion
   d. Avoid drug and nicotine use, which decreases FM
   e. Cardiff Count-to-Ten Method is one method currently available
      (1) Begin at the same time each day (usually in the morning, after breakfast) and count each FM, noting how long it takes to count 10 FMs
      (2) Expected findings are 10 movements in 1 hour or less

⚠ Warning!

Report these warning signs to health care provider within the day of the findings. Further testing may be required when less than 10 movements are felt in 12 hours, when it takes a longer time to reach 10 FM than on previous days—more than 1 hour for 10 FMs, or when movements are weaker or less vigorous. Report movement alarm signal of less than 3 FMs in 12 hours.

Text continues on p. 70

TABLE 3-2	**Common Discomforts Associated with Pregnancy and Relief Interventions**

Discomforts (trimester likely to occur)	Recommended Relief Interventions for the Pregnant Woman
Reproductive System	
Breasts:	Wear supportive maternity bra
Tenderness, pain, tingling (1st)	Use absorbent pads (change frequently)
Leakage (2nd, 3rd) (rule out mastitis)	Keep nipples and areola clean and dry; avoid soap
Leukorrhea (2nd, 3rd) (rule out infection)	Perform perineal care (washing from front to back with soap and water) daily
	Use panty liners or perineal pads (change frequently)
	Wear loose cotton underwear
	Avoid panty hose and tight pants
	Report changes in characteristics (odor, color), pruritis, dysuria
	WARNING! Never douche during pregnancy.
Braxton Hicks contractions (3rd) (rule out labor)	Change position
	Ambulate for short periods
	Practice childbirth breathing and relaxation techniques, effleurage
	Increase fluid intake
	Keep bladder empty
Oxygenation and Circulation	
Nasal stuffiness, epistaxis (1st, 2nd, 3rd)	Use humidifier, cool-air vaporizer
	Apply normal saline nasal spray or drops
Dyspnea, SOB (3rd) (rule out pulmonary edema)	Maintain good posture
	Raise arms and stretch above head
	Use extra pillows at night
	Avoid large meals
	Stop smoking cigarettes
	Balance activity and rest
	Report productive cough, increasing fatigue
Faintness or dizziness from hypotension (2nd, 3rd as uterus enlarges)	Assume side-lying position when in bed
	Place small pad under one hip when supine
	Avoid sudden position changes; move slowly and carefully
	Avoid warm and crowded areas
	Wear support stockings
	Exercise moderately to enhance venous return
	Avoid hypoglycemia by eating small, frequent meals
Varicose veins, edema of lower extremities (3rd)	Avoid long periods of uninterrupted standing or sitting
	Do not wear constrictive clothing
	Avoid crossing legs

Continued

TABLE 3-2	Common Discomforts Associated with Pregnancy and Relief Interventions—cont'd
Discomforts (trimester likely to occur)	**Recommended Relief Interventions for the Pregnant Woman**

Oxygenation and Circulation—cont'd

Maintain adequate fluid intake

Perform moderate exercise, leg and foot exercises while sitting or standing; ambulate frequently

Rest with legs and hips elevated

Wear support stockings

Assume lateral position when in bed to enhance renal blood flow and urine formation

Report worsening edema which persists after sleeping; upper body edema

Nutrition, Fluid and Electrolytes

| Nausea and vomiting (1st) (rule out hyperemesis gravidarum) | Avoid empty and overdistended stomach by eating small, frequent meals (5-6/day with snacks or every 2-3 hr); eat foods that are liked or craved, high in potassium and magnesium, easily digested
Do not brush teeth immediately after meals
Eat dry carbohydrate in morning before **slowly** getting out of bed (unsalted crackers, dry popcorn, or toast with jelly)
Eat bedtime snack of slowly digested protein food or complex carbohydrate (yogurt, milk, cheese, boiled egg, lean meat)
Avoid spicy, fried, gas-forming foods
Plan relaxed meal times and rest periods
Sit upright after meals
Drink fluids between meals not with them; herbal teas are helpful
Use acupressure; that is, put pressure on wrist points with fingers or wrist bands
Reduce stress by use of relaxation techniques and verbalization of feelings
Avoid strong, unpleasant odors; lemon scent and fresh air are helpful
WARNING! Report vomiting that is unresponsive to relief interventions, weight loss, signs of dehydration, and increased vomiting. |
| Bleeding, tender gums; epulis (3rd) (rule out gum disease) | Perform gentle and frequent oral care, especially after vomiting
Obtain appropriate dental care
Maintain good nutrition |

TABLE 3-2 Common Discomforts Associated with Pregnancy and Relief Interventions—cont'd

Discomforts (trimester likely to occur)	Recommended Relief Interventions for the Pregnant Woman
Nutrition, Fluid and Electrolytes—cont'd	
Pyrosis (2nd, 3rd)	Avoid overdistended stomach by eating small, frequent meals Limit or avoid gas-forming, fatty, spicy foods Remain upright for at least 1 hr after meals Maintain good posture Try sipping milk, herbal tea, chewing gum, low sodium antacids (Maalox)
Elimination	
Urinary frequency, urgency, stress incontinence (1st, 3rd) (rule out UTI)	Perform Kegel (pubucoccygeus or pubococcygeal muscle) exercises to strengthen pelvic muscles Drink fluids during the day but limit fluids before bedtime; limit caffeine Establish regular elimination patterns Wear panty liners **WARNING!** Report dysuria and any change in urine characteristics (clarity, odor).
Constipation (2nd, 3rd)	Maintain adequate intake of fluid (6-8 glasses) and roughage daily Exercise moderately on a daily basis Establish regular elimination patterns Use relaxation interventions Avoid over-the-counter remedies (stool softeners, laxatives, enemas) unless approved by health care provider
Flatulence, bloating, belching (2nd, 3rd)	Eat slowly, chewing foods completely Avoid gas-forming, fatty, and spicy foods Avoid large meals Exercise moderately on a daily basis Establish regular elimination patterns
Hemorrhoids (3rd)	Avoid constipation—straining at stool Use sitz baths, medicated pads (Tucks) Assume Sims position to elevate buttocks

Continued

TABLE 3-2	Common Discomforts Associated with Pregnancy and Relief Interventions—cont'd

Discomforts (trimester likely to occur)	Recommended Relief Interventions for the Pregnant Woman
Physical Activity, Rest	
Fatigue, diminished energy level, insomnia (1st, 3rd) (rule out pathologic anemia, depression, inadequate nutrition, cardiac decompensation)	Schedule rest periods (home, workplace) Perform relaxation exercises Exercise moderately on a daily basis Follow a balanced diet with iron supplementation Enlist the help of support system Support body parts when at rest and during sleep Use safe interventions to induce sleep such as warm milk or a warm, relaxing shower or bath **WARNING!** Avoid saunas and hot tubs because they can elevate body temperature, which leads to fetal damage.
Low back pain (2nd, 3rd) (rule out preterm labor)	Perform exercises: pelvic rock or tilt, tailor sit position, squatting Wear maternity girdle (abdominal support), low-heeled shoes Maintain good posture and use good body mechanics Rest on firm mattress Use local interventions such as heat, ice, and massage Avoid lifting heavy objects or climbing on ladders and step stools
Leg cramps (2nd, 3rd) (rule out thrombophlebitis, low calcium or potassium [less likely])	Extend leg and dorsiflex foot, or stand and lean forward on affected leg Apply heat over and massage affected area (only if thrombophlebitis is ruled out) Include calcium rich foods in the diet or take approved calcium supplement **WARNING!** Report unilateral pain in calf, erythema, heat, positive Homans' sign.
Integument	
Pruritis gravidarum (rule out infection, allergy)	Bathe in warm water with sodium bicarbonate or oatmeal Avoid or reduce the use of soap Wear soft, loose clothing Avoid scratching, especially if fingernails are long Use lotions that relieve symptoms **WARNING!** Report changes in skin condition and other symptoms such as fever and malaise.

TABLE 3-3   Common Laboratory Tests for Low-Risk Pregnancies

Laboratory Tests	Purpose and Scheduling	Expected Results
Blood Tests		
Hematocrit and hemoglobin Leukocytes Platelets	Detect anemia, first visit and at 26-28 wk Detect infection, as required Evaluate blood clotting mechanism, first visit and as required	32-42%, 10.5-14 g/dl 5,000-15,000/mm^3 150,000-350,000/ mm^3
Blood type, Rh, Coombs' (indirect)	Determine Rh status of mother; if mother is Rh-negative and father is Rh-positive, a Coombs' test (indirect) is done to detect if antibodies against Rh-positive blood cells have been formed; first visit, at 28 wk, and as required	Negative Coombs' test indicates sensitization has not occurred, and Rh$_o$(D) immune globulin (RhoGAM) can be given during third trimester
Sickle cell anemia screening	Detect sickle cell hemoglobin in African-American women; first visit	Negative is the desired result; if positive, further testing is required to differentiate between carrier and disease status
Rubella titre [hemagglutination inhibition test (HAI) titre]	Determine immunity to rubella; first visit	Greater than 1:10 ratio indicates immunity to rubella
Antibody screening	Screen for exposure to toxoplasmosis, rubeola, rubella, anti-rh	Negative titre
VDRL, rapid plasma regain (RPR), fluorescent treponemal antibody absorption (FTA-ABS)	Screen for exposure to syphilis; first visit, 32 wk	Negative, nonreactive
Hepatitis B surface antigen (HbsAG)	Screen for hepatitis B infection; first visit and as required	Negative

Continued

TABLE 3-3 Common Laboratory Tests for Low-Risk Pregnancies—cont'd

Laboratory Tests	Purpose and Scheduling	Expected Results
1-hour glucose	Screen for gestational diabetes: administer 50 g oral glucose and draw blood 1 hour later; 24-28 wk	Less than 140 mg/dl at 1 hour after administration of the 50 g glucose; if over 140, a 3-hr glucose tolerance test (GTT) is done
Maternal serum alpha-fetoprotein (MsAFP)	Screen for open neural tube defects, i.e., spina bifida (elevated) or Down syndrome (decreased); 16-18 wk	Desired result is within the normal range; consult with laboratory performing the test for the normal range
Screening for human immunodeficiency virus (HIV)	All women should be tested; some states mandate testing	Negative; positive test result allows for treatment with zidovudine (AZT) during pregnancy and scheduling of an elective cesarean birth to reduce transmission potential of HIV
Multiple or triple marker screening	Screen for Down syndrome usually for women over 35 years of age; determine levels of AFP, human chorionic gonadotrophin (HCG), and estriol	Desired result is within the normal range for each substance tested
Urine Tests. Use clean catch, midstream specimen, if possible, because it enhances accuracy		
Analysis	Detects cells, casts, nitrates, pH, specific gravity to determine presence of health problems from renal function; first visit and as needed	No differences in usual values are expected during pregnancy
Human chorionic gonadotropin (HGC)	Basis of pregnancy test; first visit and when pregnancy is suspected; use first voided morning urine as it is most concentrated	Positive test indicates presence of HCG

Microscopic/culture	Screen for asymptomatic bacteria; first visit and as needed, i.e., signs of urinary tract infection	Negative
Glucose, acetone, protein	Screen for signs of diabetes, ketosis, pregnancy induced hypertension (PIH); every visit using the dipstick method	Trace to 1+ for glucose and protein, and negative for acetone
Other		
Tuberculin skin [tine, purified protein derivative (PPD)]	Screen for exposure to tuberculosis, first visit	Nonreactive; if reactive, chest x-ray after 20 weeks' gestation, screen family members, discuss findings with client and family
Pap smear	Screen for atypical cells that can indicate cancer of cervix or certain types of reproductive tract infections; first visit	Negative
Testing of cervical and vaginal smears	Screen for reproductive tract infections such as gonorrhea, human papillomavirus, herpes virus, Group B Streptococcus, Chlamydia; first visit, at 37-38 wk, and as needed	Negative

TABLE 3-4 Major Nutrient Requirement Recommendations During Pregnancy and Lactation*

Nutrient and Its Importance	Requirement	Food Sources
Calories Supplies energy for Increased metabolic rate Utilization of nutrients Protein-sparing so it can be used for: Growth of fetus Development of structures required for pregnancy, including placenta, amniotic fluid, tissue growth Milk production **WARNING!** Failure to meet caloric requirements can lead to LBW and ketosis as fat and protein are used for energy. Ketosis has been associated with fetal damage.	Pregnancy: 300 cal/day above the pre-pregnancy daily requirement; adjust to meet energy requirements of activity level Begin increase in 2nd trimester Use weight gain pattern as an indication of adequacy of calorie intake Lactation: 500 cal/day above pre-pregnancy level	Foods of high nutrient value such as protein, complex carbohydrates (whole grains, vegetables, fruits) Variety of foods representing food sources for the nutrients required during pregnancy No more than 30% fat
Protein Fetal tissue growth Growth of maternal tissue, including uterus and breasts Development of essential pregnancy structures Formation of red blood cells (RBCs) and plasma proteins Formation of milk protein **WARNING!** Inadequate protein intake has been associated with onset of pregnancy induced hypertension (PIH).	Pregnancy: 60 g/day or an increase of 10 g above daily requirements for age group Lactation: 65 g/day Note. Adolescents have a higher protein requirement than mature women because adolescents must supply protein for their own growth as well as protein to meet the pregnancy requirement	Lean meat, poultry, fish Eggs, cheese, milk, yogurt Dried beans, lentils, peas, nuts Whole grains

WARNING! Vegetarians must take note of the amino acid content of protein foods consumed to ensure intake of sufficient quantities of all amino acids.

Calcium

Growth and development of fetal skeleton and tooth buds

Maintenance of mineralization of maternal bones and teeth

WARNING! Current research is demonstrating an association between adequate calcium intake and the prevention of PIH.

Pregnancy and lactation: 1000 mg/day; 1300 mg/day is recommended for women under 19 years of age

10 mcg/day of vitamin D is required because it enhances absorption of both calcium and phosphorous

Dairy products: milk, yogurt, ice cream, cheese, egg yolk
Whole grains, tofu
Green leafy vegetables (not spinach or Swiss chard)
Canned salmon and sardines with bones
Calcium fortified foods such as orange juice
Vitamin D sources: fortified milk and margarine, egg yolk, butter, liver, seafood

Iron

Expansion of blood volume, hemoglobin and RBC formation

Establishment of fetal iron stores for first few months of life

WARNING! Inadequate iron intake results in anemia and depletion of iron stores in the mother.

Pregnancy: 30 mg/day represents a doubling of the pre-pregnant daily requirement

Begin supplementation at 30 mg/day in *2nd* trimester because diet alone is unable to meet the pregnancy requirement

60 to 120 mg/day along with copper and zinc supplementation for women who have low hemoglobin values or iron deficiency anemia before pregnancy

70 mg/day of vitamin C enhances iron absorption

Lactation: 15 mg/day of iron (same requirement as pre-pregnancy) and 95 mg/day of vitamin C

Liver, red meat, fish, poultry, eggs
Enriched/whole grain cereals and breads
Dark green leafy vegetables, legumes
Nuts, dried fruits
Vitamin C sources: citrus fruits and juices, strawberries, cantaloupe, tomatoes, green peppers, broccoli and cabbage, potatoes
Iron from food sources is more readily absorbed when served with foods high in vitamin C

*Represents requirements for a healthy, well-nourished woman with a singleton pregnancy. Additional requirements, including supplementation, usually are recommended for poorly nourished women, women with multiple gestations, vegetarians, and women who are heavy cigarette smokers.

Continued

TABLE 3-4	Major Nutrient Requirement Recommendations During Pregnancy and Lactation*—cont'd		
Nutrient and Its Importance	**Requirement**		**Food Sources**
Iron—cont'd	Inadequate iron intake results in: Maternal effects: anemia, depletion of iron stores, decreased energy and appetite, cardiac stress especially during labor and birth; poor wound healing and increased risk for infection Fetal effects: decreased availability of oxygen thereby affecting fetal growth **WARNING!** Iron deficiency anemia is the most common nutritional disorder of pregnancy.		
Zinc Formation of enzymes May be important in the prevention of congenital malformations of the fetus	Pregnancy: 15 mg/day representing an increase of 3 mg/day over pre-pregnancy daily requirements Lactation: 19 mg/day		Liver, meats, shell fish Eggs, milk, cheese Whole grains, legumes, nuts
Folic Acid, Folacin, Folate Formation of RBCs and prevention of anemia DNA synthesis and cell formation Prevention of neural tube defects (i.e. spina bifida) and perhaps Down syndrome	Pregnancy: 600 mcg/day representing an increase of more than 200 mcg over the daily pre-pregnancy requirement Lactation: 500 mcg/day		Liver, kidney, lean beef, veal Dark green leafy vegetables, broccoli, asparagus, artichokes, legumes Fortified whole grains (cereals, bread, rice, pasta), peanuts Oranges, orange juice, strawberries, cantaloupe

*Represents requirements for a healthy, well-nourished woman with a singleton pregnancy. Additional requirements, including supplementation, usually are recommended for poorly nourished women, women with multiple gestations, vegetarians, and women who are heavy cigarette smokers.

TABLE 3-5	Common Nursing Diagnoses, Expected Outcomes, and Interventions for the Antepartal Period

Nursing Diagnoses, Expected Outcomes	Nursing Interventions

Altered nutrition, less than or more than body requirements related to: lack of knowledge about nutrient requirements during pregnancy; inadequate intake associated with nausea and vomiting
 	
Woman will:
Identify nutrient requirements during pregnancy
Consume a diet that reflects the nutrients required during pregnancy
Report a decrease in nausea and vomiting
Gain approximately ____ lb/wk during the second and third trimesters. (Insert weekly weight gain recommended for the woman's BMI.)
	Teach woman about the nutrient needs of the pregnant woman (see Table 3-4, p. 64)
	Discuss the relationship of nutrition to her own health, pregnancy outcome, and fetal growth. Good nutrition is a major factor in preventing LBW.
	Teach woman about the recommended weight gain for pregnancy based on her BMI; explain the distribution of weight gained
	Develop a diet **with the woman** that reflects data from the nutrition assessment, the food diary, cultural preferences, activity level, and nutritional requirements during pregnancy
	Serving suggestions:
	  Milk, yogurt, and cheese group: 3-4 servings
	  Meat, poultry, fish, dry beans, eggs, and nuts group: 2-3 servings
	  Vegetable group: 3-5 servings
	  Fruit group: 2-4 servings
	  Bread, cereal, rice, pasta group: 6-11 servings
	Discuss food preparation methods to preserve nutrient content
	Caution the woman that:
	  Vitamin supplementation with prenatal vitamins is not a substitute for a balanced, nutritious diet
	  Megadoses of vitamins, especially fat-soluble vitamins, can be toxic and result in fetal damage
	  Fat, simple carbohydrates, and caffeine intake should be limited
	  Alcohol should not be ingested during pregnancy
	Instruct client to take an iron supplement on an empty stomach if tolerated to enhance absorption; that GI upset and constipation can occur; and to try a change in preparation (e.g., switch from ferrous sulfate to ferrous fumarate)
	Teach client interventions that are helpful to diminish the nausea and vomiting (see Table 3-2, p. 57)

Constipation related to decreased peristalsis associated with elevated progesterone levels and inadequate intake of fluid and roughage	Review woman's diet for sources of roughage and amount of fluid included each day Determine usual bowel elimination patterns and interventions woman already uses to facilitate elimination

Continued

TABLE 3-5	Common Nursing Diagnoses, Expected Outcomes, and Interventions for the Antepartal Period—cont'd

Nursing Diagnoses, Expected Outcomes	Nursing Interventions

Woman will:
Report regular elimination of soft, formed feces
Follow a diet that reflects sufficient intake of roughage and fluids
	Discuss physiologic and anatomic bases for the occurrence of constipation during pregnancy and importance of roughage, fluids, and activity as safe and natural prevention interventions
	Teach client to:
	  Drink 6 to 8 glasses of fluid each day (at least 2000 ml/day)
	  Include sources of roughage (fiber) with each meal such as whole grains, fresh fruits and vegetables, nuts
	  Participate in a moderate level of activity daily, such as walking for 15 to 30 min.
	  Caution to check with health care provider before using stool softeners, laxatives, enemas
	WARNING! Pregnant women should not ingest mineral oil because it adversely affects absorption of fat-soluble vitamins.

Altered sexuality patterns related to physiologic and anatomic changes that occur during pregnancy	Describe effects of pregnancy on sexuality and sexual expression Emphasize importance of open communication of feelings and concerns about the changes from pregnancy and their effects on sexuality

Expectant couple will:
Openly discuss concerns about the effect pregnancy has on their sexuality
Identify a variety of mutually acceptable ways to express their sexuality
	Reassure couple that in a normally progressing pregnancy there is no evidence that intercourse is harmful although some vaginal spotting (from the fragility of the cervix and vagina) and mild uterine cramping may normally occur after intercourse
	Emphasize the importance of safer sex techniques to prevent infection
	Discuss the expectant couple's current sexual practices as required
	Provide information about alternative means of sexual expression:
	  More comfortable positions
	  Massage, oral sex, masturbation
	  Touch to feel bodily changes
	  Relaxation techniques
	Identify maternal problems that may limit the manner of sexual expression such as bleeding, premature rupture of membranes, history of spontaneous abortions or preterm labor. Note that intercourse and orgasm may be contraindicated.

TABLE 3-5	Common Nursing Diagnoses, Expected Outcomes, and Interventions for the Antepartal Period—cont'd

Nursing Diagnoses, Expected Outcomes	Nursing Interventions
Anxiety related to a lack of knowledge about the expected anatomic and physiologic changes of pregnancy

Woman will:
Identify the anatomic and physiologic adaptations for each trimester of pregnancy
Identify effective interventions to relieve the discomforts of pregnancy
Follow a lifestyle that reflects health habits conducive to a positive pregnancy outcome
Express feeling more prepared to cope with changes of pregnancy
Utilize appropriate interventions to facilitate family adjustment to pregnancy | Counsel couple together and separately, as appropriate
Make referrals, i.e., to sexual counseling, if needed
Use teaching approaches that take into consideration the change in concerns as the pregnancy progresses:
First trimester (egocentric, accepting pregnancy): ready to learn about adaptations of pregnancy as they are affecting her and interventions to facilitate her well-being and comfort
Second trimester (focusing on fetus, introspective): ready to learn about fetal growth and development, role changes, interventions to facilitate fetal well-being
Third trimester (separation from fetus in childbirth): ready to learn about baby care, what will be needed, and interventions to cope with the process of labor (childbirth classes)
Use a variety of methodologies:
Lectures, group discussions, role playing
Films; internet resources to consult
Demonstration, redemonstration
Written literature: pamphlets, prepared handouts, books
Tour of agency where birthing will occur
Essential topics should include the following:
Anatomic and physiologic adaptations expected during pregnancy, why they occur and how they are exhibited; warning signs of pregnancy and signs of approaching labor
Effect of pregnancy on each member of the family, including siblings and grandparents; preparation methods for siblings
Interventions to enhance well-being and optimal pregnancy outcome, i.e., nutrition, appropriate physical activity, sufficient rest and relaxation, stress reduction, lifestyle changes (eliminate smoking, alcohol, drugs)
Discomforts of pregnancy: why they occur, appropriate relief interventions (see Table 3-2, p. 57)
Preparation for childbirth
What to expect during the postpartum period
Preparation for parenting and care of newborn |

III. Methods to determine fetal health status in a high-risk pregnancy

A. Use the same methods as for low-risk pregnancy but conduct them more frequently plus specialized prenatal testing is likely to be ordered

B. More frequent prenatal visits
   1. Assess maternal-fetal unit for warning signs that can occur at any time; include assessment of emotional status because stress can adversely influence fetal health
   2. Instruct woman and her family about self-assessment interventions, warning signs, and the importance of participation in health guidance and treatment regimen

C. Specialized antepartal testing
   1. Three purposes
      a. Early detection of fetal warning signs with prompt intervention to prevent fetal morbidity and death; avoid premature intervention
      b. Identification of fetal anomalies
      c. Determination of the timing and method of birth that would present the lowest maternal-fetal risk
   2. Guidelines
      a. Discretion must be used. The advantages must outweigh the risks, cost, and maternal discomfort.
      b. Combination of tests is often required moving from simple to more complex. Examples include Daily Fetal Movement Count, then Non-Stress Test (NST), then Biophysical Profile (BPP), then Contraction Stress Test (CST).
      c. Tests may be repeated to monitor changes in status and to confirm abnormal results
         (1) Serial ultrasonography to monitor fetal growth
         (2) Weekly NST to monitor fetal health in a post-term pregnancy
         (3) Repeat of a positive CST in 24 hours
      d. Woman and her family should be prepared
         (1) Frightening issues to cope with: baby in jeopardy, pregnancy is different from expected
         (2) Testing procedures: tiring, uncomfortable, time-consuming, costly, embarrassing
         (3) Stress response can affect results including FHR pattern
      e. The role of nurse is an educator, advocate, and/or provider of emotional support
         (1) Reassure woman and family with a calm, competent, knowledgeable approach
         (2) Explain testing method and procedure
         (3) Provide time for expression of feelings

D. *Ultrasonography*—**sound waves reflect off tissue, allowing for visualization of the contents of the uterus including the fetus, placenta, amniotic fluid, and blood flow through the umbilical cord**
1. Purposes
   a. Diagnose pregnancy by visualizing gestational sac
   b. Date pregnancy by evaluating the size and volume of the gestational sac and crown-to-rump length (CRL)
   c. Detect multiple gestation
   d. Monitor fetal growth by making serial measurements of crown to rump length, biparietal diameter, femur length, abdomen, and head-to-abdomen ratio
   e. Evaluate fetal structure and function including movement, anomalies, blood flow through the umbilical cord
   f. Estimate amniotic fluid volume
   g. Evaluate placental location and efficiency of function
   h. Facilitate safe performance of other antepartal tests by location of the essential structures: placenta, chorion villi, and fetus
2. Approaches
   a. Transabdominal—use a supine position
   b. Transvaginal—use a lithotomy position
3. Specific preparation and support interventions
   a. Transabdominal approach requires a full bladder and is done when gestation period is 20 weeks or fewer
      (1) Facilitates identification of pelvic organs and the positioning of the uterus for visualization
      (2) Have woman drink 1 to 1.5 L of water approximately 1 to 2 hours before the examination
      (3) Full bladder produces discomfort
   b. Position woman: supine with transabdominal and lithotomy with transvaginal
   c. Test lasts 20 to 30 minutes; point out fetal structures to enhance reality of fetus and foster attachment; support woman if abnormalities are noted or if she does not want to look

⚠ Warning!

Be alert for signs of supine hypotension during test and postural hypotension when arising at the end of the test.

E. *Non-Stress Test (NST)*
1. Purpose—screening test performed to assess the response of the FHR to FM
   a. Testing begins after 27 to 30 weeks' gestation when the fetal autonomic nervous system is mature enough to respond effectively
   b. Performed weekly, twice a week, or daily, depending on the condition of maternal-fetal unit

  2. Indications—pregnancies at risk for placental insufficiency. Examples include postmaturity, PIH, diabetes, maternal cigarette smoking, and poor nutrition.
  3. Protocol
      a. Take into account the typical sleep-wake cycle for this fetus (ask mom) to schedule the test for time of fetal activity
      b. Maternal preparation
          (1) Refrain from smoking (2 hours before) or using sedatives before the test
          (2) Eat about 2 hours before the test
          (3) Mother is assisted into a semi-Fowler's position, with small pillow under one hip or in a lateral position
      c. Assess maternal vital signs, especially BP, before and during the test
      d. Attach external electronic fetal monitors
          (1) The tocotransducer is positioned over fundus to detect uterine contractions and FMs
          (2) The ultrasound transducer is positioned over abdominal site where most distinct fetal heart sounds are detected
  4. Interpretation of results
      a. Reactive result—indicates fetal well-being with a nervous system unaffected by hypoxia
          (1) Two or more accelerations of the FHR of 15 or more beats per minute, lasting 15 or more seconds in a 10- to 20-minute period as a result of FM
          (2) Baseline FHR between 110 and 160 beats per minute
          (3) Variability, of 10 or more beats per minute
      b. Nonreactive result—requires further evaluation with another NST, BPP, or CST
          (1) Stated criteria for a reactive result are not met within 40 minutes
          (2) Could indicate a compromised fetus. Note: There is a high false-positive rate.
F. Biophysical Profile (BPP)
  1. Purpose—the combined use of external electronic fetal monitoring and ultrasonography to assess fetal status (healthy, compromised, or at risk) and the fetus within the intrauterine environment. There are five assessment factors, which are:
      a. Non-Stress Test (NST)—see Part C.
      b. Fetal breathing movements—number and duration; first to be affected by early stress and may be predictive of preterm labor because prostaglandins that stimulate labor also decrease fetal breathing movements
      c. Fetal body movements—gross or discrete movements of the fetal body and limbs
      d. Fetal muscle tone—presence of active extension with a return to

flexion of limb, trunk (spine), hand; least sensitive to hypoxia and last sign to be affected

e. Amniotic fluid volume—presence and size of fluid pockets; **oligohydramnios** (diminished fluid volume) may indicate an extended episode of fetal stress with reduced urine formation; certain anomalies can affect the amount of amniotic fluid

2. Protocol—follow the guidelines for ultrasonography and for NST; approximately 40 to 60 minutes are required to perform the test to accommodate the fetal sleep-wake cycle

3. Indications—as for NST and CST; often used to follow-up on a nonreactive NST or warning signs found with DFMC

4. Interpretation of results: Note that there is a low incidence of false positives

   a. Each sign receives a score of 0 (abnormal) or 2 (normal)—some testing procedures use a 0, 1, 2 scoring system, with 2 being the most favorable score for each sign and a total score of 10 being perfect

   b. Total score of 8 or more is considered reflective of a healthy fetus

   c. Lower scores may indicate compromise requiring follow-up

G. *Contraction Stress Test (CST)*

1. Purpose—use of external electronic fetal monitoring and stimulation of uterine contractions to assess fetal risk for hypoxia from uteroplacental insufficiency during contractions

2. Indications—assess pregnancies at risk for placental insufficiency that could compromise the fetus, especially during labor

3. Contraindications—history or danger of preterm labor, third trimester bleeding (placenta previa)

4. Protocol

   a. Begin testing at 32 to 43 weeks' gestation

   b. Repeat at weekly intervals

   c. Maternal preparation:

      (1) Empty bladder

      (2) Position as for NST; see p. 72

      (3) Encourage mother to practice childbirth breathing techniques with contractions

   d. Assess maternal vital signs before and during test

   e. Attach external monitor as for NST, and run a baseline strip for 10 to 15 minutes; look for accelerations with FM and spontaneous occurrence of uterine contractions

   f. Obtain a pattern of at least 3 uterine contractions lasting 40 to 60 seconds each in a 10-minute period; stimulation usually is required

      (1) Administration of IV oxytocin (Pitocin) piggyback to a primary infusion, gradually increase the dosage to a desired contraction pattern

(2) Nipple stimulation to facilitate release of endogenous oxytocin from the posterior pituitary gland

> ⚠ **Warning!**
>
> Be alert for hyperstimulation of the uterus: uterine contractions lasting 90 seconds or longer, contractions that occur every 2 minutes or less, or both.

    g. Interventions for the event of hyperstimulation
       (1) Discontinue uterine stimulus immediately
       (2) Continue IV fluids
       (3) Turn the mother onto her side
       (4) Administer oxygen via mask at 8 to 10 L/min
       (5) Monitor maternal vital signs and FHR
       (6) May need to suppress uterine contractions with tocolytics (terbutaline sulfate, 0.25 mg, subcutaneously)
    h. After test is completed the woman must wait until the uterine activity subsides (less than 4 contractions in 30 minutes) and vital signs and FHR are stable and have returned to pretest baseline levels
  5. Interpretation of results
    a. Negative result—indicates good functioning of the fetal-placental unit
       (1) No late deceleration patterns
       (2) Baseline FHR between 110 and 160
       (3) Good variability
       (4) FHR accelerations with FM
       (5) *Repeat in 1 week; fetus likely to tolerate the stress of labor*
    b. Positive result—may indicate inadequate placental function and fetal risk for perinatal morbidity and mortality
       (1) Repetitive, persistent late deceleration patterns with more that 50% of the uterine contractions
       (2) More ominous if accompanied by a decrease in variability and an absence of acceleration of the FHR with FM
       (3) *Action taken may be further testing or induction of the birth*
    c. Suspicious or equivocal result—late decelerations occur but with less than 50% of the contractions; further testing required within 24 hours
H. *Amniocentesis*
  1. Purposes—to obtain a sample of amniotic fluid by inserting a needle transabdominally into amniotic sac for each of the following reasons:
    a. Genetic screening
       (1) Testing time: beginning at 14 weeks' gestation with results available in 2 to 4 weeks

(2) Performed to determine presence of such problems as
    (a) Chromosomal abnormalities (e.g., Down syndrome)
    (b) Inborn errors of metabolism (e.g., Tay-Sachs disease)
    (c) Other genetic disorders known to have genetic markers
    (d) Open neural tube defects indicated by elevated alpha-fetoprotein (AFP) levels in the fluid
  b. A diagnosis of fetal hemolytic disease based on mother's Rh-positive antibody titre; percutaneous umbilical blood sampling (PUBS) may be done instead
  c. A determination of fetal maturity; primarily the lungs
    (1) Testing time—during third trimester around 36 weeks' gestation (a little before, at, or just after) when lung maturation is likely to have occurred
    (2) Factors—both of these results should be present at approximately 36 weeks' gestation for the indication of mature lungs:
      (a) Lecithin-sphingomyelin (L/S) ratio of greater than 2:1
      (b) Presence of phosphatidylglycerol (PG)
2. Indications
  a. Family history of genetic problems
  b. Women aged 35 years or older
  c. Assurance of lung maturity before the induction of labor or the performance of an elective cesarean birth
3. Overall complication rate is under 1% primarily from the invasiveness of the procedure: infection, maternal-fetal damage, bleeding, preterm labor
4. Protocol
  a. Ultrasonography—identify placental and fetal location to avoid damage and pinpoint amniotic fluid pockets
  b. Preparation of the woman
    (1) Provide emotional support and assistance with relaxation techniques since she may be restless and frightened
    (2) Witness a signature for the informed consent
    (3) Assist woman to empty bladder (if performed before 20 weeks' gestation the bladder may be full to elevate the uterus)
    (4) Put in supine position; be alert for supine hypotensive syndrome during the procedure as the pregnancy advances and postural hypotension after the test when woman first sits up
  c. Assessment of maternal vital signs and FHR before, during, and after the procedure
  d. Preparation of site with betadine

Warning!

Surgical asepsis is critical for the preparation of the site and during the procedure.

5. After the procedure
   a. Encourage the woman to rest on her side
   b. Monitor maternal vital signs
   c. Use external monitor to assess for uterine contractions and FHR patterns
   d. Administer Rh$_o$(D) immune globulin (RhoGAM) to the Rh-negative mother
   e. Provide discharge instructions; instruct the mother to
      (1) Report
         (a) Changes in FM
         (b) Vaginal discharge—any clear fluid, blood, or thick, purulent, malodorous discharge
         (c) Presence of pain
         (d) Findings of infection (i.e., temperature over 100° F), malodorous discharge, pain, malaise
      (2) Rest for remainder of day
      (3) Avoid heavy lifting, bending, strenuous exercise for several days
   f. Discuss when results will be available and whom to call
   g. Provide emotional support during the waiting period and if results indicate fetal problems

I. *Chorionic villus sampling* **(CVS)**
   1. Purpose—removal of tissue sample from a fetal portion of the placenta (the chorionic villi) for examination to determine the presence of genetic abnormalities; a transabdominal or transcervical approach may be used
   2. Indications—genetic testing at 10 to 12 weeks' gestation with results obtained in 1 to 2 weeks
   3. Complications—primarily from bleeding, spontaneous abortion, rupture of membranes, infection, and fetal limb defects if performed before 10 weeks' gestation (missing fingers or toes)
   4. Protocol
      a. Ultrasonography is used throughout to guide the procedure
      b. Preparation of woman is similar to that for amniocentesis; full bladder may be needed to position uterus for easier catheter insertion
      c. Position depends on the approach; use a supine position for the transabdominal approach or a lithotomy position for a transcervical approach
      d. Vital signs are monitored
      e. Care after the procedure and discharge instructions are similar to those for an amniocentesis

WEB Resources

http://www.pregnancytoday.com

This website provides pregnancy, parenting, and baby related information and resources for moms by moms.

http://www.firstbabymall.com

The Expectant Mom's Resource Center of this site provides the primigravid woman and her family with articles related to pregnancy, childbirth, and parenting.

http://www.ncemch.org

National Center for Education in Maternal and Child Health—a research center of Georgetown University's Public Policy Institute.

http://www.noah.cuny.edu

NOAH is the New York online access to health. To access information related to fetal assessment during pregnancy first click on Health topics, then Pregnancy, and finally Fetal Testing in the Prenatal and Birth section.

http://www.women.com/pregnancy

This website covers all aspects of pregnancy, birth, and parenting of an infant including pregnancy complications.

REVIEW QUESTIONS

1. A woman is pregnant for the second time. Her first pregnancy ended in a spontaneous abortion at 12 weeks. The correct terms to use to describe this woman's obstetrical history would be which of these pairs of terms?
   1. Primigravida, nullipara
   2. Multigravida, primipara
   3. Primigravida, primipara
   4. Multigravida, nullipara

2. A woman is pregnant for the second time. Her first pregnancy resulted in the birth of twin boys at 35 weeks' gestation. The boys are now 3 years old. To use the 5-digit system to describe this woman's current obstetrical history, the nurse would record which of these items?
   1. 1-0-2-0-2
   2. 1-1-0-0-2
   3. 2-0-1-0-2
   4. 2-2-0-0-1

3. A woman must collect her urine and bring it to the laboratory of the prenatal clinic so that a pregnancy test can be performed. To ensure accuracy the woman should do which of these actions?
   1. Collect the urine during her last voiding of the day, and refrigerate the specimen
   2. Void immediately on arising in the morning, drink two glasses of water, and collect urine from her next voiding
   3. Before eating or drinking, collect the urine of her first voiding in the morning with the use of a clean catch, midstream technique
   4. Collect urine after breakfast in the morning and just before she leaves for the clinic visit

4. At 24 to 28 weeks' gestation, a 1-hour glucose test usually is performed as a screening test for gestational diabetes. Which of these findings would require the performance of a 3-hour glucose tolerance test?
   1. 110 mg/dl
   2. 120 mg/dl
   3. 130 mg/dl
   4. 145 mg/dl

5. A pregnant woman demonstrates understanding of the nurse's instructions about the relief of leg cramps if she report the use of which action?
   1. Wiggles and points her toes during the cramp
   2. Applies cold compresses to the affected leg
   3. Extends her leg and dorsiflexes her foot during the cramp
   4. Avoids weight bearing on the affected leg during the cramp

6. A pregnant woman, at 4 weeks' gestation, asks the nurse when she will be able to hear the baby's heartbeat. The nurse can tell her that with a special ultrasound stethoscope which amplifies sounds, the baby's heartbeat can be heard in approximately how many more weeks?
1. 2-4
2. 6-8
3. 10-12
4. 14-16

7. A pregnant woman is taught how to assess fetal status with the use of a daily fetal movement count (DFMC) that follows the Cardiff protocol. The woman exhibits a need for further instruction if she reports which of these actions?
1. Begins DFMCs at the 27th week of pregnancy
2. Performs the count in a comfortable side-lying position
3. Begins counting before getting out of bed in the morning
4. Recognizes that 10 movements in 1 hour or less is a reassuring sign of fetal well-being

8. The fetal movement alarm signal (MAS) is defined as which of these parameters?
1. More than 1 hour to reach 10 movements
2. Less than 10 movements in 12 hours
3. Less than 3 movements in 12 hours
4. Weakened, less vigorous movements

9. Which of these preparatory actions is required as part of the protocol for a nonstress test (NST)?
1. Avoid eating for at least 2 hours before the test
2. Attach both a tocotransducer and a ultrasound transducer to the woman's abdomen
3. Assist the woman into a supine position
4. Instruct the woman to begin stimulating her nipples 1 hour before the start of the test

10. A pregnant client is scheduled for a biophysical profile (BPP). She asks the nurse what this test is all about. The nurse would explain the test by which of these statements?
1. The test is designed to see how your baby's heart rate reacts to activity, to watch your baby move, and see how much amniotic fluid you have
2. The size of your baby will be measured
3. A score of 5 or greater is the expected finding that indicates that your baby is healthy
4. Uterine contractions will be stimulated for part of the test

ANSWERS, RATIONALES, AND TEST-TAKING TIPS

Rationales	Test-Taking Tips

1. Correct answer: 4

Multigravida represents two or more pregnancies, regardless of the outcome. Nullipara indicates that no pregnancy has been completed to the age of viability. Primigravida refers to the first pregnancy. Primipara indicates that one pregnancy has been completed to the age of viability.

Recall that the sequence is pregnancy, then birth. Associate this sequence with the alphabetical order of the terms *gravida* and *para*. Thus, gravida means pregnancies, and para means number of births after the age of fetal viability has been reached, regardless of the outcome. Viability is reached at about 20 to 24 weeks' gestation. Some authorities say at least 22 weeks. Narrow your choices to options 2 and 3 because two pregnancies are "multiple." With no births, select option 4—nulli means none.

2. Correct answer: 3

Gravida = pregnancy (the first number) = 2 because this woman has been pregnant twice

Para means births (next four numbers):
T: 0 Term births
P: 1 Preterm birth at 35 weeks' gestation
A: 0 Abortions
L: 2 Living children (twins)

The number of pregnancies is two, so narrow the options to either 3 or 4. The number of term births is none, so the correct option is 3. A term pregnancy is considered to be 38 to 42 weeks' gestation.

3. Correct answer: 3

Use of the first voided specimen in the morning before eating and drinking results in a concentrated urine specimen and an increased amount of human chorionic gonadotrophin (HCG) for easier detection of the pregnancy. A clean catch technique enhances the accuracy because debris in urine could interfere with the

If you are unsure of the correct answer, use a grouping or cluster approach. With the use of a cluster technique, you can use two themes to cluster three of the options. Then select the odd option as the correct answer. The first theme to cluster options 1, 2, and 4 under is "no specific collection technique" is stated. Therefore, select the option with the use of a clean catch results. Options 1, 2, and 4 will not yield the most concentrated specimen of urine.

midstream. The other theme is "the type specimen in terms of dilute or concentrated." The only concentrated specimen is option 3. Select it.

4. Correct answer: 4

The results of the 1-hour glucose test should be below 140 mg/dl. If above this level, a 3-hour glucose tolerance test should be performed to determine if the woman has gestational diabetes.

A 50-g, 1-hour glucose test at 24 to 28 weeks' gestation is the screening test for diabetes in pregnant women. A level of 140 mg/dl or higher 1 hour after oral intake of 50g of glucose requires further testing. The 3-hour glucose tolerance test is the definitive test or the diagnostic test for the determination of gestational diabetes and for diabetes mellitus in the nonpregnant population.

5. Correct answer: 3

Pointing of the toes can aggravate a leg cramp. Application of heat is recommended. An alternative to dorsiflexion is to stand with most of the weight on the affected leg and lean forward.

Think anatomy and physiology. A muscle tightens. The counteraction is to stretch it. Then act out each option at your seat if possible. If not, simply close your eyes and picture the action in your mind. The correct answer will quickly become evident.

6. Correct answer: 2

Fetal heart sounds can be detected with the use of an ultrasound stethoscope or Doppler ultrasonography by week 10 to 12 of pregnancy. Because this woman is already 4 weeks pregnant, the fetal heartbeat should be heard in 6 to 8 more weeks. Fetal heart sounds can be auscultated with a fetoscope by week 18 to 20 of pregnancy or in 14 to 16 more weeks.

When numbers of weeks are involved, read carefully and methodically. Then write down the numbers as you narrow the options down to two. The question is worded in terms of *how many more weeks* from her 4 weeks. The question is not at which weeks would you hear fetal heart sounds. Also the type of equipment is essential to note in the stem. A Doppler ultrasonography, being more specialized, can pick up sounds earlier than can a fetoscope which is similar to a regular stethoscope.

7. Correct answer: 3

Fetal movements (FM) should be counted after meals because

The clue to the correct answer is to read the question slowly and

Rationales	Test-Taking Tips

FMs are increased and more vigorous at this time from the increased glucose levels. The other options indicate correct actions with no need for further instruction.

carefully to "a need for further instruction." Then use common sense that the fetus will probably be least active before the mother gets out of bed in the morning.

8. Correct answer: 3

Options 1, 2, and 4 are warning signs that problems exist in the FM patterns. Both the MAS and the warning signs should be reported to the health care provider immediately. These often require further testing by nonstress test (NST) or biophysical profile (BPP).

The clue in the stem is the word "alarm." An alarm is associated with critical life-threatening events. Thus, use your common sense to select the option that is the worst with the least amount of movements.

9. Correct answer: 2

A woman should eat within 2 hours of the test because maternal glucose levels affect FMs to increase them. For the test the woman should be in a semi-Fowler's position, with lateral tilt or in a lateral position. Nipple stimulation is not required because uterine contractions are not a part of this test.

If you have no idea of a correct action, focus on which action is most reasonable with what you know. Recall that a NST is to assess the response of the FHR to periods of FM after 27 to 30 weeks' gestation when the fetal autonomic nervous system is mature enough to respond effectively. Thus, eliminate option 3 because you know that a supine position supports hypotension, and this is unwanted during any test event. Eliminate option 4 because nipple stimulation stimulates uterine contraction, not FMs. With options 1 and 2 left, go with what is more likely, the use of equipment during the test, option 2. Do not select option 1, which is a dietary action, if you are unsure of it.

10. Correct answer: 1

A score of 8 or higher is reassuring. The fetal size is not measured but fetal breathing,

Eliminate the options that are narrow with specific information when you have no idea of a correct answer.

body movement, muscle tone, and amniotic fluid volume are assessed. Uterine contractions are not required for this test. A BPP with a low incidence of false positives is more accurate that the NST or CST alone to detect fetal compromise and risk.

Option 1 is the most comprehensive answer and therefore makes the best educated guess.

4

High-Risk Pregnancy

FAST FACTS

1. **High-risk pregnancy** implies that the life and health of the maternal-fetal unit is in jeopardy, with a resultant impact on the pregnant woman's family.
2. The period of high-risk pregnancy is from conception through the postpartum period.
3. The greatest risk for perinatal morbidity and mortality of the mother, fetus, and newborn occurs in a high-risk pregnancy.
4. Health assessment and care must utilize a holistic approach that focuses on all aspects of a pregnant woman's life because risks arise from many sources, including psychosocial ones.
5. Any bleeding during pregnancy should be considered serious until assessment of the pregnant woman proves otherwise.
6. Vaginal examination of a woman who has fresh bleeding must never be done unless immediate delivery of the fetus can be accomplished. If placenta previa is the cause of the bleeding, further separation of the placenta may occur.
7. All cases of PIH should be considered severe and taken seriously because it is an unpredictable disease and can progress rapidly. Baseline data gathered during prenatal care is a critical factor in the early detection of signs indicative of PIH.
8. In PIH, the typical decrease in blood pressure in the second trimester does not occur; in contrast, both the systolic and diastolic BP increase in the second trimester.
9. A low salt diet or calorie restriction is not recommended for preeclampsia.
10. Most spontaneous abortions occur before 16 weeks' gestation.

CONTENT REVIEW

I. **High-risk pregnancy—assessment, diagnoses, and interventions**
   A. Early, on-going health care is critical to assess the degree and nature of risk and to intervene in a timely manner to enhance the likelihood for a positive outcome to pregnancy
   B. Preconception care must be used to help women and men achieve the best possible health state and reduce the impact of risk factors. Examples include the stopping of cigarette smoking and use of other harmful substances, reversal of nutritional deficits, and stabilization of chronic health problems before pregnancy.
   C. Comprehensive prenatal care must be accessible to all pregnant women and include ongoing assessment of risk status because risk factors can appear or worsen at any time during pregnancy
   D. Nursing diagnoses can include
      1. Alteration in nutrition (less than body requirements) related to
         a. Insufficient oral food and fluid intake associated with persistent vomiting
         b. Loss of appetite associated with activity restriction
      2. Risk for fluid volume deficit related to
         a. Excessive blood loss associated with placenta previa, abruptio placenta, spontaneous abortion, or ectopic pregnancy
         b. Persistent vomiting during or beyond the first trimester
         c. Shift of fluid to the interstitial space with preeclampsia
      3. Risk for maternal injury related to
         a. Increased CNS irritability associated with preeclampsia
         b. Muscle atrophy and orthostatic hypotension associated with prolonged activity restriction
      4. Impaired gas exchange related to fluid accumulation in the lungs (pulmonary edema) associated with cardiac decompensation
      5. Risk for fetal injury related to
         a. Increased maternal core temperature associated with infection
         b. Alteration in placental perfusion associated with preeclampsia, abruptio placenta, or decreased cardiac output (CO)
      6. Anxiety related to the unexpected need for medical intervention during pregnancy and concern for the safety of the pregnant woman and her fetus
      7. Alteration in family processes related to limitation on the pregnant woman's activity level and risk of financial strain
   E. **Nursing interventions should facilitate both the healthy coping of high-risk pregnant women and their families and safe and effective execution of the treatment plan**
      1. Provide time for meeting the needs of high-risk pregnant women and their families
         a. Meet with family members together and separately to discuss feelings, frustrations, concerns, and fears

b. Educate pregnant women and their families about the health problem and the components of the treatment plan; prepare them for the possibility of increasingly complex interventions such as hospitalization, antepartal fetal monitoring, and cesarean birth

c. Encourage participation in the plan of care with positive reinforcement for this participation

2. Reduce stress associated with medical treatment requirements

a. Arrange for home care if possible because the home environment with support from family members is generally more conducive to healing

b. Organize support groups on high-risk pregnancy units so women can share experiences and feelings and support each other; liberal visiting hours, diversional activities, and health teaching sessions may further reduce the stress of hospitalization

c. Coordinate the efforts of the interdisciplinary team to have continuity of care and formation of therapeutic relationships with women

d. Identify stressors related to such factors as finances, childcare, home maintenance; make appropriate referrals

3. Provide time for family interaction after the birth to facilitate the attachment process; use creative approaches if separation occurs as a result of treatment requirements

4. Assist the family through the grieving process if the outcome of the pregnancy is not a positive one. Examples are death of the mother, fetus, or newborn, or development of serious, long-term health problems in the mother or newborn.

5. Facilitate recovery by providing health teaching and arranging needed support in the home because recovery is often a long process that requires follow-up care

6. Help women and their families to view the high-risk experience in realistic terms: what happened, why it happened, and implications for future pregnancies

II. Risk factors that place the maternal-fetal unit in jeopardy

A. Risk factors from the woman's characteristics and lifestyle

1. Age—under 15 or over 35 years of age

2. Nutritional habits and status—less than or greater than desired weight; inadequate intake of appropriate nutrients

3. Stature—5 feet or under

4. Substance use or abuse—tobacco, alcohol, and drugs (see Box 1-1, p. 14)

5. Hostile environment at home or at work—exposure to teratogens, physical abuse, or mental abuse

B. **Risk factors from the health status and lifestyle of the father of the baby**
   1. Abuse of drugs, alcohol, and tobacco
   2. Potentially harmful sexual practices, including bisexuality and unsafe sex
   3. Exposure to environmental hazards
C. **Risk factors from pre-existing health problems**
   1. Health problems present before the onset of pregnancy
      a. Cardiovascular and renal dysfunction
      b. Diabetes mellitus
      c. Anemia
      d. Neurologic dysfunction such as epilepsy and multiple sclerosis
      e. Infections such as the herpes virus and HIV
   2. Pregnancy affects the health problem, and the health problem affects the pregnancy. Examples include medications needed to treat epilepsy that can cause congenital defects in the fetus and insulin requirement changes during the pregnancy of a woman with pre-gestational diabetes.
D. **Risk factors from health problems that arise during pregnancy**
   1. Occur as a result of ineffective adaptation to pregnancy changes. Examples include PIH, anemia, hyperemesis gravidarum, hemorrhage, and gestational diabetes.
   2. More likely to occur among women who are already at risk. Examples include women with pre-gestational diabetes, very young or older pregnant women, women with hypertension.
E. **Risk factors for obstetric and gynecologic status**
   1. Number of pregnancies (gravida) and births (para). Examples include primigravidas and grand multiparous woman (5 or more births).
   2. Pelvic and uterine abnormalities
   3. History of sexually transmitted diseases (STDs) and pelvic inflammatory disease (PID)
   4. History of complications with previous pregnancies. Examples include spontaneous abortions, hemorrhage, preterm labor, and birth.
   5. History of infertility
   6. Mother's exposure to diethylstilbestrol (DES) as a fetus
F. **Risk factors from psychosocial status**
   1. Unstable family relationships
      a. Separation or divorce
      b. Abusive relationship with partner or father of the baby
      c. Paternal lack of interest in the pregnancy
      d. Single status of mother, especially if family-support system has a negative reaction to the pregnancy
   2. Inadequate economic resources
      a. No health insurance
      b. Need to depend on public assistance for health care

c. Struggle to meet essential living needs, lowering the priority of prenatal care

3. Limited access to nearby, culturally sensitive prenatal care or high-risk pregnancy center

4. Minority status in terms of race or ethnicity; minorities experience higher rates of maternal and infant morbidity and mortality as well as LBW

5. History of mental health disorders, including depression, psychosis, and mood disorders

III. Approach to risk factors

A. **Risk factors vary as to danger level presented and intervention required. Examples include moderate obesity compared with pre-gestational diabetes, PIH with this pregnancy compared with a history of PIH with a previous pregnancy.**

B. **Risk factors can occur at any time during the pregnancy or puerperium**

C. **More that one risk factor can be present. An example is a 15-year-old single parent who smokes cigarettes and uses marijuana, is underweight, and has a history of STDs.**

D. **One risk factor can precipitate the occurrence of another. An example is a woman with diabetes mellitus who is at increased risk for PIH, infection, and abruptio placenta.**

IV. Psychosocial impact of a high-risk pregnancy on the woman and her family

A. **Stressors are magnified and increase in high-risk pregnancies. Stressors must be recognized and addressed because they can contribute to the worsening of an already difficult situation and diminish the energy needed to cope with the pregnancy. Stressors arise from a variety of situations:**

1. Changes in lifestyle and normal living patterns
   a. Family processes are altered
   b. Family members may have difficulty accepting the severity of the pregnant woman's health problem because she may not "look sick"
   c. Added health care expenses and the loss of a second income
   d. More frequent prenatal visits, antepartal testing, treatment regimens, and possible hospitalization

2. Interference with the ability to fulfill the developmental tasks of pregnancy
   a. Securing safe passage for self and fetus; the woman must follow a strict treatment regimen, which may be difficult and uncomfortable: she questions, "Is it worth it?" "Will it work?"
   b. Ensuring acceptance of the newborn by significant others, including family members and friends; the woman may fear

that the baby will not survive, or if it does, that it will not be normal

   c. Binding into her child

     (1) The woman may fear an "emotional investment" in a fetus that may not survive

     (2) The mother and infant often are separated after birth

   d. Learning to give of herself; the woman must expend energy and time to cope with the pregnancy, with little left to care for others

  B. Psychological reactions—experienced by all involved in the pregnancy

   1. Denial and disbelief

   2. Guilt and blame: parents may blame themselves, each other, or even the baby; they may ask, "What did we (I) do wrong?"

   3. Fears concerning survival of the mother and baby

   4. Grief and mourning

    a. Anticipatory grief: preparation for potential fetal or newborn loss; if fetus survives, transition must be made to relate to the newborn and its care needs

    b. Grieving the loss of the expected "normal" child; or grieving the death of the baby, mother, or both

V. Bleeding during pregnancy

⚠ Warning!

Any bleeding during pregnancy should be considered serious until assessment of the pregnant woman proves otherwise.

  A. The uterus becomes more vascular as pregnancy progresses, increasing the danger of hemorrhage (massive blood loss) and hypovolemic shock

  B. The cause of bleeding during pregnancy changes as the pregnancy progresses

  C. Common causes of bleeding in early pregnancy

   1. **Abortion**—termination of the pregnancy before the age of fetal viability. Authorities believe viability is reached after 20 to 24 weeks' gestation or when fetal weight is over 500 g

    a. Clinical manifestations vary according to the abortion type and the gestational age; influences fetal size, and size and adherence of placenta (Table 4-1, p. 92)

    b. Sonography may be used to assess the integrity of the gestational sac

    c. HCG levels determine if pregnancy is still viable. An increasing level suggests viability.

    d. Treatment approach is determined by the type of abortion; ranges from bed rest to dilation and curettage

2. **Ectopic pregnancy**—implantation occurs at a site outside of the uterus, most often the fallopian tube
   a. Incidence is increasing with pelvic inflammatory disease (PID) and intrauterine devices (IUDs) as major risk factors
   b. Clinical manifestations appear at approximately 6 to 12 weeks' gestation just before or with rupture of tube
      (1) Amenorrhea
      (2) Adnexal fullness; tender abdominal mass
      (3) Unilateral dull colicky pain (stretching of tube) to severe unilateral pelvic and abdominal pain, often referred to the shoulder (rupture of tube)
      (4) Nausea, faintness
      (5) Bleeding, which can lead to excessive blood loss and shock

 Warning!

Blood may accumulate in the abdominal cavity with only spotting or irregular bleeding apparent.

   c. Clinical manifestations may be similar to other health problems, including appendicitis and ruptured ovarian cyst. A pregnancy test facilitates the diagnosis.
   d. Treatment
      (1) Early ectopic pregnancy before rupture: methotrexate intramuscularly to dissolve the tissue
      (2) Advanced ectopic pregnancy just before or just after rupture: removal of tube and products of conception (fetus, placenta, membranes)
D. **Common causes of bleeding in late pregnancy**
   1. **Placenta previa**—placenta is abnormally implanted in the lower uterine segment rather than in the fundus
      a. Varies as to the degree of previa: marginal to complete coverage of the internal cervical os
      b. Clinical manifestations appear when placenta loosens as the lower uterine segment changes and the cervix ripens toward the end of pregnancy in preparation for labor
         (1) Bright red, *painless* bleeding
         (2) Increases as placenta continues to separate

 Warning!

Vaginal examination of a woman who has fresh bleeding must never be done unless immediate delivery of the fetus can be accomplished because further separation of the placenta may occur.

Text continues on p. 94

TABLE 4-1 Manifestations and Management of Spontaneous Abortion (Miscarriage)*

Type of Abortion	Manifestations	Management

Threatened abortion: manifestations may persist for several days or weeks, then subside with continuation of the pregnancy or progress to loss of the pregnancy; approximately 50% progress to loss	Slight bleeding, spotting
	Mild uterine cramping, backache
	Cervix closed: no effacement and dilation
	No passage of tissue
		Confirm status as a threatened abortion
		Use watchful waiting (expectant management):
		  Bed rest for 48 hours, sedation
		  Avoid stress, orgasm
		Evaluate response to management
		Provide emotional support

Inevitable or imminent abortion: pregnancy cannot be saved, abortion will occur	Moderate bleeding
	Mild to severe uterine cramping, backache
	Membranes may rupture
	Cervix is open, dilated, and soft
	No passage of tissue
		Confirm status as an inevitable abortion
		Wait for expulsion of uterine contents and examine for completeness,
		or
		Terminate pregnancy:
		  Dilation and curettage or uterine aspiration when less than 16 weeks' gestation
		  Dilation and evacuation after 16 weeks' gestation
		Provide emotional support and assist through the grieving process

Type	Signs and Symptoms	Management
Incomplete abortion: only a portion of the products of conception are expelled; usually it is the placenta that is retained, especially after 10 weeks' gestation	Heavy to profuse bleeding associated with the retained placenta Severe uterine cramping Tissue is passed with the bleeding Cervix is open and dilated	Manage as for inevitable abortion in terms of evacuation of the uterus Contents of uterus must be completely removed: Bleeding and cramping will continue if placenta is retained because adequate, sustained contraction of the uterus cannot occur Infection risk increases if placenta pieces are retained Provide emotional support and assistance through the grieving process
Complete abortion: all products of conception are expelled; uterus is fully emptied spontaneously, and tissue passed is complete and intact	Slight bleeding Mild uterine cramping Complete products of conception are passed Cervix is closed	No medical intervention is required if: Bleeding and cramping subside after passage Tissue passed is evaluated to be complete and intact Infection does not occur Provide emotional support and assistance through the grieving process
Missed abortion: fetus dies but products of conception are not passed or aborted	Slight bleeding, brownish discharge No uterine cramping No tissue is passed Cervix is closed Signs of pregnancy subside and pregnancy test is negative	Wait for approximately 1 month to allow for spontaneous emptying of uterus Terminate pregnancy using methods described for inevitable abortion Retention of decomposing fetus can Affect maternal clotting integrity leading to disseminated intravascular coagulation (DIC) Increase infection risk Provide emotional support and assist through the grieving process

*Most spontaneous abortions occur before 16 weeks' gestation.

    c. Management varies based on the amount of bleeding, the placental location in terms of the cervix, and gestational age

        (1) Watchful waiting—bed rest with close observation if pregnancy has not reached term, fetal lungs are immature, and separation and bleeding are limited; care may be home- or hospital-based

        (2) Immediate cesarean section birth—if bleeding is excessive with continued separation because fetal viability and maternal well-being are endangered

        (3) Vaginal birth—if placenta does not cover the cervical os

    d. Major postpartum complications are associated with placenta previa

        (1) Hemorrhage—limited contractility of lower uterine segment

        (2) Infection—location of healing placental site at cervical os

  2. **Abruptio placenta**—premature separation of a normally implanted placenta (fundal implantation)

    a. Separation can occur spontaneously or is related to trauma or a convulsion

    b. Clinical manifestations vary as to the degree and the location of separation

        (1) Bleeding—scant to massive, depending on the degree of separation

            (a) Concealed hemorrhage indicates separation occurs from the center, with blood forced into uterine myometrium *(Couvelaire uterus)*

            (b) Overt hemorrhage of *dark red blood* indicates that separation occurs at the margins

        (2) Pain and abdominal tenderness—occur as the placenta separates and pain increases in severity with concealed hemorrhage

    c. Management varies based on the degree of separation and severity of blood loss; ranges from watchful waiting to emergency cesarean birth; hospital-based care is recommended

    d. Hemorrhage is a major postpartum complication caused by

        (1) Diminished contractility of the uterine fundus with a Couvelaire uterus

        (2) Exhaustion of clotting factors with excessive bleeding; risk of disseminated intravascular coagulation (DIC) is present

VI. Pregnancy-Induced Hypertension (PIH)

  A. Definition—hypertensive syndrome associated with pregnancy beginning after 20 weeks' gestation through early postpartum period. PIH is characterized by hypertension, with or without edema, and proteinuria. PIH is a major cause of maternal-fetal morbidity and mortality.

B. Risk factors for PIH
1. Chronic health problems affecting the vascular system. Examples include diabetes mellitus, renal disease, and chronic hypertension.
2. Family or personal history of PIH
3. Exposure to chorionic villi, resulting in an immunologic reaction
   a. Primigravida or first pregnancy with a new partner
   b. Multiple gestation, hydatidiform mole, large fetus with a large placenta—increased number of chorionic villi
4. Age less than 20 or over 35 years
5. Poor nutrition, especially in terms of insufficient protein and calcium ingestion

C. Classifications of PIH
1. Transient hypertension—development of hypertension after 20 weeks of pregnancy in a woman who was normotensive before pregnancy

⚠ **Warning!**

Edema and proteinuria do not occur in women with transient hypertension.

2. Preeclampsia—mild or severe as determined by degree of hypertension, edema, proteinuria, and other clinical manifestations
3. Preeclampsia—with prior chronic hypertension; pregnancy adversely affects chronic hypertension. Careful monitoring and the continued treatment of the chronic hypertension are essential.
4. Eclampsia—onset of seizure activity or coma in women with preeclampsia who have no preexisting neurologic pathology
5. HELLP syndrome—severe form of preeclampsia that involves hemolysis (H), liver dysfunction (EL, elevated liver enzymes), and a low platelet count (LP), along with multisystem organ failure. The life of the maternal-fetal unit is in serious jeopardy.

⚠ **Warning!**

All cases of PIH should be considered severe and taken seriously because PIH is unpredictable and can progress rapidly. Baseline data gathered during prenatal care is a critical factor in the early detection of signs indicative of PIH.

D. Pathophysiologic basis for the clinical manifestations of PIH—venospasm increases peripheral vascular resistance, which prevents the dilation of vascular network to accommodate the increasing blood volume that occurs during pregnancy
1. The typical decrease in blood pressure in the second trimester does not occur. The systolic, diastolic BP, or both, begin to increase instead.

2. Intravascular fluid is forced into the interstitial spaces as a compensatory mechanism and as a result of an increased vascular permeability
   a. Peripheral and organ edema
   b. Hypovolemia that results in decreased tissue perfusion, including that of the placenta, and hemoconcentration with increased hematocrit level
E. **Clinical manifestations of preeclampsia**
   1. Elevation of BP
      a. BP 140/90 mm Hg or higher on two occasions, 4 to 6 hours apart (mild)
      b. BP 160/90 mm Hg or higher on two occasions, 4 to 6 hours apart with pregnant woman on bed rest (severe)
      c. Mean arterial pressure (diastolic pressure plus one third of pulse pressure) over 105 mm Hg
   2. Generalized and upper body edema
      a. Dependent edema with some puffiness of eyelids, face, fingers, and hands (mild)
      b. Generalized edema with more noticeable upper body edema; pulmonary edema may be present (severe)
      c. Edema is not responsive to 12 hours of bed rest
      d. Rapid weight gain of more than 2 kg in 1 week
      e. *Pitting edema* often is present: measures depth of depression remaining after pressing finger into edematous tissue located over a bone
   3. CNS changes from cerebral edema and venospasm; more likely with severe preeclampsia
      a. Irritability, insomnia, and altered level of consciousness
      b. Headache ranging from transient to severe and constant
      c. Changes in vision, that is, blurring, spots before eyes, photophobia
      d. Brisk deep tendon reflexes, 3+ or higher (hyperreflexia) with possible ankle clonus
      e. Convulsion (grand mal type) occurs in 5% of women with PIH
         (1) Any stimulus can precipitate a convulsion. Examples include sudden activity in or near the hospital room, a telephone ring, turning on the light or the television.
         (2) Half occur before labor, one quarter during labor, and one quarter within 48 hours of birth
   4. Pulmonary edema
   5. Hepatic dysfunction from venospasm and edema of the liver
      a. Epigastric and upper right quadrant pain from liver enlargement
      b. Nausea and vomiting
      c. Jaundice

     d. Elevated liver enzymes [alanine aminotransferase (ALT), aspartate aminotransferase (AST), lactate dehydrogenase (LDH)]

     e. Liver necrosis with bleeding; liver rupture is a possibility

6. Renal involvement from diminished perfusion and increased permeability of the glomerular membrane

     a. Proteinuria—a late-appearing sign present in two clean catch specimens taken at least 6 hours apart: 2+ to 3+, mild; 4+ or higher, severe

     b. Specific gravity—increased

     c. Oliguria—under 25 to 30 ml/hr, or under 100 ml in 4 hours

     d. Blood urea nitrogen (BUN) and serum creatinine levels—increased

7. Hemolysis and decrease in number of available platelets

     a. RBCs change in form and become easily destroyed as they are forced through narrow, contracted blood vessels *(venospasm)*

     b. Platelets adhere to endothelial lesions in blood vessels resulting from venospasm; clotting may be affected, resulting in bruising, epistaxis, and postpartum hemorrhage

8. Diminished placental perfusion from hypovolemia and venospasm

     a. Decreased placental size and earlier aging; risk for abruptio placenta

     b. Fetal effects

        (1) Intrauterine growth restriction (IUGR)

        (2) Preterm birth may be required from the severity of preeclampsia and its effects on the maternal-fetal unit because the only definitive cure is termination of the pregnancy

        (3) Increased danger of fetal distress during parturition

F. Mild preeclampsia—home care of the woman

1. Monitoring the progression of preeclampsia and fetal status

     a. Teach pregnant woman and her family how to assess health status, including BP; weight; urine (protein level); daily FM counts; and signs of worsening condition, including headache, vision changes, and epigastric pain

     b. Encourage woman to keep a record of her findings and her concerns for review during prenatal visits or during home visits by a health care provider

     c. Stress the importance of keeping prenatal appointments and participating in antepartal monitoring procedures

2. Monitoring cooperation with treatment regimen

     a. Limitations on activity level range from frequent rest periods with an emphasis on sedentary activities to bed rest with bathroom privileges. Have woman:

        (1) Maintain a lateral position (alternate between right and left sides) when in bed to enhance renal perfusion (fluid loss) and placental perfusion

     (2) Use relaxation techniques, diversional activities, and gentle range-of-motion exercises to the extremities for a decrease in complications associated with bed rest or limited activity

     (3) Involve family, friends, and home care agencies to assist with home maintenance activities

  b. Nutrition—Have woman:

     (1) Maintain a balanced diet appropriate for pregnancy

     (2) Increase protein intake to replace losses and to keep fluid within the vascular bed; 60 to 70 g/day of protein

     (3) Maintain calcium intake at 1200 mg/day

     (4) Maintain fluid intake of 2000 to 3000 ml/day

     (5) Include roughage to facilitate bowel elimination, especially because activity level is reduced; avoid alcohol, tobacco, and highly salted foods

 Warning!

A low salt diet or calorie restriction is not recommended for women with preeclampsia.

G. Moderate to severe preeclampsia—hospital care of the woman

1. Systematic, ongoing assessment of the maternal-fetal unit to detect changes indicative of an improving or worsening condition

2. Information for family of assessment findings and treatments, including purpose and potential effects

3. Keep woman on bedrest alternating between a left and right lateral position

4. Seizure precautions and care

  a. Reduce environmental stimuli with regard to noise, light, activity; consider room assignment, avoiding rooms near high activity areas such as the nurse's station or visitor's lounge

  b. Be prepared for seizures by padding side rails, keeping bed in low position, instructing woman to wear loose clothing, and keeping oxygen and suction equipment near by

  c. Implement appropriate care should a seizure occur

  d. Observe for an onset of labor, signs of fetal distress, and abruptio placenta after a seizure

5. Medications

  a. Sedatives—combined with bed rest and reduced environmental stimuli, can facilitate rest and reduce CNS irritability

  b. Magnesium sulfate—see Chapter 7, Table 7-1 p. 190 for nursing interventions required during administration of magnesium sulfate

    (1) Effects

      (a) CNS depressant; primary expected outcome of treatment is seizure prevention; relaxation effects occur

      (b) Vasodilation effect produces a slight, temporary decrease in BP and a feeling of warmth with some flushing

          (c) Smooth muscle relaxation effect reduces uterine contractions, thereby potentially interfering with the labor process and postpartum contraction of the uterus

      (2) Administration

          (a) Administer IV piggyback using an IV controller

          (b) Loading dose of 4 to 6 g/250 ml of IV fluid over 15 to 30 minutes

          (c) Mix 40 g in 1 L of Ringer's lactate to infuse at the maintenance dose of 1 to 3 g/hr

  c. Antihypertensive medications—antihypertensive of choice is hydralazine hydrochloride (Apresoline)

      (1) Administer according to BP level, for example, if systolic pressure is 160 or higher or diastolic pressure is 110 mm Hg or higher, or both

      (2) Monitor BP before and after administration (measure with a sphygmomanometer and stethoscope)

      (3) Maintain diastolic pressure between 90 to 100 mm Hg to ensure adequate placental perfusion

6. Goals—full-term, vaginal delivery; labor induction and augmentation may be required because magnesium sulfate suppresses uterine contractions

7. Postpartal care

  a. Continue treatment for preeclampsia until condition stabilizes, with a decrease in BP, edema (diuresis and diaphoresis), and proteinuria

  b. Utilize Pitocin as the oxytocic of choice to enhance fundal contraction because methylergonovine maleate (Methergine) and ergonovine maleate (Ergotrate) can further elevate BP

  c. Observe for signs of hemorrhage

  d. Provide time for interaction with newborn

  e. Caution woman to avoid another pregnancy for approximately 2 years to facilitate full recovery

VII. Hyperemesis gravidarum

  A. Definition—excessive, intractable vomiting during pregnancy, most often during the first 16 weeks but can last longer, that results in weight loss of at least 5% of pre-pregnancy weight, dehydration, and fluid, electrolyte, metabolic, and nutritional imbalances

  B. Causative factors

    1. Hormonal factors—high levels of estrogen, thyroid hormone, and HCG

    2. Gastrointestinal (GI) factors, including liver dysfunction, decrease in level of hydrochloric acid, and reduced GI motility (progesterone effect)

3. Psychological and emotional factors
   a. Continuing ambivalence about pregnancy and impending motherhood; more common when pregnancies are unplanned or unwanted
   b. Negative family responses to pregnancy, especially by the father of the baby
   c. Typical response to stressors involves GI disturbances
C. **Major concern relates to the impact of imbalances on the health status of the maternal-fetal unit**
   1. Maternal effects
      a. Weight loss—5% or more of normal weight
      b. Fluid volume deficit—dehydration and hypovolemia with resultant alteration in vital signs, including hypotension and tachycardia
      c. Acid-base imbalance—metabolic alkalosis progressing to metabolic acidosis
      d. Nutritional deficit
      e. Electrolyte deficit—hypokalemia, hyponatremia
      f. Activity intolerance—fatigue, weakness
      g. Fears—welfare of self and fetus
   2. Fetal effects
      a. Hypoxia and intrauterine growth restriction from diminished placental perfusion and limited nutrient availability from the mother
      b. Anomalies from exposure to ketosis
D. **Major and immediate goal of treatment is to restore fluid, electrolyte, and acid-base balance**
   1. Administer fluids, electrolytes, and nutrients
      a. Provide IV hydration—5% glucose in lactated Ringer's solution with added multivitamins and magnesium sulfate
      b. Provide nutrients—total parenteral nutrition (TPN)
   2. Reduce fluid losses by using sedatives and antiemetics [vitamin B_6, prochlorperazine maleate (Compazine), promethazine hydrochloride (Phenergan)]
   3. Monitor effectiveness of treatment
      a. Assess vital signs
      b. Watch for signs of fluid balance, including weight, turgor, specific gravity of urine, input and output
      c. Obtain serum electrolyte and glucose levels
E. **Additional goals of treatment**
   1. Rest GI tract by maintaining NPO status until dehydration is resolved and for 48 hours once vomiting ceases
   2. Restore ability to take and retain oral fluids and food
      a. Introduce and advance diet gradually beginning with small amounts of clear fluids such as ice chips or tea; alternate with dry carbohydrates every 2 to 3 hrs

      b. Follow fluid and food preferences

      c. Use interventions effective for morning sickness

  3. Maintain integrity of oral cavity with frequent oral care to keep mouth clean and moist; especially important after an episode of vomiting because emesis is acidic

  4. Promote rest and relaxation

      a. Create a quiet, restful environment

      b. Provide emotional support

      c. Facilitate the expression of feelings and concerns

      d. Teach stress management and relaxation techniques

  5. Prepare for discharge

      a. Educate pregnant woman and family about her condition, signs of improvement or deterioration, and treatment measures

      b. Make referrals, as appropriate, to monitor and supervise treatments such as TPN

      c. Arrange for follow-up prenatal visits

VIII. Diabetes mellitus during pregnancy

  A. Pre-gestational diabetes—diabetes mellitus present before pregnancy. It is affected by pregnancy's influence on glucose metabolism.

    1. Alteration in insulin requirements during pregnancy

      a. First trimester—insulin requirement is reduced

        (1) Fetal utilization of glucose

        (2) Decreased maternal nutritional intake from nausea and vomiting

        (3) Increased tissue response to insulin

        (4) Risk for hypoglycemia until insulin dosage is regulated

      b. Second and third trimesters—insulin requirement is increased

        (1) Higher level of cortisol that increases serum glucose level

        (2) Insulin antagonists secreted by the placenta

        (3) Increased tissue resistance to insulin

        (4) Risk for diabetic ketoacidosis until insulin is increased to required level; intrauterine fetal death and preterm labor can result

      c. Parturition—energy demands of labor and birth require a delicate balance of glucose and insulin

      d. Postpartum period—insulin requirement is reduced as insulin antagonists are removed

        (1) Up to 4 weeks are required to return to usual pre-gestational insulin requirements

        (2) Lactating women need to continue careful regulation of glucose levels and insulin requirements

    2. Maternal complications from pre-gestational diabetes

      a. Polyhydramnios increases the risk for premature rupture of the membranes, cord prolapse, preterm labor and birth, and postpartum hemorrhage

    b. Vascular changes associated with diabetes, increasing the risk for PIH, placental insufficiency, and abruptio placenta

    c. *Dystocia* (difficult labor) and increased potential for caesarian birth from fetal macrosomia

    d. Risk for genitourinary infection including *Candida,* urinary tract infection (UTI)

    e. Risk for hypoglycemia and diabetic ketoacidosis

  3. Fetal and newborn complications

 Warning!

Significant risk for morbidity and mortality exists unless pre-conception glucose-insulin balance is attained and pregnant blood glucose levels are maintained at 65 to 130 mg/dl.

    a. Alteration in size

      (1) Large for gestational age and macrosomia caused by

        (a) Exposure to high glucose levels when maternal control is poor

        (b) Increase in fetal insulin secretion as a response to high glucose levels; insulin accelerates the growth rate

      (2) Intrauterine growth restriction (IUGR) if vascular changes associated with diabetes are advanced and affect placental circulation

    b. Congenital anomalies including cardiac, CNS, neural tube (spina bifida), and skeletal defects, especially if a woman becomes pregnant in a poorly controlled state

    c. Preterm birth with a higher risk for respiratory distress because surfactant production is inhibited by increased fetal insulin levels

    d. Stillbirth

    e. Fetal hypoxia caused by

      (1) Placental insufficiency

      (2) Limitation on oxygen availability from increased level of glycosylated hemoglobin (glucose molecule attaches to hemoglobin altering its oxygen carrying capacity) in women with poorly controlled diabetes. The fetus compensates by increasing RBC production, resulting in polycythemia vera.

    f. Neonatal hypoglycemia because newborn continues to secrete high levels of insulin that are no longer balanced by maternal glucose

    g. Neonatal hyperbilirubinemia from destruction of increased number of RBCs produced during pregnancy

Warning!

Oral hypoglycemic agents cannot be used to maintain glucose control because they are teratogenic.

B. *Gestational diabetes*—**diabetic state that develops during the second half of pregnancy, usually in the third trimester, in some women who are not diabetic**

1. Diagnosis
   a. Screening
      (1) All pregnant women should be tested using a 50-g, 1-hour glucose test at 24 to 28 weeks' gestation
      (2) A level of 140 mg/dl or higher at 1 hour after oral intake of 50 g of glucose requires further testing
   b. 3-hour glucose tolerance test (GTT)—used to diagnose gestational diabetes in women with a positive glucose screening or who are at high risk for developing gestational diabetes. Examples include obesity, women with a family history of diabetes, and those with a personal history of gestational diabetes.
   c. The definitive diagnosis of gestational diabetes is made on the basis of two or more abnormal values on a 3-hour GTT
2. Glucose control is achieved with diet alone or with both diet and insulin
3. Maternal, fetal, and newborn complications are the same as those for pre-gestational diabetes, except for congenital anomalies, which are no higher than for the general population

C. **Management of pre-gestational and gestational diabetes (GDM): goal of a vaginal term birth can be met if the treatment regimen is fulfilled and euglycemia (glucose within the normal ranges) is maintained**

1. Ongoing assessment of the health status of the maternal-fetal unit
   a. More frequent prenatal visits
   b. Hospitalization—may be required to stabilize insulin-glucose balance
   c. Antepartal fetal monitoring
   d. Maternal testing
      (1) Blood glucose levels for glucose management
         (a) Laboratory testing: fasting blood glucose (65 to 95 mg/dl), 1-hour postprandial blood glucose (less than 130 mg/dl), and 2-hour postprandial blood glucose (less than 120 mg/dl)
         (b) Home monitoring before meals, 2 hours after meals (postprandial), and at bedtime (no less than 70 mg/dl)
      (2) Testing for glycosylated hemoglobin levels; a value of 7% indicates good diabetic control over the previous 4 to 6 weeks
      (3) Urine testing for ketones
2. Dietary management must take into consideration requirements of pregnancy and lactation as well as the need to maintain glucose control
   a. First trimester—from 30 to 35 cal/kg (ideal body weight without causing hypoglycemia or ketoacidosis)

b. Second and third trimesters—from 35 to 40 cal/kg (ideal body weight or pre-pregnant weight without causing hypoglycemia or ketoacidosis)

c. Balanced diet—of 50% to 60% total calories for carbohydrates with fiber, 12% to 20% protein, and 20% to 30 % fat

d. Meal distribution—three meals (25%, 30%, 30%) and three snacks (5% each) or two snacks (5% daytime snack and 10% bedtime snack) to maintain a stable blood glucose level and prevent hypoglycemia or ketoacidosis

e. Fasting during sleep—bedtime snack of complex carbohydrate and protein is especially important before the sleep period

3. Administration of insulin

a. Daily insulin dosage is based on serum glucose levels with the goal of maintaining a euglycemic state of 65 to 130 mg/dl

b. Insulin isophane suspension (NPH Iletin), which is intermediate-acting, and short-acting. Regular insulin or rapid acting Lispro (Humalog) insulin is used alone or in combination. Note: Lispro has an onset of action within 15 minutes and peaks within 40 to 60 minutes.

c. Administration patterns

(1) Combination of long- and short-acting insulin twice a day, with two thirds of the daily dosage before breakfast and one third before supper, *or* administer short-acting with dinner and long-acting at bedtime

(2) Use short-acting before each meal and long-acting at bedtime

 Warning!

Some authorities caution against the use of the leg as an administration site because of the circulatory changes that occur as pregnancy advances.

4. Health teaching and emotional support

a. A full explanation of diabetes during pregnancy, signs and symptoms of hypoglycemia and ketoacidosis, need for prenatal visits, antepartal fetal monitoring, following a healthy lifestyle during pregnancy, and the required therapeutic regimen to maintain glucose control

b. Demonstration, practice, and redemonstration are required for the psychomotor skills of home blood glucose monitoring, urine testing, and insulin administration

c. Emotional support is required to reduce the anxiety and fear experienced when changes occur in usual living patterns in terms of diet, insulin administration, and need to perform invasive procedures

5. Care during labor and birth commonly includes an IV infusion containing glucose to meet energy needs and administration of insulin (IV or SQ) according to blood glucose levels

   6. Postpartum follow-up
      a. Observation of the newborn and care is required for
         hypoglycemia, hyperbilirubinemia, and respiratory distress
         especially if preterm
      b. Care for the pre-gestational diabetic woman
         (1) Monitor blood glucose levels as during pregnancy and
             administer insulin at a dosage to maintain euglycemia until
             pre-pregnant levels return in 3 to 4 weeks
         (2) Instruct woman that breast feeding is permitted as long as
             glucose control is maintained; hypoglycemia inhibits
             lactation and the let-down reflex
         (3) Space the next pregnancy at approximately 2 years to
             allow for a full recovery
      c. Information for the gestational diabetic woman about the need
         to maintain a balance of nutrition and activity to avoid obesity
         because she is at increased risk for gestational diabetes in
         future pregnancies and diabetes mellitus later in life

IX. Cardiac disease during pregnancy

   **A. Pregnancy places stress on the cardiovascular system as a result
   of plasma volume expansion, which increases CO and cardiac
   workload**
   **B. The degree of cardiac dysfunction before pregnancy serves as the
   basis for pregnancy management. Determination of cardiac
   status is made before pregnancy, at 3 months' gestation, and
   again at 7 months' gestation when blood volume is at its
   maximum and stress on the heart is greatest. Functional
   classifications of organic heart disease (New York State Heart
   Association) along with general recommendations for
   management are as follows**
   1. Class I
      a. Asymptomatic at normal levels of activity
      b. Management recommendations include:
         (1) Do not limit activity; however, some limitations may be
             needed as pregnancy progresses to maintain functional status
         (2) Limit stress
         (3) Take additional rest periods at night (8 to 10 hours of
             sleep) and after meals (30 minutes)
         (4) Instruct woman that close health supervision during
             pregnancy is needed, with prompt treatment of infection
   2. Class II
      a. Symptomatic with increased activity
      b. Management recommendations same as for Class I along with
         some activity limitations in terms of heavy exertion and
         stopping activity that causes even minimal signs of cardiac
         decompensation

      c. Hospitalization for evaluation and treatment is likely as pregnancy reaches term

  3. Class III

      a. Symptomatic with ordinary activity

      b. Approximately 30% of pregnant women in this class will experience cardiac decompensation

      c. Management recommendations include moderate to marked activity limitations and bed rest for most of the day

      d. Hospitalization is likely as pregnancy reaches the 7th to 8th month

  4. Class IV

      a. Symptomatic at rest

      b. Pregnancy is not recommended but if it occurs, cardiac status must be improved early. Early therapeutic abortion with regional anesthesia and prophylactic antibiotics may be required for the safety of the mother.

C. Effects of cardiac disease on pregnancy

  1. Women with Class I or II cardiac disease generally experience an uneventful pregnancy as long as health supervision is provided and recommendations are followed

  2. Women with Class III or IV are at risk for severe cardiac decompensation, resulting in adverse effects on the maternal-fetal unit

  3. Problems that are encountered:

      a. Cardiac decompensation

      b. Spontaneous abortion and stillbirth

      c. Preterm labor and birth

      d. Intrauterine growth restriction (IUGR)

D. Ongoing assessment of health status is required throughout pregnancy, labor, birth, and the postpartum period

  1. Observe for signs of cardiac decompensation, especially during

      a. 28 to 32 weeks' gestation when vascular volume reaches its peak and when CO and cardiac workload are greatest

      b. Labor and birth when a woman must cope with the added stressors of pain and the work of giving birth

      c. The first 48 hours postpartum when vascular fluid volume increases with the reabsorption of extravascular fluid

  2. Signs indicative of cardiac decompensation and pulmonary edema—may appear gradually or suddenly

      a. Decreasing energy level; fatigue increases with difficulty performing usual activities

      b. Irregular, weak, and rapid pulse (100 beats per minute or higher); palpitations

      c. Alteration in respiratory pattern

        (1) Increase in respiratory rate (25 breaths per minute or higher)

(2) Dyspnea with usual activities; orthopnea

(3) Moist, frequent cough; crackles (rales) on auscultation

(4) Cyanosis of lips and nail beds

   d. Progressive, generalized edema noted as weight gain, upper body and pitting edema of legs and feet

  3. Antepartal monitoring to assess fetal status

E. Management of the pregnant woman with cardiac disease

  1. Pharmacologic interventions

   a. Cardiac medications such as propranolol, lidocaine, digoxin to strengthen activity of the heart and enhance CO

   b. Thiazide diuretics and furosemide (Lasix) to reduce fluid retention

   c. Anticoagulant therapy with heparin to reduce clot formation

> **⚠ Warning!**
>
> Heparin, as a large molecule drug, does not cross the placenta, whereas warfarin sodium (Coumadin) does cross the placenta to affect the fetus.

   d. Antibiotics such as penicillin, ampicillin, gentamicin, or amoxicillin to prevent infections, including endocarditis; infections result in added strain on the heart and increase its rate

  2. Nutrition

   a. Balanced diet with calorie and nutrient increases to gain approximately 24 pounds; excessive weight gain will further increase cardiac workload

   b. Roughage to prevent constipation and straining at stool

   c. Sodium restriction may be required to reduce fluid retention; observe for signs of hyponatremia because sodium requirements increase with pregnancy

   d. Iron supplementation to prevent anemia because anemia increases stress on cardiac function

  3. Stress reduction, relaxation, and rest

   a. During pregnancy—actions for the mother

    (1) Relaxation and stress management techniques

    (2) Involvement of family, friends, and home care agencies to reduce household workload

    (3) Periods of rest in the lateral position balanced with periods of activity

    (4) Attend childbirth classes

   b. During labor

    (1) Regional anesthesia and comfort interventions

    (2) Lateral position to enhance circulation

    (3) Limitation on bearing down effort by using lateral position, episiotomy, low forceps/vacuum extractor

c. During the postpartum period, healthy recovery is the goal
  (1) Gradually increase activity from bed rest to ambulation, as tolerated; observe effect of activity on woman's vital signs, color, and stability
  (2) Employ interventions to prevent hemorrhage, infection, and constipation
  (3) Provide time for interaction with newborn, including a gradual increase in opportunities to care for newborn
  (4) Implement discharge planning that includes arrangements for help with household and infant care responsibilities, thus enhancing recovery
  (5) Evaluate effect of breast feeding; usually discouraged for women in Classes III and IV
  (6) Encourage use of birth control to space or prevent future pregnancies; sterilization may be recommended women in Classes II, III, and IV

X. Infection during pregnancy

A. **There is an increased risk for infection and the impact may be greater during pregnancy**
  1. Risks arise from suppression of the immunological system to prevent rejection of the fetus as foreign tissue and from the genitourinary (GU) adaptations to pregnancy
  2. Risk for infection and severity of resulting complications increase among women who already exhibit physical and psychosocial risk factors before pregnancy. Examples include diabetes, limited access to health care, inadequate hygienic practices, unsafe sexual practices, nutritional deficits, stressful lifestyle, use of tobacco and drugs, and previous history of infections.
  3. Impact of systemic infections
    a. Elevation of maternal core temperature—fever
      (1) Increases fetal temperature, heart rate, basal metabolic rate, and oxygen consumption
      (2) Fetal anomalies, spontaneous abortion, IUGR, prematurity, and stillbirth are possible
    b. Pneumonia may be a complication with a resultant effect on oxygenation
    c. Organisms causing the infection can cross the placenta and directly infect the fetus. Viruses are especially harmful (Table 4-2, p. 109)
      (1) First half of pregnancy—spontaneous abortion and anomalies
      (2) Second half of pregnancy—IUGR, stillbirth, preterm birth, and neonatal infection

Text continues on p. 112

TABLE 4-2   Common TORCH (Teratogenic) Infections*

Infection and Mode of Transmission	Selected Care Management, Approaches, and Considerations

Toxoplasmosis
A protozoan infection transmitted by:
  Handling raw meat, cat litter, or soil contaminated with cat feces.
  Eating raw or inadequately prepared meat or animal products.
  Eating inadequately washed vegetables that have come in contact with contaminated soil.
	Sulfadiazine, erythromycin, spiramycin are the anti-infectives of choice during pregnancy.
	Teach woman to:
	  Practice good hand washing technique.
	  Cook meat thoroughly.
	  Wash vegetables carefully.
	  Wear gloves or have someone else handle cat litter, soil, or raw meat.

Other
Hepatitis A (infectious hepatitis)
A viral infection transmitted by:
  Droplets.
  Hands contaminated with oral or fecal material while eating.
  Eating food handled by persons with contaminated hands.
	Administration of gamma globulin is recommended as a prophylactic measure after exposure.
	Adherence to asepsis and good hygiene must be strict.

Hepatitis B (serum hepatitis, HBV)
A viral infection transmitted by contact with blood or body substances containing blood, for example:
  Use of or injury by contaminated needles and syringes
  Sexual intercourse
  Handling of materials containing blood including transfusions, dressings, and drainage
  Exposure during a splash or spray of blood as may occur during birth or surgery
	Knowledge of and strict adherence to standard precautions are the major preventive interventions.
	Hepatitis B vaccine may be given to protect all persons, including those at risk for HBV such as health care workers.
	May be given to newborns and to high-risk pregnant women.
	Administration of Hepatitis B immune globulin is recommended as a prophylactic measure after exposure.
	Breast feeding is permitted.

Human Immunodeficiency Virus (HIV) A retrovirus transmitted by contact with contaminated body fluids, including blood and semen.	No known cure exists for HIV but many treatment interventions are available to prolong life and well-being.

Characteristics: **TORCH** (**T**oxoplasmosis, **O**ther, **R**ubella, **C**ytomegalovirus, **H**erpes simplex virus) is a group of infections caused by organisms that can cross the placenta or ascend through birth canal and adversely affect fetal growth and development. These infections often are characterized by vague influenza-like signs and symptoms, rashes and lesions, enlarged lymph nodes, and jaundice (hepatic involvement). In some cases the infection may go unnoticed in the pregnant woman yet have devastating effects on the fetus.

Continued

Table 4-2   Common TORCH (Teratogenic) Infections*—cont'd

Infection and Mode of Transmission	Selected Care Management, Approaches, and Considerations
HIV—cont'd Infected pregnant women can infect the fetus or newborn Transplacentally. By contact with maternal blood or body fluids during labor and birth. By ingestion of breast milk. **WARNING!** Pregnant women infected with HIV have an increased susceptibility to other dangerous infections, including other TORCH infections and reproductive tract infections.	Antiviral therapy with AZT has been found to decrease the fetal transmission rate from approximately 25% without AZT to approximately 8% with AZT. Prevention of transmission by using standard precautions is critical. Currently, testing of all pregnant women is recommended and in some states may be mandated by law, because treatment during pregnancy with AZT and performing a cesarean birth before the onset of labor and rupture of membranes have significantly decreased the transmission of HIV to the newborn.
Rubella (German or 3-day measles) Viral infection that is transmitted by droplets.	Rubella titres to determine immunity should be done before each pregnancy, with vaccine given if woman is not immune. Women must avoid getting pregnant within 3 months of receiving the rubella vaccination. Pregnant women who are not immune must be: Cautioned to avoid persons at risk for rubella, especially young children without immunity. Given rubella vaccine *after* the birth of the neonate. Cautioned to avoid pregnancy for at least 3 months after being vaccinated.

Characteristics: **TORCH** (**T**oxoplasmosis, **O**ther, **R**ubella, **C**ytomegalovirus, **H**erpes simplex virus) is a group of infections caused by organisms that can cross the placenta or ascend through birth canal and adversely affect fetal growth and development. These infections often are characterized by vague influenza-like signs and symptoms, rashes and lesions, enlarged lymph nodes, and jaundice (hepatic involvement). In some cases the infection may go unnoticed in the pregnant woman yet have devastating effects on the fetus.

TABLE 4-2   Common TORCH (Teratogenic) Infections*— cont'd

Infection and Mode of Transmission	Selected Care Management, Approaches, and Considerations
Cytomegalovirus (CMV) Viral infection transmitted by contact with contaminated saliva, respiratory secretions, urine, semen, breast milk, blood, and cervical or vaginal secretions. Most often the mother is asymptomatic but this virus produces severe fetal and neonatal effects, including hemolytic anemia, jaundice, hydrocephaly or microcephaly, pneumonitis, and mental retardation.	Strict adherence to aseptic principles, which include standard precautions, is of vital importance. Health care workers are at increased risk. No treatment currently exists.
Herpes Simplex Virus (HSV-2; genital herpes) A sexually transmitted viral infection that occurs when contact is made with contaminated genital secretions. Infected women can infect the fetus: Transplacentally, especially during a primary infection when systemic signs and symptoms occur and are most severe. By contact with active lesions and contaminated secretions during passage through the birth canal.	Pregnancy may increase the risk for and severity of infection, especially a primary infection. Risk for recurrent infections increases as pregnancy progresses (25% risk for recurrence during the last month of pregnancy). Cesarean birth is performed if prodromal symptoms or lesions are present and membranes have not ruptured. If no evidence of infection exists, vaginal birth is allowed. Acyclovir (Zovirax) is safe to use during pregnancy when the infection is active.

4. Impact of genital tract infections
   a. Origin of genital tract infections
      (1) Sexually transmitted diseases
      (2) Organisms normally present in the female genital tract, for example, Group B *Streptococcus* (GBS)
         (a) Most common cause of neonatal sepsis and meningitis in the United States
         (b) Present in the reproductive tract of as many as 20% of women and is most likely to cause problems among those women already exhibiting risk factors
         (c) IV antibiotics administered during labor to women with positive results of cultures, especially if at risk, have been found to be helpful in preventing neonatal infections
   b. Potential for direct infection of fetus as a result of
      (1) Transmission during passage through the birth canal as the fetus comes in contact with infected body substances: blood, vaginal secretions, and feces
      (2) Intrauterine infection
         (a) Infectious organisms weaken amniotic membranes and lead to premature rupture of the protective amniotic membranes
         (b) Infectious organisms can then ascend into the uterus
      (3) Transplacental transmission
   c. Labor and birth are often complicated
      (1) Preterm birth may be precipitated by premature rupture of the membranes
      (2) Cervix may be blocked by or fail to dilate adequately as a result of genital lesions and scarring
      (3) Cesarean birth is often the method of choice when culture results are positive, lesions are present, and membranes are intact

> ### ⚠ Warning!
> Birth must take place as soon as possible once membranes rupture to prevent ascent of organisms into the uterus.

      (4) Invasive procedures must be kept to a minimum
         (a) Limit number of vaginal examinations and avoid the use of internal monitoring
         (b) Cleanse newborn immediately after birth, before any invasive procedure is performed
   d. Neonatal infection, with early or late onset, can result in septicemia, CNS (meningitis), respiratory (pneumonia), and sensory (blindness and deafness) involvement, mental retardation, chronic infection, and even death
5. Treatment options are limited by the potential for adverse effects on fetal well-being

B. **Diagnosis of infections during pregnancy**
1. Specific clinical manifestations may be limited, go unnoticed, or be attributed to another cause or pregnancy changes
2. Testing, including cultures of vaginal, cervical, and rectal secretions and serum antibody titres, can determine if exposure or infection has taken place or is present
3. The presence of infection must be assessed throughout the pregnancy to determine if high-risk behaviors continue with re-exposure to infectious organisms and if treatment interventions have been effective

C. **Prevention of infection is the best and safest approach**
1. Preconception care
    a. Testing to determine exposure and immunity
    b. Immunizations
    c. Treatment without concern for fetal damage
    d. Reduction of high-risk behaviors, including unprotected sexual intercourse with multiple partners
2. Protective interventions during pregnancy
    a. Hygiene and asepsis—hand washing, genital care, precautions when handling body substances
    b. Safe food preparation (washing and cooking) and storage
    c. Avoidance of high-risk situations or use of appropriate precautions (hygiene, standard precautions, safer sex practices) from exposure to
        (1) Contaminated cat litter, soil, and meat
        (2) Persons known to be infected or at risk for infection, such as sexual partner(s) and young children especially if not immunized

D. **Treatment approaches utilized are determined by the type of infection present with consideration given to the effect of such treatment on fetal well-being**

 Warning!

Counseling and emotional support is of great importance if infection occurs and results in a strong possibility of congenital anomalies and fetal-newborn infection.

WEB Resources

http://www.noah.cuny.edu

NOAH is the New York online access to health. To access information related to high-risk pregnancy, first click on Health Topics, then on Pregnancy, and finally click on your topic of interest in the Problems and Risks section.

http://www.son.wisc.edu/~son/bedrest/index.html

This website is related to pregnancy bed rest and provides information and support for high-risk pregnant women and their families and caregivers. It is produced by Judy Maloni, PhD, RN, FAAN who is noted for her contributions to pregnancy bed rest research.

http://www.sidelines.org

Sidelines National Support Network for women experiencing high-risk pregnancies.

http://www.pc101186.med.cornell.edu

This is the website of the Hypertension Center of the New York Presbyterian Hospital Joan and Sanford Weill Medical College of Cornell University. Click on the Hypertension in Pregnancy section for information and resources related to pregnancy-induced hypertension.

http://www.diabetes.org

American Diabetes Association. Using the "search our site" tool, type in pregnancy, gestational diabetes, or pre-gestational diabetes to access information related to the care management of pregnant women diagnosed with diabetes.

REVIEW QUESTIONS

1. Which of these actions would be least effective in the reduction of the stress associated with a high-risk pregnancy?
   1. Educate the woman and her family about the health problems that complicate the pregnancy and the components of the treatment plan
   2. Encourage participation of both the woman and her family in the plan of care
   3. Arrange for home care if possible
   4. If hospitalization is required, reduce the number of visiting hours to facilitate rest and relaxation

2. Signs of a threatened abortion are noted in a woman at 8 weeks' gestation. Which of these actions is an appropriate management approach for this type of abortion?
   1. Prepare woman for a dilation and curettage
   2. Explain the need for bedrest of at least 1 week and re-evaluate
   3. Prepare woman for a sonogram to determine the integrity of the gestational sac
   4. Comfort the woman by telling her that if she loses this baby she can try to get pregnant again in about 1 month

3. A woman has been diagnosed in the emergency room with a ruptured ectopic pregnancy. She is crying about the sudden change in her pregnancy status and states that she is in a great deal of pain. Which would be the primary nursing diagnosis at this time?
   1. Risk for infection
   2. Fluid volume deficit
   3. Pain
   4. Anticipatory grief

4. During the assessment of a pregnant woman, the nurse must be alert for risk factors associated with pregnancy induced hypertension (PIH). A risk factor for PIH would be which of these findings?
   1. Status as a multigravida
   2. Age between 25 and 32 years
   3. Diabetes mellitus
   4. Dietary deficiency of iron and magnesium

5. To prevent infection by the Hepatitis B virus for herself and her fetus, the pregnant woman should do which of these actions?
   1. Receive gamma globulin during the first trimester
   2. Carefully wash hands before eating or preparing food
   3. Receive the Hepatitis B vaccine
   4. Take Zidovudine (AZT) during the second and third trimester

ANSWERS, RATIONALES, AND TEST-TAKING TIPS

Rationale	Test-Taking Tips

1. Correct answer: 4

Women with a high-risk pregnancy often need the diversion and support that visitors can offer. Therefore, visiting hours should be individualized to meet the needs of the high-risk pregnant woman.

Avoid overlooking the obvious clue: *least* effective action. To ensure your clarity of thought reread the question one last time with the option that you have selected.

2. Correct answer: 3

A HCG level along with the sonogram are used to determine the status of the gestational sac. Dilation and curettage are not considered until the signs progress to an inevitable abortion or the expulsion of the uterine contents is incomplete. Bedrest is recommended for 48 hours initially. Telling a woman she can get pregnant again soon is not a therapeutic response because to do so discounts the importance of this pregnancy. If the pregnancy is lost, she must be helped through the grieving process.

Use the nursing process as the guide for the best action. The client has a problem that threatens the pregnancy. Because it has not yet affected the pregnancy, further assessment of the situation is required based on the information given in the stem. When further assessment is required the best timeframe to use as a guide is 48 to 72 hours, then re-evaluate the situation. This can be a general rule applied to many situations.

3. Correct answer: 2

While options 1, 3, and 4, are appropriate nursing diagnoses, fluid volume deficit takes the highest priority. In this situation with the rupture of the tube excessive bleeding occurs into the abdominal cavity. Immediate action must be take to prevent hemorrhage and shock.

The result of rupture of an internal part—intestine, appendix, or ectopic pregnancy—is physiologic crisis in the form of shock. Therefore, with the use of Maslow's hierarchy, stabilization of circulation takes precedence over pain relief or emotional needs.

4. Correct answer: 3

Diabetes presents a risk from the vascular changes associated with it. PIH is more common with

If you have no idea of a correct answer, focus on what you know and go with it. Of the given

first exposure to chorionic villi (primigravida) or increased amount of chorionic villi as with multiple gestations. The age of risk is under 20 or over 35 years. Protein and calcium deficiencies have been associated with PIH, not iron and magnesium.

options, diabetes mellitus is definitely associated with hypertension across the life span; the other options may or may not be. Select diabetes, which mainly effects the blood vessels and in return effects multiple systems—eyes, kidneys, and heart.

5. Correct answer: 3

Hepatitis B is a bloodborne infection. Hepatitis B vaccine is safe to use in pregnancy, especially if the woman is at high risk. Options 1 and 2 are actions for hepatitis A. AZT is used to reduce the risk for fetal transmission of HIV if the mother is infected with HIV.

If you have no idea of a correct answer, simply match the focus in the stem, hepatitis B, to an option that has the same focus, option 3. Only use this approach if you have no idea of what the answer is.

5

Nursing Process Applications and the Process of Labor and Birth

FAST FACTS

1. Labor *(parturition)* usually begins between 38 to 42 weeks' gestation.
2. Multiple factors are responsible for the onset of labor: limited uterine stretch, change in the estrogen-progesterone ratio, increase in prostaglandin activity, and fetal maturation.
3. Uterine stretch is limited and results in increased irritability, with contents expelled once capacity is reached.
4. The estrogen-progesterone ratio changes. Estrogen becomes more dominant to enhance uterine contractility by increasing oxytocin receptors. The uterus is more sensitive to oxytocin and prostaglandin, increasing myometrial contractility.
5. Prostaglandin activity increases and enhances **cervical ripening,** which is the softening and thinning of the cervix in preparation for labor. False labor contractions may enhance cervical ripening. Passage of the cervical mucous plug (operculum) accompanies cervical ripening.
6. Fetal maturation plays a role to increase prostaglandin activity and to produce substances that contribute to uterine contractility.
7. **Premonitory signs of labor** signal the approach of the parturition and appear in varying degrees from several days to weeks before labor begins.
8. The premonitory signs of labor are (a) lightening; (b) a 1- to 3-lb weight loss from reduction in fluid retention; (c) an energy burst; (d) false labor

contractions, and (e) a bloody, pink show from the passage of the cervical mucous plug *(operculum)*.

9. False labor contractions (exaggeration of Braxton Hicks contractions) are irregular and not progressive in terms of intensity, frequency, and duration and can be relieved by activity such as ambulation or a change in position. These contractions are strong and uncomfortable for the woman.

10. There are four stages of childbirth. In the first, the cervix effaces and dilates in preparation for passage of the fetus. In the second, the fetus descends through the birth canal and is born. In the third, the placenta separates and is expelled. In the fourth, the first 1 to 2 hours after birth, the mother recovers and stabilizes.

11. The five Ps of labor are the powers, passenger, passage, position of the mother, and psychological (emotional) status of the mother.

12. **Powers of Labor** (the five Ps) are the forces that facilitate cervical changes and fetal descent and birth.

13. The primary powers are the uterine contractions. The secondary powers are the contractions of the abdominal muscles.

14. The nursing process is used to manage the care of the laboring woman: use a holistic approach to assess the physical and psychosocial responses to childbirth, and use a variety of sources to facilitate data collection, including prenatal records, laboring woman, coach, and family members.

15. Prioritize data collection by evaluating the laboring woman's condition and the phase of labor: use an organized approach to admit the laboring woman, and assess maternal-fetal unit with increasing frequency as the labor progresses because vulnerability to complications becomes greater (see Box 5-1, p. 133).

16. A nursing approach that projects calmness, confidence, and concern enhances the laboring woman's confidence in the nursing care she is receiving and facilitates the ability of her coach to provide support and guidance in childbirth techniques.

17. Documentation is a critical nursing responsibility. All data collected, nursing actions taken as a result of data analysis, and the results must be fully and accurately documented.

CONTENT REVIEW

I. Primary power is uterine contractions

A. Regular, progressive uterine contractions that signal the onset of true labor (Figure 5-1)

B. Characteristics of uterine contractions
1. Four phases
   a. Increment—pacemaker cells near the tubes are activated; contraction begins in the fundus and radiates over the body of the uterus
   b. Acme—maximum intensity of the contraction
   c. Decrement—gradual decrease in uterine activity

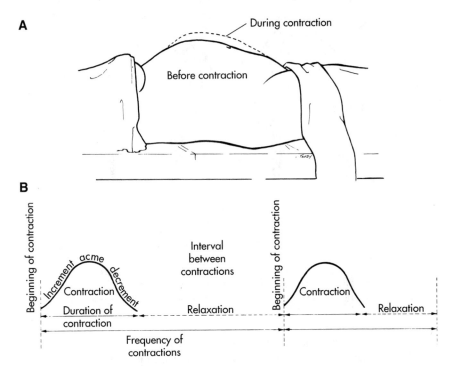

Figure 5-1 Assessment of uterine contractions. **A,** Abdominal contour before and during uterine contraction. **B,** Wavelike pattern of contractile activity. (From Lowdermilk DL, Perry SE, Bobak IM: *Maternity and women's health care,* ed 7, St. Louis, 2000, Mosby.)

    d. Rest—reduction in uterine tone between contractions; essential for restoration of blood flow through the uterus and placenta

  2. Fundal dominance: contractions begin, are most intense, and end in the fundus

  3. Progressive nature: frequency, intensity, and duration increase as a result of a positive feedback cycle

    a. During a contraction, fundal force pushes the fetus downward against the cervix; cervical impulses are sent to pituitary gland; oxytocin is secreted; and an increase in the intensity and the duration of the next contraction occurs

    b. This cycle is enhanced by an upright maternal position and activity as a result of gravity

  4. Discomfort: begins in the lower abdomen and back, then radiates over the entire abdomen; increases as contractions progress

C. Effects of uterine contractions

  1. Division of the uterus into two segments (Figure 5-2)

    a. Fundus—the upper, thickening, contracting portion of the uterus provides force to push the fetus downward

    b. Lower uterine segment—thinner, relaxed portion expands to allow fetal descent

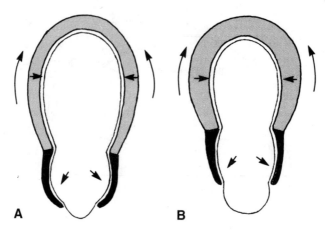

Figure 5-2   Lower uterine segment and cervix are pulled up (retracted) as the fetus and amniotic sac are pushed downward by the force of the fundus. **A,** Lower uterine segment is thinned and the cervix is effaced and partially dilated. **B,** Cervical dilation is complete. Cervix is being pulled upward as presenting part descends. Intrauterine space is decreasing. (From Wilson JR, Carrington ER: *Obstetrics and gynecology,* ed 8, St. Louis, 1988, Mosby.)

2. **Effacement:** thinning and shortening of the cervical canal as the lower uterine segment is pulled upward by uterine contractions and the descending fetus (see Fig. 5-2)
   a. Progress is expressed as a percent—25% effaced, 50% effaced, 75% effaced, 100% effaced
   b. Primigravida—effaces before dilation
   c. Multipara—effaces and dilates simultaneously
3. **Dilation:** widening of the cervix from less than 1 to 10 cm as a result of the upward pull from the fundus and the downward pressure of fetus during uterine contractions (see Fig. 5-2)
   a. Amniotic membranes and fluid (bag of waters) act as a dilating wedge before rupture of the membranes
   b. Fetal presenting part acts as a dilator after the membranes rupture; fetal head is a more effective dilator than the fetal buttocks or bag of waters
   c. Pattern of dilation
      (1) The progress of dilation is influenced by parity, for example, nullipara dilates more slowly than the multipara
      (2) The rate of dilation is influenced by the efficiency and progress of contractions, and maternal activity and position (Table 5-1, p. 124)
4. Progress of fetal descent
   a. Station—measurement of descent in centimeters above or below the pelvic ischial spines
   b. Rate of descent—influenced by parity, maternal activity and position, effectiveness of uterine contractions, and bearing down efforts (BDEs)

5. Rupture of membranes can occur spontaneously (spontaneous rupture of membranes, SRM) or can be induced by the use of an Amnihook or other sharp instrument guided through the cervix to the membranes (**amniotomy** or artificial rupture of membranes, AROM)
    a. SRM usually occurs at the acme of an intense contraction during the active or transition phase of the first stage of labor or it may occur before the onset of labor
        (1) Premature rupture of the membranes (PROM) occurs at term; labor usually begins within 12 to 24 hours
        (2) Preterm premature rupture of the membranes (PPROM) occurs before 38 weeks' gestation
    b. The expected outcome of AROM is the stimulation of uterine contractions to enhance the progress of labor
    c. Rupture of membranes increases the risk for
        (1) Prolapse of the cord with compression; gush of fluid carries the cord past the presenting part
        (2) Risk of intrauterine infection increases as amount of time between rupture and birth lengthens
6. Diminished uteroplacental blood flow during contractions: limits the exchange of oxygen and carbon dioxide between the mother and the fetus
7. Separation and expulsion of placenta: contractions decrease uterine size to squeeze the placenta off the implantation site. The placenta is pushed and lifted out.
8. Prevention of postpartum hemorrhage: contracted uterus constricts to seal off blood vessels at the implantation site

II. Secondary power is abdominal muscle contractions

A. **Pushing or bearing down effects (BDEs) involve the contraction of the abdominal muscles to increase intraabdominal pressure. Abdominal muscle contractions are combined with uterine contractions to enhance fetal descent and birth.**

B. **Begin during the second stage of labor when the cervix is fully dilated and effaced and the urge to bear down (Ferguson reflex) is experienced**

III. *Passage* is composed of the bony pelvis and soft tissues of lower uterine segment, cervix, vagina, and muscles of the pelvic floor

A. **Bony pelvis: the shape, type, and size play a critical role in the ability of the fetal skull and shoulders to pass through the birth canal**

1. Gynecoid, female pelvis: the rounded shape with adequate diameters accommodates the fetal skull and shoulders. This is the most common and most favorable pelvic type for a vaginal birth

Text continued on p. 128

TABLE 5-1	The Process of Labor and Birth		

Stages and Duration of Labor	Expected Events	Assessment
First Stage Focus: cervical effacement and dilation Powers: uterine contractions		
1. Latent Phase Average of 6-8 hr Nullipara: maximum of 20 hr Multipara: maximum of 14 hr	Effacement: progressing Cervical dilation: 0-3 cm Uterine contractions: Intensity: mild to moderate Irregular Frequency: every 5-30 min Duration : 30-50 sec Show: brownish discharge progressing to pinkish mucous; scant Descent: station 0 Mood, behavior: excited, anxious, alert, follows directions	FHR: every 30-60 min Maternal vital signs: Pulse, BP, respirations: every 30-60 min Temperature: every 4 hr until membranes rupture, then every 2 hr Uterine contractions: every 30-60 min Vaginal show: every 30-60 min
2. Active Phase Average of 3-6 hours	Effacement: progressing Cervical dilation: 4-7 cm Uterine contractions: Intensity: moderate to strong Regular Frequency: every 3-5 min Duration: 40-70 sec Show: pink to bloody mucous; scant to moderate Station: +1 to +2 Mood, behavior: serious, increased anxiety, introspective, tired, some difficulty in following directions	FHR: every 15-30 min Maternal vital signs: Pulse, BP, respirations: every 30-60 min Temperature: every 4 hr until membranes rupture, then every 2 hr Uterine contractions: every 15-30 min Vaginal show: every 30 min

3. Transition Phase
   Average of 20-40 min
   Nullipara: maximum of 3 hr
   Multipara: maximum of 1 hr

Effacement: to 100%
Cervical dilation: 8-10 cm
Uterine contractions:
   Intensity: strong
   Some irregularity may occur
   Frequency: every 2-3 min
   Duration: 45-90 sec
Fetal descent: accelerates to
   Nullipara: 1 cm/hr
   Multipara: 2 cm/hr
Show: bloody mucous: copious
Rupture of membranes usually occurs
Station: +2 to +3
Mood, behavior: frustrated, loss of control, irritable, nausea and vomiting, hyperventilation, great difficulty following directions

FHR: every 15-30 min
Maternal vital signs:
   Pulse, BP, respirations: every 15-30 min
   Temperature: every 4 hr until membranes rupture, then every 2 hr
Uterine contractions every 10-15 min
Vaginal show: every 15 minutes

Second Stage

Focus: fetal descent and birth
Powers: uterine contractions coupled with abdominal muscle contractions
Average of 15-60 min
Nullipara: maximum of 2 hr
Multipara: maximum of 1.5 hr

1. Early, Latent: First Phase
   Average of 10-30 min

Progressive descent of fetus along with the cardinal movements of labor
Rate of descent
   Nullipara: 1 cm/hr
   Multipara: 2 cm/hr

Transient decrease in intensity and frequency of contractions
Time to rest and conserve energy until the urge to push is felt
Urge to push: slight to absent
Mood, behavior: relief, sleepy, resumes control

FHR: every 5-15 min
Maternal vital signs: pulse, BP, respirations: every 5-30 min
Uterine contractions: assess every contraction
BDE: assess each effort
Vaginal show: every 15 minutes

*Frequency of assessment is determined by the risk status of the maternal-fetal unit. More frequent assessment is required in high-risk situations (i.e., if the range is every 30-60 min, then frequency for the high-risk maternal-fetal unit would be every 30 min). The frequency of assessment and method of documentation also are determined by agency policies, which usually are based on the recommended standards of medical and nursing organizations. Always check the protocols of your agency.   *Continued*

TABLE 5-1   The Process of Labor and Birth—cont'd

Stages and Duration of Labor	Expected Events	Assessment
Second Stage—cont'd		

2. Active, Descent: Second Phase
Average duration varies according to:
Parity
Efficiency of BDE
Use of spinal or epidural anesthesia
Maternal level of energy
Fetal size
	Ferguson reflex is noted: rhythmic urge to bear down stimulated by fetal pressure against pelvic floor
	Active BDEs begin
	Uterine contractions:
	  Intensity: increasing
	  Frequency: every 2 to 2.5 min
	  Duration: 90 sec
	Show: dark red, bloody mucous, increased amount
	Perineal bulging
	Crowning, burning sensation	

3. Transition, Perineal: Third Phase
 	
Average of 5-15 min
	Birth
	Uterine contractions:
	  Frequency: every 1-2 min
	  Duration: 90 seconds
	Mood, behavior: overwhelmed with effort to give birth, powerlessness, excited after birth of head
	Use of interventions to facilitate birth
	  Episiotomy
	  Forceps-assisted or vacuum-assisted	

Third Stage

Focus: placental separation and expulsion

Powers: uterine contractions and abdominal muscle contractions

Average of 15-30 min

Signs of placental separation:
Bleeding: gush or trickle
Fundal elevation to umbilicus
Fundal shape: globular
Cord advances, ceases pulsation

Placental expulsion:
Separated placenta falls into lower uterine segment
Gentle pushing facilities expulsion
Placenta is lifted out
Episiotomy repair

Maternal vital signs: pulse, BP, respirations: every 15 min

Uterine contractions: palpate fundus to:
Determine changes that indicate separation
Ensure fundus remains firm to prevent hemorrhage; massage if bogginess (uterine atony) is noted

Placental assessment:
Completeness: fragments left in uterus could lead to hemorrhage and infection
Condition: size, weight, presence of ischemic areas and signs of infection

Fourth Stage

Focus: physiologic stabilization of the woman after birth, and bonding of the family with the newborn

WARNING! Major concern of this stage is the prevention of hemorrhage and hypovolemic shock.

Average of 1 to 2 hr; continues if vital signs do not stabilize and if bleeding is profuse

Vital signs: stabilized
Fundus: remains firm
Bleeding: moderate
Mood, behavior: excited and eager to celebrate birth of baby; exhausted with limited interest in newborn other than to validate its health status

Maternal vital signs:
Pulse, BP, respirations: every 15 min first hour, and every 30 min second hour
Temperature: once or twice
Postpartal check every 15 min, then every 30 min just as for vital signs:
Fundus
Lochia
Perineum: episiotomy, lacerations
Bladder for fullness
Lower extremities: return of sensation and movement after an epidural or spinal block anesthesia

*Frequency of assessment is determined by the risk status of the maternal-fetal unit. More frequent assessment is required in high-risk situations (i.e., if the range is every 30-60 min, then frequency for the high-risk maternal-fetal unit would be every 30 min). The frequency of assessment and method of documentation also are determined by agency policies, which usually are based on the recommended standards of medical and nursing organizations. Always check the protocols of your agency.

2. Diameters are measured in first or third trimester by manual or ultrasound techniques
   a. Inlet—upper border of true pelvis
      (1) Anteroposterior diameter at least 11 cm
      (2) Transverse diameter at least 13 cm
   b. Midplane—curved pelvic cavity
      (1) Anteroposterior diameter at least 11.5 cm
      (2) Transverse diameter between the ischial spines at least 10.5 cm
   c. Outlet—lower border of true pelvis
      (1) Anteroposterior diameter at least 11.9 cm from the lower border of the symphysis pubis to the tip of sacrum; the coccyx can be pushed backward to increase available space
      (2) Transverse diameter between ischial tuberosities is at least 8 cm
3. Enhancement factors facilitate pelvic accommodation to the fetus
   a. Relaxin—corpus luteal hormone that facilitates slight expansion and mobility of pelvic joints
   b. Maternal position—squatting or sitting slightly increases the pelvic diameters

B. Soft tissues
1. Tissues of the lower uterine segment, cervix, and vagina soften and become more stretchable
2. Cervix effaces and dilates during the first stage of labor
3. Pelvic floor muscles guide the fetus during its descent through the passage

IV. The *Passenger* (fetus) descends through the passage. The descent is influenced by seven factors.

A. Size of the fetal skull
1. Diameters: average size at term is indicated
   a. Biparietal diameter—largest (widest) transverse diameter of the skull, an average of 9.25 cm
   b. Anteroposterior diameter—determined by the degree of extension or flexion of the fetal head
      (1) Suboccipitobregmatic—smallest diameter is presented when the head is fully flexed; an average of 9.5 cm (vertex presentation)
      (2) Occipitomental—presented when the head is in full extension; an average of 13.5 cm (face presentation)
2. Molding: skull bones can overlap slightly to allow the fetal skull to adjust to the diameters of the maternal pelvis
B. Fetal lie: relationship of fetal spine to maternal spine (Figure 5-3)
1. Longitudinal-vertical lie: fetal spine and maternal spine are parallel; cephalic and breech presentations

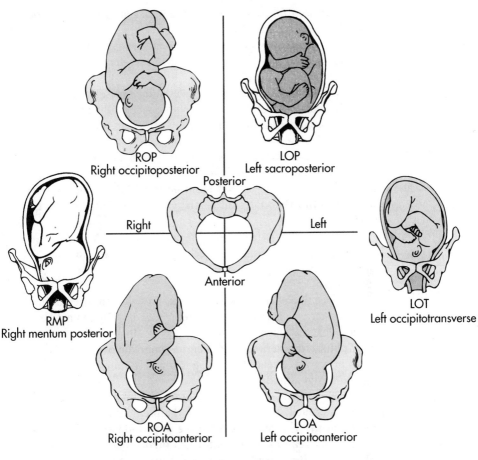

ROP
Right occipitoposterior

LOP
Left sacroposterior

Posterior

Right

Left

Anterior

LOT
Left occipitotransverse

RMP
Right mentum posterior

ROA
Right occipitoanterior

LOA
Left occipitoanterior

Lie: Longitudinal or vertical
Presentation: Vertex, breech, face
Reference point: Occiput, mentum, sacrum
Attitude: Complete flexion, extension

Figure 5-3 Examples of fetal presentations and positions in relation to front, back, and side of the maternal pelvis. (From Lowdermilk DL, Perry SE, Bobak IM: *Maternity and women's health care,* ed 7, St. Louis, 2000, Mosby.)

2. Transverse-horizontal lie: fetal spine and maternal spine are perpendicular (at right angles); seen with shoulder presentation

C. **Fetal attitude: relationship of the fetal parts to one another** (see Fig. 5-3)
   1. General flexion: fetus accommodates to uterine size and shape by assuming a flexed oval shape
   2. Extension: fetal extension of the head inhibits descent and may result in the need for cesarean birth

D. *Fetal presentation (presenting part):* **the fetal part that enters the pelvic inlet first** (see Fig. 5-3)
1. Cephalic: head enters first; most common
    a. Vertex—head is fully flexed, and the area over the parietal bones presents first
    b. Face—head is fully extended, and the face presents first
2. Breech: buttocks, foot, or feet enter first; more difficult vaginal birth because the head is delivered last, allowing less time to accommodate to the pelvis
3. Shoulder: shoulder enters first; vaginal birth is impossible because the fetus is in a transverse lie

E. *Fetal position:* **location of a set point on the fetal presenting part in a quadrant of the maternal pelvis; changes as fetus descends** (see Fig. 5-3)
1. The set points are for the vertex (occiput—O), for the face (mentum, chin—M), for the breech (sacrum—S), and for the shoulder (scapula—Sc)
2. Examples
    a. Left occipitoanterior (LOA)—vertex presentation, occiput in left anterior quadrant of the maternal pelvis, longitudinal lie, and flexed attitude
    b. Right sacroposterior (RSP)—breech presentation, sacrum in right posterior quadrant of maternal pelvis, longitudinal lie, and flexed attitude

F. *Cardinal Movements of Labor* **(mechanism of labor): the powers of labor combined with resistance of the birth canal and changes in maternal pelvis diameters force the fetus to change the position of its head as it moves toward birth; movements occur concurrently with a gradual downward progress** (Figure 5-4)
1. Engagement: fetal biparietal diameter passes through pelvic inlet and reaches the level of the ischial spines (zero station)
2. Descent: fetus moves downward as a result of pressure from the powers of labor and stretching of the lower uterine segment, cervix, and vagina; progress designated in terms of station, for example -1, 0, $+1$, $+2$, and so on
3. Flexion: fetal head flexes to allow the smallest anteroposterior diameter to pass through the pelvis
4. Internal rotation: fetal head turns to allow the biparietal diameter to pass between the ischial spines
5. Extension: fetal head extends upward when it reaches the perineum; occiput pivots beneath the symphysis pubis
6. External rotation, restitution: fetal head turns, realigning with shoulders, on emerging from the pelvis; shoulders move through pelvis and are delivered from under the symphysis pubis (anterior) and then from over the perineum (posterior)

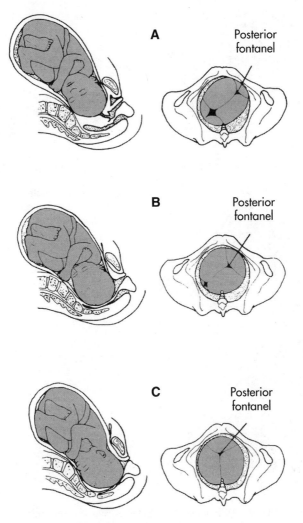

Figure 5-4   Mechanism of labor in left occipitoanterior (LOA) presentation. **A,** Engagement and descent. **B,** Flexion. **C,** Internal rotation to OA. (From Lowdermilk DL, Perry SE, Bobak IM: *Maternity and women's health care,* ed 7, St. Louis, 2000, Mosby.)   *Continued*

       7. Expulsion: delivery of the fetal trunk follows the birth of its head and shoulders

  G. **Operative interventions to facilitate birth**

       1. **Episiotomy:** perineal incision performed to enlarge the vaginal outlet; controversy exits about the routine use of an episiotomy

       2. Instruments

          a. Forceps-assisted birth: metal instruments applied around the fetal skull

          b. Vacuum-assisted birth: suction cup is attached to the fetal skull at the occiput

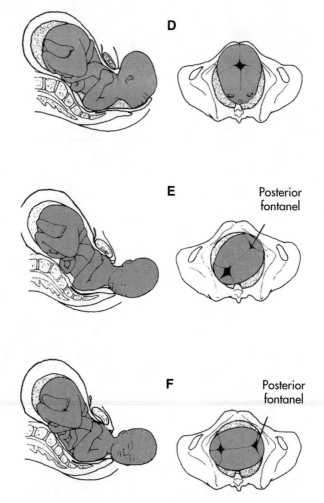

Figure 5-4, cont'd   D, Extension. E, External rotation (restitution). F, External rotation (shoulder rotation). (From Lowdermilk DL, Perry SE, Bobak IM: *Maternity and women's health care,* ed 7, St. Louis, 2000, Mosby.)

    c. Instruments facilitate birth
       (1) By assisting in the internal rotation and descent, especially when immediate birth is required in the presence of maternal or fetal distress
       (2) By augmenting ineffective maternal pushing efforts as a result of regional anesthesia, fatigue, and cardiovascular disorders

V. Assessment of the laboring woman: Health history
(Box 5-1, Table 5-1 pp. 124-127)
   A. **Current labor events**
       1. Onset
       2. Show, passage of mucous plug

Box 5-1
Critical Data for the Admission of the Laboring Woman

Questions to Ask

When did your labor begin?
How have your contractions been progressing? How frequently do they occur? How
  long do they last? How strong are they?
Has your water broken? When did it happen? What did the fluid look like?
Have you had any discharge from your vagina? When? What is it like? How much is
  there?
Have you noticed any change in your baby's movements recently?
When was the last time you ate or drank? What did you eat or drink?
How many times have you been pregnant? What was the result of each pregnancy?
What is your birth plan? Do you have a coach or someone with you?
What type of health care did you have during your pregnancy?
Did you have any health problems during pregnancy? Do you have any now?
Is there anything else you think I should know?

Assessment Techniques

Inspect external genitalia and perform vaginal examination to determine the following:
  Presence of lesions and signs of reproductive tract infections
  Presence of vaginal show or bleeding; if no active bleeding, continue with the
    vaginal examination
  Cervical changes: consistency, effacement, dilation, and position
Fetal presentation, position, and station
Condition of membranes; if ruptured, test fluid (**nitrazine test,** ferning) and assess
  characteristics
Perform maternal vital signs: pulse, BP, respirations, and respiratory effort, chest
  sounds, and temperature
Attach external electronic fetal monitor to determine:
  Pattern of uterine contractions
  FHR pattern
Obtain specimens of blood and urine for laboratory testing, as required
Determine the overall emotional status of the laboring woman, her coach, and her
  family

     3. Rupture of membranes—when, characteristics of fluid
     4. Uterine contractions—intensity, frequency, and duration
     5. FMs—changes in character
     6. Time and nature of most recent meal or oral intake
  **B. Birth plan: consider cultural implications and whether plan is
     realistic**
     1. Childbirth techniques to be used, for example, the Lamaze
       method (Box 5-2, p. 134)
     2. Anticipated support-group participation in the process of labor:
       coach, doula, persons to be present at the birth
     3. Expectations about parturition events
       a. Analgesia and anesthesia
       b. Comfort interventions and nonpharmacologic interventions to
         enhance progress

Box 5-2
Prepared Childbirth

Prepared childbirth techniques are taught at the beginning of the third trimester when motivation is highest and repeated practice of techniques and exercises is possible

Purpose
Provides information to reduce fear of the unknown
Teaches childbirth techniques, thus
  Reducing stress and tension
  Conserving energy and enhancing rest
  Reducing the perception of pain
  Decreasing the need for pharmacologic pain relief interventions in terms of type, amount, and frequency
  Creates a satisfying childbirth experience that enhances cooperation among the laboring woman, her coach, family, and health care providers

Relaxation Exercises
Consciously relaxing tense body parts as directed by touch of a coach
Rhythmic breathing
Guided imagery: use of mental pictures to perceive:
  Events of labor, such as the cervix opening or contractions pushing the fetus downward
  Pleasant places or experiences that are special and relaxing to the laboring woman

Pain Management Techniques
Reduce the perception of pain through the use of increasingly complex distracting activities:
  Breathing techniques: deliberate, conscious breathing methods that require concentration; techniques become more rapid, shallow, and complex as labor progresses
  Focal point: focusing on a favorite picture or object to enhance concentration while performing breathing techniques
  Effleurage: rhythmic stroking of the abdomen by the woman—or coach—while she is performing breathing techniques and focusing on a focal point

    c. Role of the nurse; use of a *doula,* a supportive female labor attendant
    d. Monitoring: external, internal, none at all
    e. Invasive techniques such as IVs and episiotomy
    f. Position for birth and where the birth will take place
  C. Prenatal history
    1. Current pregnancy
      a. Prenatal care received or no care rendered
      b. Effectiveness of physical and psychosocial adaptations to pregnancy with baseline health status information
      c. Difficulties encountered during pregnancy
      d. Expected date of birth (EDB); number of weeks' gestation
      e. Results of laboratory and diagnostic testing performed during pregnancy
      f. Childbirth classes attended or not attended

2. Previous experiences with pregnancy and parturition including outcomes, complications encountered, and interventions required
3. Presence of current risk factors such as diabetes, anemia, cardiovascular disorders, hypertension, reproductive tract infections, PIH, and limited or nonexistent support group

VI. Physical assessment of changes that occur during parturition

A. **Uterine contractions**
1. Characteristics (see Figure 5-1, p. 121)
   a. Frequency—timing from the onset of one contraction to the onset of the next indicates how often the contractions are occurring
   b. Duration—timing from the onset of the contraction until it ends indicates how long the contraction lasts
   c. Intensity—determine the strength of the contraction
   d. Resting tone—determine the degree of fundal relaxation during the rest phase between contractions and the duration of the rest period
2. Assessment techniques
   a. Assess a series of several contractions and rest periods to the determine an overall pattern
   b. Frequency of assessment is determined by stage of labor, condition of maternal-fetal unit, and labor events (see Table 5-1, pp. 124-127)
   c. Palpation method—place hand over fundus and use fingers to assess:
      (1) Intensity by assessing changes in tone: degree fingers can be indented into fundus; for example, a boardlike fundus with no indentation reflects a strong intensity
      (2) Frequency and duration
      (3) Occasionally palpate entire uterus to note differences in tone from fundus to lower uterine segment
   d. Electronic assessment using a tocotransducer (external method) or intratuterine pressure catheter (internal method)
3. Expected findings
   a. Gradual progression in frequency, duration, and intensity
   b. Regular pattern established but may become irregular during the transition phase
   c. Average frequency of every 2 to 5 minutes; rarely more frequently than every 2 minutes because adequate rest periods will not occur
   d. Duration of no longer than 90 seconds
   e. Rest periods of at least 30 seconds
   f. Intensity
      (1) During a contraction, less than 100 mm Hg
      (2) During rest, resting pressure of 15 mm Hg or less

4. Warning signs
   a. Failure to progress or establish a regular pattern
   b. Contractions are more frequent than every 2 minutes
   c. A duration of more than 90 seconds
   d. Limited or no relaxation of the fundus palpated during the rest period
   e. Rest periods of less than 30 seconds
   f. Intensity during a contraction of over 100 mm Hg; resting pressure of over 15 mm Hg

B. Cervical changes and fetal progress through the birth canal
   1. Vaginal examination assessment
      a. Signs of reproductive tract infections
      b. Cervical characteristics
         (1) Soft or firm consistency
         (2) Degree of effacement and dilation
         (3) Posterior, midline, anterior position
      c. Condition of amniotic membranes—intact, bulging, or ruptured
      d. Fetal characteristics—presentation, position, station, and molding
   2. Vaginal examination technique (see Figure 5-5)
      a. Explain procedure and results
      b. Follow strict asepsis to prevent infection
         (1) Cleanse vulva and perineum before and after the examination as needed; wear clean gloves for cleansing
         (2) Use sterile gloves and water-based lubricant to perform the examination
      c. Note maternal and fetal responses during and after the examination
   3. Frequency: perform examination only as needed to reduce danger of infection and limit maternal discomfort
      a. On admission
      b. After the rupture of membranes once the fetal condition is assessed
      c. Before administration of an analgesic or anesthetic to determine degree of dilation and progress of labor

A   B

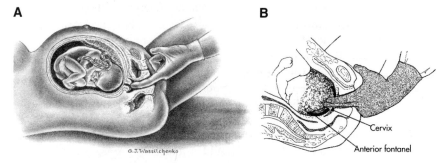

Figure 5-5 Vaginal examination. **A,** Undilated, uneffaced cervix. Membranes are intact. **B,** Palpation of the sagittal suture line. Cervix is effaced and partially dilated. (From Lowdermilk DL, Perry SE, Bobak IM: *Maternity and women's health care,* ed 7, St. Louis, 2000, Mosby.)

d. The presence of fetal heart rate (FHR) pattern indicative of distress, for example, variable deceleration or to check for cord prolapse

e. When the contraction pattern and maternal behavior indicate progress in labor has been made, for example, increased frequency and intensity of contractions, perineal pressure, and urge to bear down

⚠ Warning!

Vaginal examinations are not performed when frank bleeding is present. The bleeding may be the result of a **placenta previa.** Notify the physician and prepare for the possibility of an immediate birth.

4. Partogram is a labor graph used to compare a woman's progression in relation to dilation and fetal descent with the expected pattern for a nulliparous or multiparous woman
   a. Data gathered during vaginal examinations about dilation and descent—superimposed on an appropriate graph (Figure 5-6, p. 158)
   b. Expected finding—progress reflects norms for nulliparous or multiparous woman
   c. Warning signs—progress deviates from the expected norm
      (1) Prolonged latent phase
      (2) Protracted or arrested active phase: dilation and descent
      (3) Precipitous labor
5. Condition of amniotic membranes
   a. Determine status (intact, bulging, or ruptured)—by performing
      (1) Vaginal examination
      (2) Nitrazine test to distinguish between urine and amniotic fluid by using test paper to determine the pH of the fluid expelled
         (a) Dark blue, positive: alkaline result indicates amniotic fluid
         (b) Remains yellow, negative: acidic result indicates urine
      (3) *Ferning* check: smear fluid onto a glass slide and use microscope to detect presence of amniotic fluid crystallization, which results in a characteristic fernlike pattern
   b. Determine the time of occurrence—birth should take place within 24 hours of rupture to reduce the risk of exposure of the fetus and uterine cavity to infection
   c. Determine the characteristics of the amniotic fluid expelled—amount, color, clarity, consistency (thick or thin), odor
      (1) Expected findings—clear, slightly yellow, resembling very dilute urine and a faint fleshy, musty odor

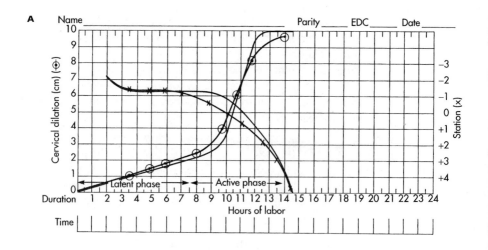

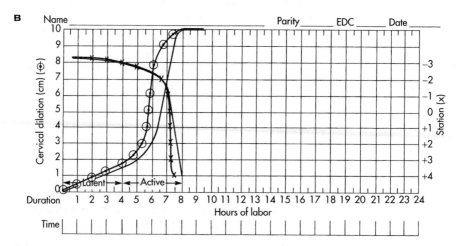

Figure 5-6   Partogram for assessment of patterns of cervical dilation and descent. Individual woman's labor patterns (marked lines) are superimposed on prepared labor graph (smooth lines) for comparison. **A,** Nulliparous labor. **B,** Multiparous labor. (From Lowdermilk DL, Perry SE, Bobak IM: *Maternity and Women's Health Care,* ed 7, St. Louis, 2000, Mosby.)

      (2) Warning signs
         i. Thick and cloudy with a foul odor indicates infection
        ii. Thick and green indicates recent passage of meconium by the fetus from recent hypoxia or a breech presentation
       iii. Yellow indicates bilirubin or hypoxia over 36 hours ago
       iv. Wine color indicates bleeding
    d. Nursing actions for rupture of membranes
      (1) Assess FHR pattern: immediately and 5 minutes later; FHR pattern should continue to exhibit reassuring characteristics

(2) Perform vaginal examination after assessment of fetal status to determine the presence of cord prolapse and the progress in effacement, dilation, and descent

(3) Assess characteristics of the fluid

(4) Monitor maternal temperature orally every 2 hours between contractions; increased danger of infection exists after membranes rupture

(5) Provide comfort interventions by keeping the woman clean and dry with reassurance about her condition and that of her fetus

C. **Characteristics of vaginal discharge** *(show)* (see Table 5-1, pp. 124-127)

1. Expected findings
   a. Pink to blood-tinged, sticky, mucoid-type discharge
   b. Faint fleshy, musty odor
   c. Gradual increase as cervical changes and fetal descent progress

2. Warning signs
   a. Frank bleeding
      (1) Bright red blood may be indicative of **placenta previa**
      (2) Dark red blood may be indicative of **abruptio placenta**
   b. Foul odor indicates infection

D. **Assess pain and discomfort experienced during the process of labor and birth**

1. The source and the location of pain experienced

> ⚠ **Warning!**
>
> Never assume that pain experienced by the woman in labor is originating from the labor process. For example, chest pain might occur from cardiac problems or a pulmonary embolism.

2. Expected characteristics of pain experienced during childbirth
   a. Pain from contractions
      (1) Intermittent
      (2) Begins in lower back and radiates over the entire abdomen as blood vessels are compressed and uterine muscle cells become hypoxic; diminishes during rest period
      (3) Intensifies as contractions become more frequent, longer, and intense
   b. Pain from compression and stretching of nerves, organs, and tissues of cervix, vagina, and perineum; intensifies and extends into rest period as fetal descent progresses
   c. Pain from occiput posterior position of fetal head results in "back labor"; back pain is intense as the occiput presses against the sacrum
   d. Effects of pain on the maternal-fetal unit
      (1) Alteration in maternal vital signs: increase in BP, pulse, and oxygen use; hyperventilation

          (2) Anxiety, fear, and muscular tension occur: may impede labor, uteroplacental perfusion, descent, and magnify the pain sensation

          (3) Impressions of labor are formed from her assessment of her ability to cope effectively with labor pain

    3. Effectiveness of relief interventions

    4. Factors that influence the pain experience

      a. Availability of a partner, coach, or doula influences a woman's pain experience and her ability to cope to the degree that they support her and her willingness to accept their support

      b. Unique pain threshold and cultural patterns in response to pain

      c. Physical condition at the onset of labor

      d. Personal expectations about the pain of labor

          (1) Primigravida: fear of unknown, stories heard, expects the worst

          (2) Previous positive or negative experiences with parturition

          (3) Relief interventions learned in childbirth education classes; realistic and effective

      e. Unique character of labor including length, ease of birth, and need for medical intervention openness to a variety of interventions to relieve pain (Table 5-2, p. 124)

E. Assess status of oxygenation and circulation during parturition

    1. Maternal BP, pulse, respirations: use a consistent technique and assess between contractions

      a. When to assess

          (1) Recommended frequency: according to stage of labor and risk status (see Table 5-1)

          (2) Increased frequency: maternal vital signs deviate from her baseline range, nonreassuring FHR patterns occur, and medications that can affect vital signs are administered

      b. Expected findings

          (1) Remain close to baseline range established during pregnancy

          (2) Slight elevations may be noted as a result of pain, fatigue, stress, and dehydration

          (3) Slight decreases may occur with relaxation after the use of pain relief interventions

      c. Warning signs

          (1) Increasing rate and decreasing volume of the pulse (rapid, thready) and decreasing BP are associated with hemorrhage

          (2) Increasing BP could be indicative of PIH: over 140/90 mm Hg

          (3) Decreasing BP may occur as a result of spinal block anesthesia

          (4) Decreasing respiratory rate (RR) and depth of respirations (hypoventilation) may occur after analgesic or anesthetic administration and may restrict oxygenation

(5) Dyspnea, crackles, and cough could be indicative of pulmonary edema accompanying cardiac decompensation

2. Effectiveness of breathing techniques used during contractions
   a. Ability to effectively use techniques with contractions to reduce pain
   b. Occurrence of hyperventilation—rapid, deep respiratory pattern leads to a decrease in carbon dioxide and respiratory alkalosis. The woman experiences lightheadedness, dizziness, and tingling in her extremities. The remedy is to increase the carbon dioxide level by rebreathing exhaled air using a paper bag, a cupped hand, or a rebreather mask

3. Circulatory status to extremities including signs of thrombophlebitis

4. Laboratory tests
   a. Review test results from the antepartal period
   b. Complete blood count (CBC) for serum levels of hematocrit and hemoglobin (H&H), leukocytes (WBCs), and platelets
   c. Type and crossmatch as indicated

F. **Nutritional, fluid and electrolyte status during parturition: gastric motility and emptying time are decreased during labor, which increases the risk for nausea and vomiting that can limit oral intake. Assess these factors:**
   1. The amount of oral and IV fluid intake
   2. Presence of nausea, vomiting, and epigastric distress
   3. Extent of diaphoresis; expect an increase during the transition phase of the first stage of labor and during the second stage of labor
   4. Body temperature is taken every 4 hours then every 2 hours after membrane rupture; temperature elevation may indicate dehydration or infection
   5. Signs of dehydration
      a. Dry, sticky, oral mucous membranes, and thirst
      b. Decreased urinary output; urine is concentrated with a specific gravity of over 1.030
      c. Elevated body temperature
      d. Decreased turgor

G. **Elimination patterns during parturition**
   1. Bowel: character and time of last bowel movement. An empty rectum
      a. Facilitates the fetal descent and BDEs
      b. Minimizes passage of fecal material that can contaminate birth canal and inhibit BDEs
   2. Urinary: a distended bladder can inhibit fetal descent and suppress uterine contractions
      a. Obtain a clean catch midstream specimen for analysis and culture if indicated; use dipstick to test urine for protein, acetone, and glucose, repeating as indicated every 2 to 4 hours

Text continued on p. 147

TABLE 5-2   Pharmacologic Interventions to Manage Discomfort of Labor and Birth

Pharmacologic Measure	Effects on Maternal-Fetal Unit	Nursing Considerations
I. Systemic Analgesics Types: Meperidine (Demerol): narcotic analgesic, 50 mg (IM) or 25 mg (IV) Fentanyl (Sublimaze): narcotic analgesic, 50-100 mcg (IM) or 25-50 mcg (IV) Nalbuphine (Nubain): mixed agonist antagonist analgesic, 10-20 mg (IM) or 10 mg (IV) **WARNING!** IV administration is preferred to IM because a smaller dose is required, with faster onset and more reliable effect. **WARNING!** Tranquilizers when administered in combination with analgesics potentiate the analgesic's action, requiring a smaller analgesic dose. (Examples: promethazine (Phenergan), hydroxyzine (Vistaril))	Maternal effects: CNS depression: BP and respirations decrease Slowing of uterine contractions if given before labor is well-established in the active phase and cervix is dilated at least 4 cm Takes edge off of pain and sedates to allow the woman to: Regain control Rest between contractions Reduce anxiety and tension Experience a more positive and comfortable labor Maternal relaxation can enhance labor and facilitate fetal descent Fetal, newborn effects: Direct effect of analgesic: drug crosses placenta and is metabolized slowly CNS depression of fetus and of newborn if given within 2 hr of expected birth Transitory decrease in variability from mild hypoxia Respiratory depression after birth Decreased alertness and responsiveness of newborn that may persist for 24 hr or more Indirect effect of analgesic is associated with a fetal response to a decrease of maternal BP, respirations, or both	Assess need for analgesic and effectiveness of non-pharmacologic pain relief interventions Assess before and after administration Maternal-fetal vital signs Phase of labor Need and effectiveness Do not give if Labor is not established or birth is anticipated in 2 hr or less Signs of fetal hypoxia are noted Maternal BP or respirations is decreased Enhance effectiveness by: Reducing environmental stimuli Providing comfort interventions and an opportunity to rest Explaining beneficial effects of analgesia for the mother, fetus, and labor Institute safety interventions of bed rest, bed in the low position, side rails up, call light within reach Keep a narcotic antagonist such as nalaxone (Narcan) in readiness for administration to the mother or to the depressed neonate if birth occurs sooner than expected

II. Local Infiltration Anesthesia

Anesthetic agent is injected into perineal tissue during the second stage of labor just before birth or during the third stage of labor

Maternal effects:

Interrupts conduction of pain impulses from the perineum before the incision for an episiotomy and during the repair of the episiotomy and lacerations

No relief of pain associated with contractions

Allergic (systemic or local) reaction can occur

Fetal, newborn effects: none

Determine the presence of maternal allergies to local anesthetic agents

Provide support and explanations

Assess for signs of allergic reactions

Assess perineal area for ecchymosis, edema, erythema

III. Pudendal Block

Administered between contractions

Anesthetic agent is injected near the ischial spines to anesthetize the pudendal nerve during the second stage of labor just before birth

Maternal effects:

Pain relief in clitoris, labia majora and minora, perineum

No effect on pain associated with uterine contractions

Bearing down reflex may be reduced

Effective pain relief for use of low forceps or vacuum extractor, for performance of episiotomy, and repair of episiotomy and lacerations

Allergic reaction (systemic or local) may occur

Fetal, newborn effects: none

Assist with BDEs

Assess for hematoma formation

Assess perineal area for ecchymosis, edema, erythema

Assess for signs of allergic reactions

Provide client support and explanations

IV. Epidural Block

Administered between contractions

Anesthetic agent is injected into the *epidural space at level L-2 to L-4*

Anesthetic agent such as bupivacaine can be administered alone or in combination with a narcotic analgesic such as fentanyl

Maternal effects:

Hypotension: most common complication; a systolic BP of <90 mm Hg results in a BP that would be inadequate to maintain placental perfusion

Respiratory depression may occur when given with narcotic or if dura mater is punctured; profound depression, even arrest of respirations may occur

Assess maternal-fetal status before procedure

Prepare woman for and support her during the procedure:

Explain what to expect

Have woman void before the procedure

Assist into position

Sitting on side of bed or delivery table with feet on a stool and back curved by leaning forward and supported by nurse or coach

Continued

TABLE 5-2   Pharmacologic Interventions to Manage Discomfort of Labor and Birth—cont'd

Pharmacologic Measure	Effects on Maternal-Fetal Unit	Nursing Considerations
Onset occurs within 10-20 min Single injection can be used during the second stage for vaginal or cesarean birth Continuous infusion can be accomplished by inserting a catheter into the epidural space and connecting it to an infusion pump during active phase when: Contractions are well-established Cervix is dilated at least 4 cm Level of analgesia, anesthesia achieved is dose-dependent Duration of action ranges from 30 min to 4 hr, depending on agent used; bupivacaine has the longest duration of 2-4 hr	Reduced or loss of sensation to uterus, bladder, and perineum Depression of contractions, especially if given too early, can prolong labor Decreased sensation and motor function to lower extremities Relaxation of muscles, including the perineum Limitation of urge to bear down and ability to push effectively may occur Dosage may be decreased or stopped in second stage to facilitate BDEs Local anesthesia is used when an episiotomy is performed Allergic (systemic or local) reactions Fetal, newborn effects: primarily an indirect effect from the fetal response to maternal respiratory depression and hypotension, and to a prolonged labor that requires invasive medical procedures	Modified Sims position, with head supported on small pillow, back curved, and legs flexed Assist to maintain position without movement during procedure, use touch, keep her informed of what is occurring, what she will feel Monitor maternal-fetal effects: Electronic monitoring of maternal HR and BP is often used for continuous epidural infusions Respiratory effort and respirations: every 15 min Electronic monitoring of FHR pattern and contractions: continuous Effectiveness of pain relief; watch for breakthrough pain Bladder function for distention: every 30 min Sensation, motor function in lower extremities: every hour Site of infusion, line, pump: at frequent intervals Maintain IV infusion to ensure adequate hydration; woman who is adequately hydrated and receives a loading IV infusion is less likely to experience hypotension Intervene if hypotension occurs: increase rate of IV to 100 up to 200 ml/hr, turn on side or place a wedge under hip, raise legs (10-20 degrees), give oxygen via mask (8-10 L/min), prepare to administer a vasopressor such as ephedrine IV

V. Low Spinal (Saddle) Block

Administered between contractions

Anesthetic agent is *injected into the subarachnoid space at level L-3, L-4, or L-5 where it mixes in the spinal fluid and settles into the lower spine*

Induced during the second stage when birth is imminent and fetal head is at the perineum

Onset in 1-2 min with a duration of 1-3 hr

Effective for vaginal or cesarean birth

Maternal effects:

Hypotension

Respiratory depression if anesthetic agent rises in spinal fluid

Loss of sensation to uterus, bladder, perineum

Loss of sensation and motor function to lower extremities

Loss of bearing down reflex, which increases the use of forceps, vacuum extractor, episiotomy

Spinal headaches as a result of leakage of spinal fluid during induction; an autologous blood patch can be used to prevent or reduce leakage of spinal fluid at site of puncture

Allergic reactions (systemic or local)

Intervene if respiratory depression occurs (respirations slow to 12 or less) give oxygen via mask (8-10 L/min), prepare to administer Narcan if depression is from use of a narcotic analgesic, and raise head of bed approximately 30 degrees to facilitate breathing; resuscitation is initiated if woman is unresponsive to above interventions

Prepare to augment labor if progress slows by giving Pitocin, using nipple stimulation, and assisting with pushing

Change the woman's position from side to side every hour to equalize effect and avoid reduction in BP

Protect the woman's legs from injury

Encourage voiding every 2 hr; catheterize prn

Assess maternal-fetal status before procedure

Prepare woman for and support her during the procedure

Explain what to expect

Assist into sitting position as for epidural block; sometimes lateral position is used

Assist to maintain position without movement

Maintain an upright position for time prescribed to lower the level of anesthesia for a vaginal birth or maintain a supine, semi- or low-Fowler's position to achieve higher level for cesarean birth

Return the woman to a supine position with small pillow under shoulders and under hip

Continued

TABLE 5-2 Pharmacologic Interventions to Manage Discomfort of Labor and Birth—cont'd

Pharmacologic Measure	Effects on Maternal-Fetal Unit	Nursing Considerations
V. Low Spinal (Saddle) Block—cont'd		
	Fetal, neonatal effects: primarily indirect effects from the fetal response to maternal hypotension, respiratory depression, and invasive procedures required for birth	Raise the woman's legs together and carefully place into stirrups if used to protect them from injury Monitor maternal-fetal effects: Maternal pulse, BP, respirations FHR pattern every 2 min (for first 10 min) then every 5-10 min Urinary function, comfort level, and legs Maintain IV infusion as for epidural Take action for hypotension and respiratory depression as recommended for epidural anesthesia
VI. General Anesthesia		
Inhalation or IV induction of anesthesia results in loss of body sensation and consciousness	Maternal effects: Vomiting with aspiration from decreased gastric emptying time and loss of gag reflex	Record time and nature of recent oral intake Maintain NPO status; establish IV infusion as per orders of primary health care provider
Used primarily for emergency cesarean birth or vaginal birth requiring emergency intervention	Loss of consciousness; unable to participate in the birth Uterine relaxation increases risk of postpartum hemorrhage	Complete and ongoing assessment of maternal-fetal status Administer an alkalinizing agent such as Bicitra by mouth to decrease the acidity of gastric contents to minimize pneumonitis if aspiration should occur
Administered just before birth to limit fetal exposure because anesthetic agent crosses placenta rapidly	**Fetal, newborn effects: effects and their duration depend on depth of anesthesia, dosage, and length of time under anesthesia** CNS depression; hypoxia; altered FHR pattern Respiratory depression Decreased responsiveness, limits interaction, sucking	Place wedge under hip, tilt to side

    b. Observe for signs UTI

    c. Assess throughout labor to ensure that bladder is being emptied

       (1) Frequency: at least every 2 hours

       (2) Amount and characteristics of urine: expect at least 100 ml of clear yellow urine at each voiding

       (3) Bladder distension: evaluate by palpation and percussion over the lower abdomen above the symphysis pubis

> ⚠ **Warning!**
>
> Greater emphasis on urinary assessment should occur when sensitivity to bladder fullness is diminished during one of two events: the use of regional anesthetics such as a low spinal or epidural block, and the time of advanced labor in which contractions and pelvic pressure intensify and fetus descent occurs.

  H. Physical activity and rest during parturition

    1. Energy level: assess for signs of fatigue and exhaustion, which can slow progress of labor and interfere with effective pushing

    2. Degree of muscular tension or relaxation

    3. Ability to maintain positions that facilitate CO, uteroplacental perfusion and progress of labor (Box 5-3, p. 148)

    4. Desire to participate in activities that reduce tension and conserve energy

      a. Diversional activities and ambulation in early labor

      b. Relaxation interventions to rest between contractions

  I. Integument: note alterations in integrity: rashes, lesions, lacerations, bruises, and track marks indicative of physical or drug abuse

VII. Assessment of psychosocial reactions to childbirth; emotional state affects the overall progress

  A. Ongoing assessment is required because the maternal emotional status and mood change as labor progresses

    1. Latent phase: excited, anxious, talkative, and ambivalent about the ability to cope with labor; "in control"

    2. Active phase: introverted, less responsive, decreased attention span, intense concentration on "work of labor"; some loss of control may occur along with a growing irritability

    3. Transition phase: decreased confidence, loss of control, desire to give up and go home, fear of death for self and fetus; does not want to be touched and rejects help of the coach

    4. Second stage: renewed energy and purpose, "second wind," rewarded with perception of progress in fetal descent with each BDE

  B. Maternal assessment

    1. Mood and affect, including fear and anxiety levels

    2. Attention span and ability to follow directions; alertness and orientation level

Box 5-3
Maternal Positions During Labor and Birth

Semi-Recumbent Position

Woman sits with upper body elevated to at least a 30-degree angle. A wedge or small pillow is placed under the hip to prevent vena caval compression and reduce the incidence of supine hypotension.

The greater the angle of elevation, the more gravity and pressure are applied to enhance fetal descent, progress of contractions, and widening of pelvic dimensions.

This position is convenient for care interventions and external fetal monitoring.

Lateral Position

Woman alternates between left and right side-lying positions. Abdominal and back support should be provided as needed to enhance her comfort in the lateral position.

Removes pressure from the vena cava and back to enhance uteroplacental perfusion, and relieve backache

Makes it easier to perform back massage or counterpressure

Is associated with less frequent, more intense contractions

May be used as a birthing position

May make external fetal monitoring more difficult

WARNING!   Current research indicates there is no significant difference in cardiac output (CO) between the right and left side-lying positions.

Upright Position

The effect of gravity enhances the contraction cycle and fetal descent. The fetus increases pressure on the cervix, and the cervix is pulled upward, facilitating effacement and dilation. Impulses from the cervix to the pituitary gland increase. Oxytocin is secreted in a greater amount. Contraction intensifies, with a more forceful downward pressure on fetus.

The fetus is aligned with the pelvis, and pelvic diameters are widened

Effective upright positions include:

Ambulating

Standing and leaning forward with support from the coach, end of bed, or back of chair; relieves backache and facilitates counterpressure and back massage

Sitting up in bed or on a chair, birthing chair, or birthing ball

Squatting with the use of a support bar or birthing ball

Hands and Knees Position

Woman assumes an "all fours" position in bed or on a covered floor; birthing ball can be used for support

Relieves backache characteristic of "back labor"

Ideal for posterior positions of fetal presentation

Facilitates internal rotation of the fetus: increases mobility of the coccyx, increases pelvic diameters, and applies the force of gravity to turn the fetal back and rotate the head

WARNING!   Assess the effect of each position on the laboring woman's comfort and anxiety level, progress of labor, and FHR pattern. Alternate positions every 30 to 60 minutes.

  3. Body posture and movements indicative of tension
  4. Ability and desire to work with the labor process rather than against it; degree of effectiveness in use of childbirth techniques and willingness to participate in techniques designed to enhance the process of labor and ensure a positive outcome
 C. **Assessment of support person(s): coach, partner, doula**
  1. Effectiveness in the provision of support and encouragement in the use of childbirth techniques
  2. Ability to work together with the laboring woman and the health care team
  3. Response to labor events and behaviors of the laboring woman

VIII. Common nursing diagnoses encountered during parturition, along with selected client outcomes, nursing interventions, and evaluation criteria are described in Table 5-3, pp. 150-153

IX. Nursing responsibilities during the third stage of labor focus on the mother and newborn

 A. **Mother**
  1. Assessment: vital signs, fundus, blood loss, and signs of placental separation (see Table 5-1, pp. 124-127)
  2. Assist with pushing to expel separated placenta
  3. Administer oxytocic medications, which stimulate the uterus to contract thereby limiting blood loss, as directed by the primary health care provider
   a. IV oxytocin (Pitocin), 10 to 20 U, mixed in IV solution
   b. Methylergonovine maleate (Methergine), 0.2 mg, IM or PO; assess BP before and 5 to 15 minutes after administration because hypertension can occur; it is not given to women who are hypertensive (BP over 140/90)
  4. Inform woman and support person(s) about the progress of recovery
  5. Facilitate bonding between newborn and parents
 B. **Newborn**

⚠ Warning!

Wear clean gloves when handling newborn until fully cleansed of body fluids and substances.

  1. Immediately assess the newborn's adaptation to extrauterine life using the **Apgar score** (Table 5-4, p. 155)
   a. Determine the Apgar score at 1 and 5 minutes; the 5-minute score usually is considered more reflective of the newborn's ability to adapt to extrauterine life
   b. Continue at 10 minutes after birth if condition is unstable and first two scores are low

Text continued on p. 156

TABLE 5-3 Common Nursing Diagnoses Encountered During Parturition

Nursing Diagnoses, Expected Outcomes	Nursing Interventions
A. Acute pain related to the process of labor and birth Woman will: Cooperate with interventions offered to enhance her level of comfort Use techniques learned in childbirth classes to cope with the pain and discomfort of labor and birth Experience pain reduction with the use of relief interventions	Provide comfort interventions to enhance relaxation, reduce anxiety, and increase effectiveness of pharmacologic relief interventions: Back massage and counterpressure at sacrum using tennis balls, fist, heel of hand Cold packs at sacrum, warm packs at lower abdomen and sacrum Cold moist cloth on forehead Frequent change of position, ambulation Hygienic care: perineal cleansing, shower, sponge bath Oral care Encourage use of techniques learned in childbirth classes, and provide praise and positive reinforcement for her efforts (see Box 5-2, p. 134): Relaxation techniques, guided imagery, focal points *Effleurage,* that is, gentle stroking of abdomen to soothe and distract Breathing techniques Demonstrate simple breathing and relaxation techniques if no prior instruction Institute alternative interventions for pain relief, relaxation, and stress reduction as appropriate to woman and facilities available including: Biofeedback, hypnosis Acupressure, aromatherapy, music Transcutaneous electrical nerve stimulation (TENS) Water therapy such as warm showers, whirlpool bath Administer analgesics safely (see Table 5-2, pp. 142-146) Employ appropriate assessment and supportive interventions during anesthesia (see Table 5-2, pp. 142-146)

B. Fatigue related to ineffective progress of labor

Woman's labor will progress according to expected standards

Woman will participate in interventions designed to enhance the process of labor and birth

Woman's energy level will be sufficient for effective BDEs during the second stage of labor

Employ interventions to enhance rest and conserve energy:
  Create a calm and restful environment
  Encourage relaxation techniques, visual imagery, music
  Provide opportunities for enjoyable diversional activities
  Use water therapy such as warm showers, whirlpool baths
  Use interventions to reduce anxiety

Employ interventions to facilitate progress of labor
  Frequent periods of ambulation:
    Gravity pushes fetus against cervix to facilitate fetal rotation, cervical dilation, progress of contractions
    Pelvic diameters increase slightly when upright
    Diversion and relief of discomfort are enhanced
  Alternate positions: every 30 to 60 minutes with an emphasis on upright positions: take into consideration the woman's comfort level and wishes (see Box 5-3, p. 148)
  Use birthing ball to facilitate alternative positions and to stretch perineum
  Use nipple stimulation to increase secretion of endogenous oxytocin; consult unit protocol
    Stimulate only one nipple to avoid hyperstimulation
    Stimulate for short periods between contractions
    Stop when contraction begins and when pattern is established

Maintain caloric and fluid intake
  Provide easily digested light foods and a variety of fluids; woman will usually reduce her intake as labor becomes more active
  Use IV fluids only if oral intake is insufficient and signs of fluid deficit appear; infuse at 100-150 ml/hr as needed
  Assess fluid balance, intake and output, urine concentration

Ensure that active labor is established before analgesics or spinal block anesthetics are administered (see Table 5-2, pp. 142-146)

Assist woman to push effectively; woman:
  Begins to push when fully dilated and urge to push is perceived
  Pushes during uterine contractions using open-glottis technique
  Assumes position that facilitates descent
  Relaxes and rests between contractions

Continued

TABLE 5-3   Common Nursing Diagnoses Encountered During Parturition—cont'd

Nursing Diagnoses, Expected Outcomes	Nursing Interventions
C. Altered pattern of urinary elimination and retention related to effects of childbirth process on urinary tract Woman will: Void at least 100 ml every 2-3 hr Experience no bladder distension	Assist woman to void every 2 hr Measure urine and observe characteristics: color, clarity, odor, amount, level of protein, glucose, ketones Use interventions to facilitate voiding, including an upright position, privacy, running water, warm water over the vulva and perineum, blowing bubbles with a straw into a glass of water Palpate and percuss bladder for distension Catheterize as needed Perform perineal care before procedure Insert catheter at a time between contractions Place fingers in vagina and press fetal part upward if passage of catheter is impeded
D. Risk for infection related to process of labor and rupture of amniotic membranes Woman will progress through labor and birthing without the development of an infection	Use standard precautions and regular hand washing because the risk of exposure to blood and body fluids is high Limit frequency of vaginal examinations Perform perineal care with greater frequency as show increases and membranes rupture; cleanse from front to back Use principles of asepsis when performing vaginal examinations Use surgical asepsis for insertion of internal monitors and rupture of membranes Wear clean scrub clothing when working in labor Use interventions to decrease number of invasive procedures such as facilitating voiding, assisting with BDEs, and enhancing labor progress

E. Moderate level of anxiety related to lack of childbirth experience and knowledge

Woman's level of anxiety will be maintained at a mild or moderate level

Woman and coach will work together effectively as a team

Woman will participate in interventions designed to reduce anxiety and enhance relaxation

Encourage and guide the couple in their use of childbirth techniques

Provide positive reinforcement; review techniques they have learned as needed

Help them to get started and to advance techniques as labor progresses

Do not interrupt during a contraction

Review birth plan with woman and partner; ensure staff awareness of and respect for their birth plan

Facilitate relaxation with the use of comfort measures and relaxation techniques

Administer medications as needed for pain relief

Use a calm, confident approach; implement interventions that reflect a sensitivity to the woman's culture and wishes

Touch: physical contact reassures, comforts, and implies caring

Maintain privacy and modesty

Allow woman to be herself, to express herself, to deal with pain, to make sounds during pushing

Support and encourage coach

Keep woman and coach informed of progress and events

Explain procedures, equipment, routine; orient to room

Simple teaching as needed during early labor especially if unprepared for childbirth

Give progress reports in positive terms

Box 5-4
Bearing Down Efforts (BDEs), or Pushing

What are BDEs?

BDEs, or pushing, is the effective use of abdominal muscle contractions—the secondary force or power of labor—combined with uterine contractions to facilitate descent and birth of the fetus during the second stage of labor. Emphasis is placed on the woman responding to her natural urge to push.

When are BDEs done?

Phase one of the second stage of labor—early, latent (10 to 30 minutes):
   Transient decrease in intensity and frequency of uterine contractions
   Assist laboring woman to rest in a position of comfort and conserve energy until the natural urge to push is felt; changing positions, especially to an upright position, can stimulate onset of an urge to push
   Provide emotional support and encourage the use of relaxation techniques
Phase two of the second stage of labor—active, descent:
   Ferguson reflex occurs: fetal presenting part descends; pelvic floor is distended; stretch receptors are stimulated; rhythmic urge to push or bear down is felt
   Assist the laboring woman into position and coach the BDEs with contractions
Phase three of the second stage of labor—transition, perineal (5 to 12 minutes):
   Birth is imminent as perineal bulging and crowning (vulva surrounds largest diameter of the fetal head) occur
The laboring woman should be encouraged to reduce or equalize forces during delivery of the fetal head by:
   Panting to avoid abdominal muscle contractions during a uterine contraction
   Keeping the BDEs gentle and steady between contractions

How are BDEs performed?

The laboring woman assumes a position that facilitates BDEs and birth during phases two and three; changing positions will enhance effectiveness:
Upright: squatting on bed or side of bed; sitting on toilet, birthing chair, or birthing bed
Semi-recumbent: knees and legs lower than the heart and assuming a "C" posture with shoulders curved forward and knees pulled up when BDEs begin
Lateral: raise and support the upper leg during BDEs; descent is slower but the perineum is more relaxed
Lithotomy: both legs are raised and placed in stirrups; least effective position because the effect of gravity is not realized and cardiac workload is increased
Breathing techniques during the BDEs:
   Two deep "cleansing" breaths taken at the onset of the contraction to allow it to reach its acme, or peak
   One breath is taken and held for a couple of seconds at the start of the push; pushing becomes vigorous while exhaling (open glottis pushing); push for short periods, about 7 seconds
   Breaths are taken between BDEs
   At the end of the contraction the laboring woman takes two deep cleaning breaths and assumes a position of rest and comfort
WARNING!   Prolonged holding of breath while pushing (Valsalva maneuver) for periods of more than 6 seconds can decrease maternal BP and reduce uteroplacental perfusion, leading to fetal hypoxia.

TABLE 5-4   Assessment of Newborn and Interpretation of Results Using the Apgar Score*

I. Assessment Criteria

Sign Assessed	Score Assigned** = 0	Score Assigned** = 1	Score Assigned** = 2
Heart rate (HR)	Not present	Less than 100 beats per min	Greater than 100 beats per min
Respiratory effort	Not present	Weak, slow, irregular respirations	Cries vigorously
Muscle tone	Flaccid, limp	Some flexion of arms and legs, limited movement	Actively moving, good range of motion
Reflex irritability	Unresponsive when stimulated	Minimal response or grimace when stimulated	Cries, coughs, sneezes in response to stimulation
Color	Cyanotic, pale	Body pink with blue hands and feet (acrocyanosis)—the acrocyanosis diminishes during the first 24 hours after birth but slight cyanosis may reappear for as long as 7 to 10 days after birth, if the newborn is chilled or exposed to the cold: it should disappear quickly once the newborn is warm	Fully pink, including hands and feet

II. Interpretation and Recommended Actions

Score	Interpretation	Recommended Action
8-10	Reassuring—good initial response to birth	Basic newborn care Suction to maintain patent airway with a bulb syringe Prevent heat loss Facilitate bonding with parents
3-7	Mild to moderate depression, asphyxia	Support respiratory effort as indicated: Gentle stimulation; ventilation with bag, oxygen administration Oro-nasopharyngeal suction with a suction catheter and mechanical device Administer narcotic antagonist
0-2	Severe depression, asphyxia	Insert endotracheal tube, oxygenate Initiate cardiopulmonary resuscitation Administer medications as directed: narcotic antagonists, sodium bicarbonate, epinephrine, glucose

*Apgar Score assessment is performed at 1 and 5 minutes after birth and is repeated in 10 minutes from the birth if problems occur.
**Score assigned for each sign assessed for a total of 10 if each sign is normal.

    c. Apgar score, cardiopulmonary and thermoregulatory status, and the circumstances of labor and birth guide the care of the newborn immediately after birth and the need for resuscitation interventions

2. Maintain airway patency
    a. Suction mouth, then nose, as required using bulb syringe
        (1) Use for initial suction at birth of head and after birth if newborn is stable, with a good Apgar score, no meconium in amniotic fluid, and airway patency is achieved
        (2) Compress bulb, then insert along the side of the mouth and release compression slowly; follow by suctioning each nostril
        (3) Continue until the airway is patent, that is, breathing and crying sounds are clear
    b. Suction oro-nasopharynx (mouth first then nose) using mechanical suction with a catheter when
        (1) Apgar scores are low and respirations are depressed
        (2) Amniotic fluid was stained with meconium: danger if meconium is aspirated because it destroys lung tissue and increases the risk for infection
        (3) Airway secretions are copious and cannot be cleared adequately with the bulb syringe
        (4) Set at low suction: 80 mm Hg or lower
            (a) Lubricate sterile catheter (8 to 12 F) with sterile water
            (b) Insert with suction off
            (c) Apply suction as tube is removed
            (d) Limit each suction attempt to under 5 seconds and oxygenate well between attempts
        (5) Limit frequency and perform gently to prevent trauma to delicate mucous membranes
    c. Use modified Trendelenburg position (15 to 30 degrees) to facilitate drainage of lung fluid by gravity

3. Administer oxygen as required by newborn's condition
    a. Mildly depressed—whiffs of oxygen over nose
    b. Moderately depressed—tight mask
    c. Severely depressed—endotracheal tube is inserted to facilitate administration of oxygen

4. Initiate cardiopulmonary resuscitation (CPR) interventions for the severely depressed neonate

5. Maintain body temperature
    a. Institute heat conservation interventions
        (1) Dry skin with an absorbent towel
        (2) Use warming interventions during assessment of the newborn and the provision of care, including during any resuscitation interventions, by placing the newborn under a radiant heat warmer, skin-to-skin contact with mother, or in warm blankets

    b. Assess body temperature by the use of the thermistor probe from the radiant heat warmer

6. Assess general health status
    a. Vital signs
    b. Cord
        (1) Obtain cord blood samples for blood type and Rh, direct Coombs' test, serologic testing (syphilis exposure), and acid-base status
        (2) Determine presence of two arteries and one vein
        (3) Check the placement and security of the cord clamp
    c. Measure head and chest circumference, length, and weight
    d. Posture and movement
    e. Condition of integument regarding color, injuries, and peeling
    f. Presence of visible anomalies such as cleft lip and palate, absent or deformed limbs, and spinal defects
    g. Bowel or bladder elimination
    h. Gestational age

7. Institute identification procedures by the attachment of matching maternal and newborn ID bands; footprint newborn, and fingerprint mother

8. Administer medications
    a. Prevent ophthalmia neonatorum—infection of the eyes from exposure to gonorrhea or *Chlamydia* infection during the passage through the birth canal. Eye prophylaxis can be delayed for 1 hour to facilitate eye-to-eye contact for bonding.
        (1) Cleanse eyes from inner to outer canthus with sterile water
        (2) Instill erythromycin or tetracycline ointment into conjunctival sac of each eye; do not flush eyes after instillation
    b. Inject IM vitamin K [phytonadione (AquaMEPHYTON)], 0.5 to 1 mg, into lateral aspect, middle third of vastus lateralis muscle of thigh to prevent clotting problems associated with absence of intestinal bacteria needed to synthesize vitamin K

X. Nursing responsibilities during the fourth stage of labor: the first 1 to 2 hours after birth (see Table 5-1, pp. 124-127)

A. Assess recovery status: first hour every 15 minutes; second hour every 30 minutes; third hour and thereafter as indicated by maternal status

1. Vital signs: BP, pulse, and respirations
2. Fundus: consistency (firm or boggy), height (above, below, at umbilicus), location (midline or deviated to the right or left) (Figure 5-7, p. 158)
3. Lochia (Figure 5-8, p. 158)
    a. Amount (degree of pad saturation and time elapsed since pad was changed)—scant, light, moderate, profuse
    b. Characteristics—type and stage, presence of clots, and odor

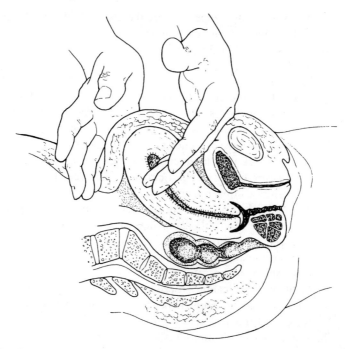

Figure 5-7   Palpating fundus of the uterus during the first hour of delivery. Note that the upper hand is cupped over the fundus; the lower hand dips in above the symphysis pubis and supports the uterus while it is massaged gently. (From Lowdermilk DL, Perry SE, Bobak IM: *Maternity and women's health care,* ed 7, St. Louis, 2000, Mosby.)

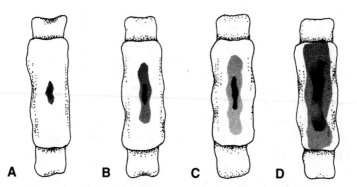

Figure 5-8   Peripad saturation volumes. **A,** Scant. **B,** Light. **C,** Moderate. **D,** Heavy or profuse. (From Lowdermilk DL, Perry SE, Bobak IM: *Maternity and women's health care,* ed 7, St. Louis, 2000, Mosby.)

Warning!

Always check under the buttocks for pooling of lochia.

4. Perineum: episiotomy and lacerations check is called "REEDA"
   a. R—redness
   b. E—ecchymosis
   c. E—edema
   d. D—drainage
   e. A—approximation

⚠ Warning!

Indications of hematoma formation are the presence of swelling, intensifying perineal pain or pressure, the sensation of a need to defecate, and the alteration in vital signs that reflect blood loss. A narrowing of the pulse pressure is often the first change in vital signs that is noted.

5. Signs of hypovolemic (hemorrhagic) shock; may be delayed since the increase in blood volume that occurs with pregnancy temporarily protects the woman from the effects of blood loss after birth.
   a. Alteration in vital signs
      (1) Narrowing of the pulse pressure (often the first sign noted) followed by hypotension
      (2) Increasing pulse rate with decreasing strength and volume
      (3) Increasing respiratory rate and effort, with a decreasing depth
   b. Profuse blood loss
      (1) Lochia: saturation of one peripad in less than 1 hour
      (2) Sensation of intense pain and pressure in the perineum, with or without swelling
   c. Cool, pale integument
   d. Altered sensorium —anxious, restless, irritable, light-headed, "feels funny, nauseous," "sees stars"
6. Additional assessments for the fourth stage of labor
   a. Urinary elimination
      (1) Amount of urine should be at least 100 ml per voiding
      (2) Bladder distention elevates the fundus above the umbilicus and pushes it off midline to result in inhibition of uterine contractions (boggy or soft uterus) and an increased blood loss
   b. Progress in recovery from anesthesia
      (1) Spinal block: the return of movement to the lower extremities occurs first and then the return of sensation occurs, at which time sensation of bladder fullness may occur
      (2) General anesthesia: return of consciousness and the gag reflex

     c. Presence of pain—severity and location
     d. Temperature—elevation usually indicates dehydration, especially after long labors
     e. Level of fatigue
     f. Hunger and thirst
     g. Responses to the experience of birth and to the newborn

B. Implement interventions to prevent hemorrhage
   1. Massage fundus when boggy; massage only until firm then stop
   2. Administer **oxytocic** medications as ordered, such as Pitocin and methylergonovine maleate (Methergine), which stimulate the uterus to contract
   3. Keep the woman's bladder empty

C. Take action if signs of hemorrhage and shock are noted (follow your agency's protocol)
   1. Stay with woman, and call for help
   2. Massage fundus if boggy, expel clots with downward pressure on firm fundus, and administer oxytocics
   3. Raise legs from hip with the head of the bed flat or in a low Fowler's position
   4. Start or increase rate of IV infusion
   5. Administer oxygen via mask at 8 to 10 L/min.

D. Provide for client comfort and safety
   1. Assist with hygienic interventions
     a. Oral care and sponge bath
     b. Perineal care, including cleansing, ice packs, and topical anesthetics
     c. Clean, dry clothing and bedding
   2. Administer analgesics as needed
   3. Facilitate rest
   4. Provide food and fluids when physiologic stability is firmly established
   5. Institute safety interventions
     a. Raise side rails if indicated and keep the bed in low position
     b. Assist with ambulation until woman can move safely on her own
       (1) Determine that sensation and motor function have been restored
       (2) Move to upright position slowly
       (3) Dangle feet at side of bed for several minutes; assess for dizziness
       (4) Assist to a standing position if dizziness is not present
       (5) Support during ambulation
   6. Provide opportunities for newborn-parent interaction

WEB Resources

http://www.efn.org/~djz/birth/birthindex.html

The Online Birth Center (OBC). It presents detailed information related to midwifery, pregnancy, birth, and breast feeding. There is extensive coverage of complementary and alternative therapies.

http://www.wenet.net/~karil/index.html

This is the water birth website. It provides information about water birth: benefits, preparation, stories, and photographs.

http://www.childbirth.org

The primary focus of this website is childbirth but it also provides access to information related to pregnancy and the postpartum periods.

http://www.dona.com

Doulas of North America (DONA). This website fully describes the role of the doula during childbirth, how to find one, and even how to become one.

http://www.birthcenters.org

National Association of Childbearing Centers.

http://www.gentlebirth.org

This site focuses on pregnancy, childbirth, and well woman care from a midwifery perspective.

http://www.virtualbirth.com

The Virtual Birth Center. In addition to a major emphasis on midwifery-managed childbirth, the site includes a multimedia section that provides photographs, interviews, and video related to the birth process.

http://www.childbirth.org/CEP.html

Sponsored by the Cutting Edge Press, this website provides a wide variety of information and photographs related to nonpharmacologic measures to support the laboring woman and enhance the labor process, including nurturing touch and use of the birthing ball and other labor support tools.

REVIEW QUESTIONS

1. Cervical ripening refers to which of these physiologic changes?
1. Softening and thinning
2. Progressive dilation
3. Increasing vascularity
4. Development of oxytocin receptors and gap junctions

2. The nurse should tell a primigravida that the definitive sign indicating the beginning of labor is which of these findings?
1. Regular, progressive uterine contractions that increase in intensity with activity
2. Lightening
3. Rupture of membranes
4. Passage of the mucous plug *(operculum)*

3. Which of these items most accurately describes the discomfort expected with true labor contractions? The discomfort
1. Begins in the fundus and then radiates downward to the cervix
2. Centers in the fundus of the uterus during the entire contraction
3. Begins in the lower back and abdomen and then radiates over the entire abdomen
4. Radiates outward from the umbilicus

4. The results of a vaginal examination of a woman in labor included the note of: LST, +1. Which of these items represents a correct interpretation of this piece of data as it relates to the fetus?
1. Transverse lie
2. Shoulder presentation
3. Sacrum is located in the left side of the maternal pelvis
4. Head is 1 cm above the ischial spines

5. The cardinal movements of labor facilitate fetal progress through the birth canal. Which of these statements correctly describes the cardinal movements of labor as they relate to a cephalic presentation?
1. Engagement—head reaches the pelvic inlet
2. Flexion—chin touches chest to allow the smallest transverse diameter to pass through the pelvis
3. Internal rotation—head turns to allow the anteroposterior diameter to pass between the ischial spines
4. External rotation—head turns after it emerges from the birth canal to realign itself with the shoulders

6. A nullipara experienced a normal pregnancy and has exhibited no risk factors. It is recommended that during the latent phase of the first stage of labor the nurse follow which assessment guideline?
   1. FHR every 30 to 60 minutes
   2. Maternal BP, temperature, pulse, and respirations every 2 to 4 hours
   3. Uterine contractions every 2 hours
   4. Vaginal show every 2 hours

7. To determine the frequency of uterine contractions, the nurse should follow which time frame?
   1. The onset of the contraction until it ends
   2. The beginning of one contraction until the end of the next
   3. The onset of one contraction until the onset of the next
   4. The end of one contraction until the end of the next

8. When the nurse performs vaginal examinations on laboring women, which of these principles should guide the nurse?
   1. Cleanse the vulva and perineum before and after the examination as needed
   2. Wear a clean glove lubricated with tap water to reduce discomfort
   3. Perform the examination every hour during the active phase of the first stage of labor
   4. Perform immediately if bleeding is present

9. A laboring woman's amniotic membranes have just ruptured. The immediate action of the nurse would be to do what?
   1. Assess the FHR pattern
   2. Perform a vaginal examination
   3. Inspect the characteristics of the fluid
   4. Assess maternal temperature along with pulse, BP, and RR

10. Which of these childbirth positions during labor would be the most effective to facilitate the internal rotation of a fetus whose position is ROP?
    1. Left lateral
    2. Right lateral
    3. Hands and knees
    4. Squatting

ANSWERS, RATIONALES, AND TEST-TAKING TIPS

Rationales	Test-Taking Tips

1. Correct answer: 1

Progressive dilation occurs once the cervix is ripe. An increase in vascularity occurs earlier in pregnancy and prepares the cervix for ripening as labor approaches. Oxytocin receptors and gap junctions are formed in the myometrium of the uterus.

Recall the sequence of events in a reverse alphabet: *V*ascularity increases, *R*ipening of the cervix, *D*ilation of the cervix progresses. Compare ripening of fruit when it becomes soft with ripening of the cervix, which also becomes soft.

2. Correct answer: 1

Progressive uterine contractions are the definitive sign of labor. Options 2 and 4 are premonitory signs to indicate that the onset of labor is getting closer. Rupture of membranes, option 3, usually occurs during labor itself.

Option 1 has the most information and has clues in the terms "regular," "progressive," and "increased intensity."

3. Correct answer: 3

Radiation of discomfort from the lower abdomen and back to the entire abdomen is characteristic for most labors. For occiput posterior positions of the fetus, "back labor" with pain centered in the lower back is the expected finding.

If you narrowed the options to 1 and 3, reread the question that asks for a "most accurate" description. Note that option 1 is a more narrow anatomic description of the event compared with option 3, which is broader or global. Make an educated guess. Option 3 is more accurate.

4. Correct answer: 3

An "S" for sacrum refers to a breech presentation in which the buttocks, foot, or feet are presenting. Therefore it is described as a longitudinal lie. The information indicates that the buttocks are 1 cm below the ischial spines, with a station of +1.

A transverse lie is where the fetal spine is perpendicular to the mother's spine or in a horizontal position. This occurs with a shoulder presentation where the scapula "Sc" is the presenting part. The clue is to interpret the data as they relate to the fetus, not the mother. Therefore, option 3 is the best answer.

5. Correct answer: 4

Engagement occurs when the biparietal diameter passes through the inlet and reaches the ischial spines. Flexion affects the anteroposterior diameters, and thereby allows the smallest or suboccipitobregmatic diameter to pass through the pelvis. Internal rotation occurs when the head turns to allow the biparietal diameter to pass between the ischial spines.

Avoid reading pelvic inlet in option 1 as the pelvic ischial spines. This can happen if you are tired or nervous.

6. Correct answer: 1

In a low-risk woman in labor the following are assessed at least every 60 minutes until a change in status occurs: FHR, uterine contractions, vaginal show, and maternal pulse, BP, and respirations. Temperature for an elevation is checked every 4 hours until the membranes rupture, then every 2 hours.

If you have no idea of a correct answer, look at the clue of time. Options 2, 3 and 4 are in hours. Option 1 is in terms of minutes, which most likely is the best answer.

7. Correct answer: 3

Option 1 refers to duration. Options 2 and 4 do not reflect the timing of uterine contraction characteristics.

The clue in the question is "frequency." This is from the onset to the onset of an event. Associate this with other types of events such as frequency of angina in cardiac clients.

8. Correct answer: 1

Sterile gloves and lubricant must be used to prevent infection. Vaginal examinations are only performed as needed to limit maternal discomfort and reduce the risk of infection. The nurse never performs examinations if vaginal bleeding is present because it could result in further separation of a placenta previa.

Clues in the options to make them incorrect are as follows. In option 2, "clean tap water" contradicts the goal to prevent infection. In option 3 the words "examination every hour" contradicts the guideline to intervene based on client need. In option 4, "if bleeding perform immediately" defies common sense to refrain from further stimulation if bleeding occurs as in this situation.

Rationales	Test-Taking Tips

9. Correct answer: 1

Although options 2, 3, and 4 are important, they should be done after the FHR pattern is assessed. Compression of the cord could occur after rupture. Compression of the cord leads to fetal hypoxia as reflected in alterations in the FHR pattern, characteristically variable decelerations in which the pattern is a V- or U-shape with no consistency occuring at the onset or end of the contractions.

A theme can be given to each option. Option 1 is the fetus, option 2 is the outlet passage evaluation, option 3 is the fluid type, and option 4 is the mother's vital signs. Of these the fetus takes precedence at any time a change occurs in the laboring process.

10. Correct answer: 3

The hands and knees position increases the mobility of the coccyx and applies the force of gravity to turn the fetal back and rotate the head. This position is effective to relieve back pain. The other positions would not be helpful.

ROP is the abbreviation for right occiputoposterior fetal position in which the occiput is in the right posterior quadrant of the maternal pelvis.

6

Assessment of Fetal Responses to Labor and Birth

FAST FACTS

1. Major stressors of the labor and birth process alter placental perfusion to inhibit gas exchange, leading to fetal hypoxia, hypercapnia, and acidosis. As a result, the fetal heart rate (FHR) patterns change.
2. Major stressors of the labor and birth process are uterine contractions, medications administered during labor, maternal position, the maternal stress response, ineffective pushing technique, and impaired placental development and function.
3. Uterine contractions cause stress during the labor process because blood flow through the placenta decreases or stops, especially at the acme of the contraction, and blood pooled in intervillous spaces provides a limited reserve for fetal gas exchange.
4. Stress increases as the duration, intensity, and frequency of the contractions progress.
5. The rest phase between contractions restores blood flow and efficient gas exchange, and rest periods become shorter with advancing labor.
6. Regional analgesics and anesthetics (epidural, spinal) administered during labor may lower maternal BP to interfere with placental perfusion. Narcotic analgesics also can lower the maternal BP and RR to reduce placental perfusion and oxygen available to the fetus.
7. A supine position during the labor and birth process puts pressure on the vena cava and aorta, leading to decreased cardiac output (CO) and hypotension that reduce placental perfusion.
8. Cord compression may occur from the cord location, maternal position, or oligohydramnios.

9. The maternal stress response, fear and anxiety, may impede labor and interfere with maternal respirations (hyperventilation).
10. An ineffective pushing technique may cause prolonged breath holding *(Valsalva maneuver)*, altering maternal oxygenation and inhibiting circulation. As a result placental perfusion may be impaired, reducing the amount of oxygen available to the fetus.
11. Maternal health problems and habits during pregnancy can affect placental development, for example, PIH, diabetes, smoking, and inadequate nutritional intake.
12. Natural aging of the placenta begins at approximately 36 weeks' gestation, creating a problem when the pregnancy is post-term. Postmaturity syndrome can result.
13. Management of labor and birth must emphasize assessment of (a) FHR patterns throughout the labor and birth process to facilitate early detection and prompt treatment of hypoxia and (b) maternal vital signs and the progress of labor to identify the degree of stress experienced by the fetus and interventions to prevent fetal hypoxia.
14. Interventions to prevent fetal hypoxia are (a) maternal relaxation techniques and frequent position changes, (b) nonpharmacologic interventions to enhance the progress of labor, (c) safe and effective administration of drugs, and (d) BDEs using open-glottis pushing.

CONTENT REVIEW

I. **Assessment of FHR pattern: primary method for determining fetal health status and response to the labor and birth process**
   A. **Intermittent auscultation: use of fetoscope or Doppler ultrasonography**
      1. Determine the point of maximum impulse (PMI) of fetal heart sounds using Leopold's maneuvers to locate the fetal back (Figures 6-1 and 6-2, p. 170)
      2. Place fetoscope or Doppler over PMI, adjusting placement until the most distinct sounds are heard
      3. Assess the maternal pulse to differentiate between uterine souffle and funic souffle
      4. Count FHR
         a. During a uterine contraction and for 30 seconds afterward to determine the effect of the uterine contraction on the FHR pattern
         b. Between contractions for 30 to 60 seconds to determine the baseline rate
      5. Adjust recommended frequency according to
         a. Phase of labor and condition of maternal-fetal unit (Table 5-1, pp. 124-127)
         b. Labor events—FHR pattern should be assessed before and after
            (1) Procedures: catheterization, vaginal examinations

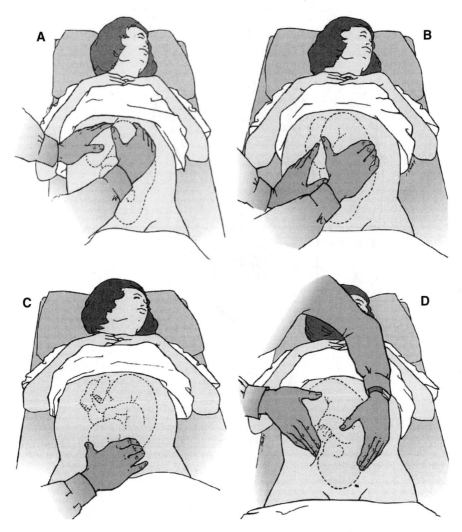

Figure 6-1   Leopold's maneuvers. (From Lowdermilk DL, Perry SE, Bobak IM: *Maternity and women's health care,* ed 7, St. Louis, 2000, Mosby.)

(2) Medication administration such as tranquilizers, analgesics, and anesthetics
(3) Labor suppression, induction, or augmentation interventions: at initiation and at each increase in dose
(4) Maternal activity: position change, ambulation, emesis, and voiding
(5) Spontaneous or artificial membrane rupture: immediately afterward and then 5 minutes later

B. *External fetal monitoring*
   1. Definition—noninvasive method of continuous or intermittent

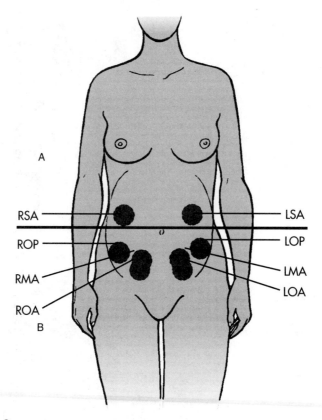

Figure 6-2 Areas of maximum intensity of FHR for differing positions: right sacrum anterior (RSA), right occipitoposterior (ROP), right mentum anterior (RMA), right occipitoanterior (ROA), left sacrum anterior (LSA), left occipitoposterior (LOP); left mentum anterior (LMA), and left occipitoanterior (LOA). **A,** presentation is breech if FHR is heard above the umbilicus. **B,** Presentation is vertex if FHR is heard below the umbilicus. (From Lowdermilk DL, Perry SE, Bobak IM: *Maternity and women's health care,* ed 7, St. Louis, 2000, Mosby.)

    monitoring of uterine contractions and FHR pattern: commonly used in low-risk pregnancies (Figure 6-3*A*)
2. Types
  a. **Tocotransducer**—device placed on abdomen over uterine fundus to assess duration and frequency of uterine contractions; intensity or resting tone is not measurable using this method
  b. **Ultrasound transducer**—device placed on abdomen over point of maximum intensity to assess FHR pattern; apply conductive gel to the transducer surface
3. Method of use (Figure 6-3*A*)
  a. Transducers are attached to the maternal abdomen using belts
  b. Placement is readjusted as needed because maternal and fetal position changes may interfere with accurate monitoring
  c. Assessment is performed for signs of skin irritation and maternal discomfort as labor progresses

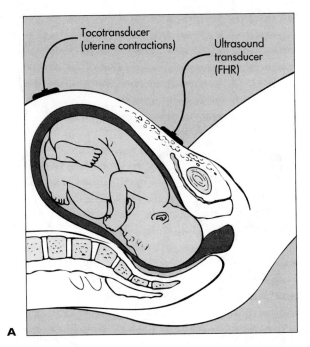

A

Figure 6-3   Electronic fetal monitoring. **A,** External fetal monitoring with tocotransducer and ultrasound transducer, with ultrasound transducer placed below umbilicus and tocotransducer placed on uterine fundus. (From Lowdermilk DL, Perry SE, Bobak IM: *Maternity and women's health care,* ed 7, St. Louis, 2000, Mosby.) *Continued*

   d. Reddened areas are massaged and cleansed; transducers are reapplied every 1 to 2 hours
   e. Portable monitors and intermittent monitoring may be used to reduce time spent in bed; maternal activity, including ambulation and frequent position changes, enhance the process of labor
C. Internal fetal monitoring
  1. Definition—invasive method of continuously monitoring uterine contractions and FHR pattern; commonly used in high-risk pregnancies or when problems are detected with external monitoring (Figure 6-3*B*, p. 172)
  2. Types
   a. Intrauterine pressure catheter (transducer)—inserted into the amniotic fluid to sense changes in intrauterine pressure during and between contractions; assesses intensity (in mm Hg), duration, and frequency of uterine contractions and resting tone
   b. Spiral electrode (cardiotachometer)—attached to the fetal presenting part for continuous assessment of FHR pattern

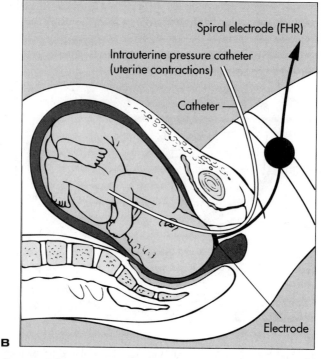

Figure 6-3, cont'd **B,** Internal fetal monitoring with intrauterine pressure catheter and spiral electrode in place (membranes ruptured and cervix dilated). (From Lowdermilk DL, Perry SE, Bobak IM: *Maternity and women's health care,* ed 7, St. Louis, 2000, Mosby.)

 3. Method of use
   a. Insertion of transducer and spiral electrode requires ruptured membranes, sufficient fetal descent, and sufficient cervical dilation
   b. Risk for infection increases; use prevention interventions and assess for signs of infection
 D. **External and internal fetal monitoring**—can be used in combination, for example, tocotransducer and spiral electrode

> ### ⚠ **Warning!**
> **Monitor strips must be evaluated and findings documented using the same frequency guidelines recommended for intermittent auscultation.**

 E. **Support interventions are required because monitoring can be frightening:**
   1. Discuss the rationale for monitoring and equipment used
   2. Describe the data collected by using the monitor strip to show the FHR pattern and uterine activity

3. Encourage the coach to use the monitor strip to facilitate guidance of prepared childbirth breathing techniques by noting the beginning, peak, and end of a contraction

II. Baseline FHR
A. **Average baseline FHR at term: 110 to 160 beats per minute; determination is made when there is no stress or stimulation affecting the fetus**
   1. During prenatal evaluation of FHR pattern
   2. During labor, between uterine contractions
B. **Variability: irregular fluctuations in baseline FHR of two or more cycles per minute as a result of mature functioning of the autonomic nervous system, which can balance cardiodeceleration (parasympathetic) and cardioacceleration (sympathetic); variability can be:**
   1. Absent or undetected; significance: nonreassuring because may be from fetal hypoxemia, acidosis, or drugs that depress CNS
   2. Minimal: less than 5 beats per minute
   3. Moderate: 6 to 25 beats per minute
   4. Marked: more than 25 beats per minute
C. **Alterations in the baseline FHR**
   1. Bradycardia
      a. FHR less than 110 beats per minute for more than 10 minutes
      b. Causes
         (1) Late hypoxia
         (2) CNS depressants and regional anesthetics (spinal, epidural)
         (3) Alteration in perfusion through cord or placenta from such factors as maternal hypotension and cord compression
      c. Significance: nonreassuring if associated with loss of variability and late deceleration
   2. Tachycardia
      a. FHR more than 160 beats per minute for more than 10 minutes
      b. Causes
         (1) Early hypoxia
         (2) Drugs such as ritodrine, terbutaline, atropine, and street drugs (cocaine, amphetamines)
         (3) Elevated maternal temperature usually associated with infection such as chorioamnionitis
         (4) Maternal hyperthyroidism
      c. Significance: nonreassuring if associated with late decelerations, severe variable decelerations, or absence of variability
   3. Alterations in variability
      a. Reduction in variability may result from:
         (1) Fetal sleep (20 to 30 minutes' duration) or first sign of hypoxia
         (2) Continued hypoxia with acidosis
         (3) Use of CNS depressants

(4) Congenital anomalies; cardiac arrhythmias

(5) Extreme prematurity (less than 24 weeks' gestation)

b. Significance: nonreassuring if caused by hypoxia and associated with late deceleration; fetal acidosis may be present

III. Periodic changes in FHR patterns are changes defined in terms of their relationship to uterine contractions, namely, timing, shape, and repetitiveness; episodic changes in FHR patterns are changes not associated with uterine contractions (Figure 6-4)

A. Acceleration of FHR: abrupt increase in FHR above baseline of 15 or more beats per minute, lasting 15 seconds or more, with return to baseline in less than 2 minutes from onset

1. Periodic: occurs with uterine contractions, often encountered with breech presentations as a result of pressure applied to fetal buttocks

2. Episodic: occurs with fetal movement and vaginal examination

3. Significance: fetal well-being

B. Early deceleration (Figure 6-4A)

1. FHR decrease (rarely below 100 beats per minute) as a result of fetal head compression, which stimulates the vagus nerve to slow the heart

2. Onset: early in contraction before the acme

3. Duration: short, with recovery to baseline by end of contraction

4. Shape: uniform; mirrors contraction shape

5. Occurrence: repetitious; occurs with each contraction between 4- and 7-cm dilation and in the second stage of labor

6. Significance: reassuring pattern

C. Late deceleration (Figure 6-4B)

1. FHR decrease (rarely below 100 beats per minute) as a result of interference with uteroplacental blood flow from such factors as maternal hypotension, analgesic or anesthetic use, placental abnormalities, uterine hyperactivity, and postmaturity

2. Onset: late in the contraction, after the acme

3. Duration: long with recovery to baseline extending into the rest period

4. Shape: uniform; mirrors contraction shape

5. Occurrence: repetitious; occurs with each contraction; influenced by intensity, duration, and frequency of contractions

6. Significance: nonreassuring because it is associated with fetal hypoxemia and acidosis, especially if combined with baseline changes

D. Variable deceleration (Figure 6-4C)

1. Abrupt FHR decrease as a result of cord compression from cord prolapse, maternal position, cord around fetal neck, short or knotted cord, or oligohydramnios

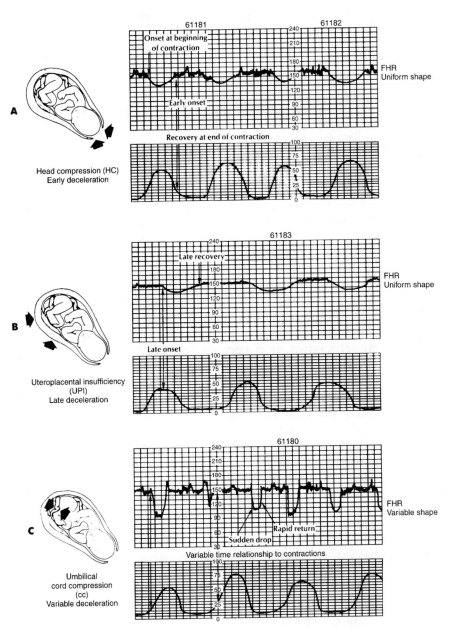

Figure 6-4 **A,** Early decelerations caused by head compression. **B,** Late deceleration caused by uteroplacental insufficiency. **C,** Variable deceleration caused by cord compression. (From Lowdermilk DL, Perry SE, Bobak IM: *Maternity and women's health care,* ed 7, St. Louis, 2000, Mosby.)

2. Onset, duration (length of time from onset to recovery), and depth of deceleration: variable depending on degree and duration of the compression (partial, complete, brief, prolonged); classified as mild, moderate, or severe

3. Shape: variable usually with sudden decrease in FHR (U-, V-, or W-shaped)

4. Occurrence: late in labor with rupture of membranes (ROM), fetal descent, pushing

5. Significance: mild are reassuring; moderate to severe are nonreassuring, especially if associated with baseline changes

E. Prolonged decelerations

1. Decrease in FHR below baseline of 15 or more beats per minute lasting more than 2 and less than 10 minutes caused from pelvic examination, application of spiral electrode, rapid fetal descent, prolonged Valsalva maneuver, progressive or severe variable deceleration, hypotension, tetanic uterine contractions, or maternal hypoxia

2. Significance: usually isolated and self-limiting; nonreassuring if associated with severe variable decelerations or with a prolonged series of late decelerations

IV. Characteristics of a *reassuring FHR pattern*

A. Baseline FHR of 110 to 160 beats per minute
B. Moderate baseline variability
C. Accelerations of FHR with fetal movement
D. Early decelerations and mild variable deceleration

V. Characteristics of normal uterine activity patterns

A. Frequency of 2 to 5 minutes
B. Duration of less than 90 seconds
C. Moderate to strong intensity of less than 100 mg Hg
D. Resting phase of at least 30 seconds; decreased tone of 15 mm Hg or less

VI. Assessment findings indicative of fetal distress

A. Characteristics of *nonreassuring FHR patterns;* warnings of mild to severe hypoxia and worsening fetal distress
1. Progressive increase or decrease in baseline
2. Tachycardia
3. Progressive decrease in baseline variability
4. Moderate to severe variable decelerations
5. Late decelerations
6. Absence of FHR variability
7. Prolonged decelerations
8. Severe bradycardia of less than 70 beats per minute

⚠️ **Warning!**

Amniotic fluid stained with meconium (thick, dark-green fecal substance found in fetal intestines) may occur in cephalic presentations and commonly occurs in breech presentations. Hypoxia increases intestinal peristalsis and relaxes the anal sphincter, causing passage of meconium.

VII. Interventions effective in the prevention and treatment of fetal distress

A. **Prevention**
   1. Alter the maternal position regularly, every 30 to 60 minutes
   2. Use nonpharmacologic measures to enhance the progress of labor, reduce anxiety, enhance relaxation, and maintain effective natural respiratory pattern
   3. Use pharmacologic measures judiciously to reduce pain or stimulate labor
   4. Teach and encourage effective pushing techniques that emphasize upright positions, cleansing breaths, and open-glottis pushing with catch breaths

B. **Treatment interventions: measure(s) used depend on the underlying cause of fetal distress; follow established protocol and professional standards**
   1. Enhance CO and uteroplacental circulation
      a. Turn to side-lying position to decrease pressure on vena cava and aorta
      b. Change maternal position to remove pressure on the cord
   2. Increase circulating blood volume: raise legs, start or increase rate of IV fluids
   3. Oxygenate blood; administer oxygen using a facemask at 8 to 10 L/min
   4. Reduce uterine hyperactivity:
      a. Discontinue oxytocin (Pitocin) infusion
      b. Administer tocolytics (medications that suppress contractions) as needed, for example, terbutaline, 0.25 mg, SQ
   5. Initiate prompt intervention for cord prolapse
      a. Reduce pressure on cord
         (1) Elevate presenting part with gloved hand
         (2) Change maternal position to elevate hips: modified Sims, Trendelenburg, or knee-chest position
      b. Maintain cord integrity
         (1) Wrap protruding cord in sterile compress of warm normal saline
         (2) Never attempt to reinsert cord
      c. Administer oxygen, start or increase IV fluids

6. Administer narcotic antagonist [naloxone hydrochloride (Narcan)] to mother if birth is imminent, to neonate after birth, or both
7. Reduce cord compression from oligohydramnios by instilling warm, sterile normal saline into uterus (amnioinfusion)
8. Reduce maternal fever and treat infection

VIII. Documentation about the fetal health status

A. **For assessment findings about FHR pattern**
   1. According to recommended frequency for low- and high-risk pregnancies and policy or protocol of the agency (see Table 5-1, pp. 124-127)
   2. Before and after significant labor events
B. **For intermittent auscultation, description of the FHR pattern in terms of:**
   1. Rate and rhythm
   2. Presence or absence of changes from uterine contractions or significant labor events
C. **For electronic monitoring (follow agency protocol)**
   1. Documentation in nurses' notes: description of monitor tracings, including average baseline FHR, degree of variability, and presence of accelerations or decelerations
   2. Documentation directly on tracing: maternal vital signs, status, and position changes, pushing, fetal movement, significant labor events, and adjustments in monitor or transducers
   3. Attach tracing to woman's chart because it is a legal component
D. **All actions taken in terms of identified fetal distress patterns and outcomes of the actions taken**
E. **Follow hospital or agency policy when documenting FHR patterns**
   1. What to document
   2. When to document: frequency
   3. Where to document: nurses' notes, tracings
   4. Handling of tracings after birth: these stay with the woman's chart or are filed on labor unit

WEB Resources

http://www.obgyn.net
   OBGYN.net is the Universe of Women's Health. Begin by clicking on the Medical Professionals Section, then click on Fetal Monitoring in the left-hand column.

http://www.med.umich.edu
   University of Michigan Health System. Begin by clicking on Health Topics A to Z, then click on Women's Health. From this point, you can access a variety of topics and sites related to pregnancy, childbirth, postpartum, and the newborn—low risk and high risk. Clicking on Tests and Procedures gives you access to fetal monitoring information.

REVIEW QUESTIONS

1. The point of maximum intensity (PMI) of the fetal heart rate (FHR) should be identified to facilitate accurate placement of the ultrasound stethoscope, fetoscope, or ultrasound transducer. Which of these methods should be used to identify the point of maximum intensity?
   1. Vaginal examination
   2. Leopold's maneuvers
   3. Ritgen's maneuver
   4. Effleurage

2. When caring for a laboring woman with external fetal monitoring, the nurse should take which action?
   1. Apply contact gel to the surface of the tocotransducer and ultrasound transducer before placement on the abdomen
   2. Place the tocotransducer over the point of maximal impulse (PMI)
   3. Keep the woman in a semi-recumbent position to ensure accuracy of the tracings
   4. Reapply the transducers and massage reddened areas at least once every 1 to 2 hours

3. The nurse caring for a woman in labor should recognize that fetal tachycardia is most likely the result of which factor?
   1. Fetal movement
   2. Maternal hypotension
   3. Elevation in maternal core temperature, i.e., fever
   4. Administration of narcotic analgesics

4. On review of a fetal monitor tracing, the nurse notes that for several contractions the FHR decelerates as a contraction begins but returns to baseline just before it ends. The nurse should
   1. Document the finding in the nurse's notes
   2. Reposition the woman onto her side, either right or left
   3. Call the physician for instructions
   4. Administer oxygen at 8 to 10 L/min with a tight facemask

5. The membranes of a woman in labor have just ruptured. During fetal heart rate (FHR) pattern assessment the nurse must be alert for which changes that are characteristic for cord compression?
   1. Baseline tachycardia
   2. Early deceleration
   3. Late deceleration
   4. Variable deceleration

ANSWERS, RATIONALES, AND TEST-TAKING TIPS

Rationales	Test-Taking Tips

1. Correct answer: 2

Leopold's maneuvers are a system of abdominal palpations to identify fetal presentation, position, and location of fetal parts. PMI usually is found over the curved back of the fetus. Ritgen's maneuver is used to control the birth of the head. *Effleurage* is the rhythmic stroking of the abdomen for relaxation and distraction during a contraction.

First eliminate the obvious incorrect answer, option 1. Then recall what you know—option 4 is a stroking technique—to eliminate option 4. Of the remaining options, select the one you are most familiar with, which is most likely option 2, Leopold's maneuvers. Let the letter P in Leopold be the clue—the Parts, Presentation, and Position of the fetus are Palpated.

2. Correct answer: 4

Only the ultrasound transducer requires contact gel before application over the PMI. The tocotransducer is placed over the fundus. Maternal position should be changed every 30 to 60 minutes and the transducers can be readjusted as needed.

The clue is "when caring for." Options 1 and 2 are associated with the setup of the monitoring equipment. Option 3 is less likely to be appropriate for all women, especially because the position would be changed for comfort or circulation purposes.

3. Correct answer: 3

Fetal movement should result in an acceleration of FHR, which is limited in duration and remains within the normal range. Options 2 and 4 result in bradycardia. Fetal tachycardia is a classic sign of maternal fever related to infection.

Recall that the FHR response to maternal hypotension is the opposite of what the mother's heart rate does. The mother's HR increases and the fetal heart rate decreases. Make an educated guess by application of a general concept, that is, fever results in an increased heart rate.

4. Correct answer: 1

An early deceleration pattern from head compression is described. No further action is required. Options 2, 3, and 4 would be implemented when nonreassuring changes

Important terms to guide you to select the option with no further action are "several contractions," and "returns to baseline." Early deceleration patterns are always reassuring. They can happen with every contraction

are noted. The sequence of actions is to reposition to the side, give oxygen, and call the physician.

until the cervix is wide enough and the pressure on the head is decreased.

5. Correct answer: 4

Variable deceleration patterns occur when compression inhibits circulation through the cord. The risk factors are oligohydramnios, cord prolapse, maternal position, short cord, or cord around the fetal neck. The degree of compression and when it occurs in relation to the contraction influence the pattern established. Early decelerations usually are benign and only require continued monitoring. Late decelerations, most commonly caused by placental insufficiency, are nonreassuring to require the three essential actions (in this order) of reposition, administer oxygen, and call the physician.

Associate decelerations with your work pattern. If you consistently arrive at work early, you are in no trouble and this fact might go to your head—you think you can do no wrong. Similarly, early decelerations caused from head compression typically cause no harm or trouble in the delivery process. In contrast, if you consistently arrive at work late, you will get into trouble. Late decelerations are the same and are caused from placental insufficiency; associate the Ls in late and placenta. Finally, if you are sometimes late, early, or on time in getting to work, your pattern is variable and you will get into trouble. It is the same with variable decelerations in which the cord becomes compressed. Depending on the degree of compression, this can lead to moderate or severe variable deceleration patterns that are nonreassuring and require the three essential actions. Note that *mild variable deceleration patterns* are often interpreted as reassuring.

7

Complications of Childbirth

FAST FACTS

1. A labor that does not conform to expected norms increases maternal stress, which may result in (a) feelings of powerlessness as labor becomes more managed and medically oriented, (b) diminished self-confidence and self-esteem as the woman feels unable to secure safe passage, (c) fear and anxiety as concern for the safety of the maternal-fetal unit begins to increase, and (d) stress response by the body that interferes with the progress of labor.
2. The nursing process is the organizing framework for the care management of the laboring woman and her support system.
3. Thorough, ongoing, and frequent assessments of the maternal-fetal unit and the progress of labor determine (1) baseline data before initiation of labor suppression, augmentation, or induction; (2) expected effects and identification of side effects during treatment; and (3) psychosocial effects of the treatment plan on the woman and her family (see Box 7-1, p. 189).
4. Nursing diagnoses reflect the physical and psychosocial effects of complications of childbirth (see Box 7-2, p. 201).
5. Nursing interventions and evaluations emphasize (1) interventions to facilitate the labor process: comfort, nutrition, hydration, activity, and positioning; (2) safe, knowledgeable implementation of ordered treatment protocols, (3) emotional support of the pregnant woman and family with explanations of interventions and descriptions of progress; and (4) detailed, ongoing documentation of observations made, actions taken, and results of actions.

CONTENT REVIEW

I. *Dystocia*
A. Definition—an abnormal, dysfunctional, or difficult process of labor resulting primarily from ineffective uterine contractions *(powers of labor)*, fetal problems *(passenger)*, or pelvic inadequacy *(passage)*
B. Uterine dystocia
  1. Contributing factors
    a. Pharmacologic interventions—analgesics or anesthetics administered too early or in too large a dose; oxytocin (Pitocin) is improperly regulated
    b. Activity level during labor: limitations on position change and activity
    c. Limitations on fluid and nutrient intake during labor lead to dehydration and energy depletion
    d. Bladder and bowel distention
    e. Uterine factors
      (1) Overdistention from macrosomia, multiple gestation, or hydramnios
      (2) Repeated stretching as with grand multiparity
      (3) Rigid cervix (older primigravida)
    f. Fetal factors—malpresentation, cephalopelvic disproportion, fetal anomalies such as hydrocephalus
  2. Types of contractions characteristic of dystocia
    a. Hypotonic uterine contractions—infrequent (less than 3 but within 10 minutes), irregular pattern; mild or low intensity
      (1) Typically occur during the active phase after a normal latent phase among multiparous women
      (2) Result in a protracted, arrested active phase
    b. Hypertonic uterine contractions—painful, strong, ineffective uterine contractions lacking fundal dominance; short rest periods, with increased resting tone
      (1) Typically occur during the latent phase of a nulliparous woman; may be from a higher level of anxiety in first-time labors
      (2) Results in a prolonged latent phase
  3. Patterns of dysfunctional labor are classified according to latent and active phases of the first stage of labor and are determined and evaluated by plotting the labor progress on a partogram
    a. Prolonged latent phase
      (1) Duration of more than 20 hours (nullipara) or more than 14 hours (multipara)
      (2) Typically noted in combination with *hypertonic* contractions
      (3) Management commonly involves therapeutic rest with use of narcotic analgesics, comfort measures and relaxation

techniques to facilitate a rest period of 4 to 6 hours; after a rest period the active phase of labor usually begins

b. Protracted active phase
   (1) Duration of the active phase of labor is prolonged from the slowing of dilation, fetal descent, or both
   (2) Nullipara: dilation less than 1.2 cm/hr, fetal descent less than 1 cm/hr, or both
   (3) Multipara: dilation less than 1.5 cm/hr, fetal descent less than 2 cm/hr, or both
   (4) Typically noted in combination with *hypotonic* contractions
   (5) Management involves ruling out *cephalopelvic disproportion (CPD)*, that is, when the fetal head is too large to fit though the pelvis, the pelvis is too small, or both. Institute labor augmentation methods if the pelvis is adequate.

c. Arrested active phase
   (1) Progress stops in terms of dilation, descent, or both
   (2) Absence of progress in dilation for more than 2 hours during the active phase
   (3) Absence of progress in fetal descent for 1 hour or more (nullipara) or 30 minutes or more (multipara)
   (4) Frequently associated with cephalopelvic disproportion (CPD)
   (5) Management involves the same interventions as for a protracted active phase. Cesarean birth is more likely since CPD is most likely the cause.

d. Precipitous labor
   (1) Rapidly paced labor; birth occurs 3 hours or less after labor onset
   (2) Often associated with intense frequent contractions that may occur with Pitocin administration or cocaine use, with low resistance of maternal tissues, resulting in a more rapid pace of dilation or descent or both
   (3) May result in a precipitous unattended birth accompanied by tearing of maternal tissue, early placental separation, and fetal cranial damage
   (4) Management includes slowing of labor with the use of tocolytics or planned induction of labor at term to control the onset and the progress of labor

C. Passenger dystocia
1. Fetal injury is a major concern from
   a. Trauma associated with medical interventions to accomplish birth such as external versions, forceps, vacuum extractor, or cesarean birth
   b. Hypoxia associated with cord compression

2. Contributing factors
   a. Fetal size
      (1) Skull: excessively large or hard associated with hydrocephalus or postmaturity syndrome; limits molding during passage
      (2) Macrosomia: large fetus for gestational age from increased intrauterine growth; associated with maternal diabetes
   b. Multiple gestations
   c. Fetal presentation or position
      (1) Occipitoposterior position: increased internal rotation arc to align occiput with symphysis pubis
      (2) Face presentation: extension of neck presents larger cephalic diameter for passage; facial bruising and edema result with vaginal birth
      (3) Shoulder presentation: fetus in transverse lie with shoulder presenting
      (4) Breech presentation: fetal buttocks, feet, or foot present: associated with
         (a) Prolonged labor from slow dilation; buttocks are less effective as a dilator
         (b) Hypoxia from cord compression; prolapse is more common
         (c) Passage of the head with less time to mold or accommodate the pelvis
         (d) Passage of meconium is more common with compression of abdomen and buttocks
         (e) Meconium aspiration because breathing can begin with emergence of the body
D. **Management of passenger dystocia: the size of maternal pelvis and the condition of maternal-fetal unit are major determining factors:**
   1. Maternal pelvis is adequate for passage of the fetus
      a. Forceps- or vacuum-assistance to facilitate internal rotation and birth of the head
      b. Maternal positioning to facilitate rotation and descent, for example, the hands and knees position facilitates internal rotation when the head is in occipitoposterior position
      c. External version attempted after 37 weeks' gestation to change presentation from breech or shoulder to cephalic by gentle pressure over the abdomen
   2. Maternal pelvis is inadequate, borderline, or doubtful (nullipara): cesarean birth is the method of choice

II. Preterm labor

A. **Definition—labor begins after 20 to 24 weeks' but before the end of 37 weeks' gestation; preterm birth is a major cause of perinatal morbidity and mortality**

B. Contributing factors
1. Previous history of preterm labor or birth
2. Demographic factors
   a. Age less than 17 or over 34 years
   b. Race (African-American)
   c. Low socioeconomic status
   d. Inadequate prenatal care
   e. Unmarried
   f. Low level of education
3. Lifestyle factors
   a. Inadequate nutrition, anemia, and hyperemesis
   b. Poor hygienic practices and unsafe sex practices
   c. Substance abuse—tobacco, alcohol, or cocaine
   d. Stress and difficulty resting
4. Health problems
   a. Infections of genitourinary tract or systemic infections, especially accompanied by fever
   b. Chronic health problems such as diabetes and hypertension
5. Uterine factors
   a. Abnormalities, for example, incompetent cervix, short cervix, or fibroids
   b. Conditions that interfere with myometrial blood flow such as overdistention with multiple gestation or *hydramnios,* which is an excessive amount of amniotic fluid; also called polyhydramnios
   c. Uterine trauma associated with surgery, childbirth injuries, or accidents
   d. Preterm premature rupture of the membranes

C. Detection of preterm labor
1. Early detection of preterm labor is important because labor suppression methods are more successful if major cervical changes have not occurred
2. Biochemical markers—fetal fibronectin is present in the cervical mucous and estriol in the saliva; detection at 24 to 34 weeks' gestation could predict the onset of preterm labor
3. Signs of preterm labor—vague and nonspecific; diagnosis of preterm labor is based on contraction pattern and cervical changes
   a. Uterine contractions:
      (1) Frequency of 1 every 10 minutes or less (six or more in one hour)
      (2) Regular pattern of increasing intensity, duration, and frequency develops
      (3) Often painless, with a sensation of tightening or tingling
   b. Cervical changes: ripening, effacement (up to 80%), and dilation (up to 2 cm)
   c. Discomfort
      (1) Dull, low, backache
      (2) Abdominal or menstrual-like cramping, with or without diarrhea
      (3) Pelvic pressure; feels like fetus is pressing down

    d. Vaginal discharge—sudden change in characteristics or increase in amount

  4. All pregnant women, especially those at high risk, must be taught how to detect the early signs of preterm labor

D. Conservative interventions to suppress preterm labor are more successful if cervical changes are minimal

  1. Home: when signs of labor are detected, woman should
    a. Empty bladder
    b. Drink 3 to 4 glasses of water, with each being 6 to 8 ounces
    c. Lie down in a lateral recumbent position
    d. Continue to count contractions
    e. If contractions are not suppressed within 1 hour the woman is to notify the physician and is usually admitted for evaluation

  2. Hospital
    a. Bed rest in the lateral recumbent position
    b. Adequate hydration without hypervolemia; combination of oral and IV intake limited to 2400 ml/day, or 100 ml/hr
    c. Regular voiding at 2-hour intervals to prevent bladder distension
    d. Interventions to enhance relaxation: emotional support, relaxation techniques, and explanations of procedures and progress
    e. Gather baseline data about maternal, fetal, and labor status in anticipation of tocolytic therapy (Box 7-1)

E. Pharmacologic approaches for preterm labor: If conservative interventions are unsuccessful, *tocolytics* are administered to suppress contractions; antenatal glucocorticoids are administered to stimulate fetal lungs to produce surfactant in anticipation of birth.

  1. Criteria to be met
    a. Fetus—healthy at 20 to 36 weeks' gestation, with no signs of distress, severe intrauterine growth restriction, or major anomalies incompatible with life
    b. Mother—must be relatively healthy without significant bleeding, intrauterine infection, severe PIH, or health problems incompatible with the tocolytic drug being used, for example, heart disease with ritodrine or terbutaline
    c. Definitive signs of preterm labor have been confirmed

  2. Tocolytic medications
    a. Beta-sympathomimetics and magnesium sulfate—the most common tocolytics used today (Table 7-1, p. 190)
    b. Other tocolytic drugs that can be used—indomethacin (prostaglandin inhibitor) and nifedipine (calcium channel blocker)

  3. Antenatal glucocorticoids such as betamethasone benzoate when pregnancy is 24 to 34 weeks'gestation
    a. Intramuscular administration of 12 mg twice; 12 hours apart
    b. Requires 24 hours to become effective

Box 7-1
Assessment Actions to Determine Maternal-Fetal Unit Status and the Progress of Labor

Maternal Status:

Circulatory status: BP, apical and radial pulse, signs of thrombophlebitis
Respiratory status: effort rate, regularity, and depth of respirations, chest sounds
Hydration status: input and output, weight, edema, signs of fluid excess or deficit
Health status including signs of infection: fever, maternal and fetal tachycardia, malodorous vaginal discharge, malaise
Comfort status: level of pain or discomfort and effectiveness of relief interventions
Emotional status: expressions of fear, anxiety, and stress
CNS status: level of consciousness, orientation, deep tendon reflexes
Laboratory and diagnostic testing as needed: electrocardiogram, CBC, urinalysis, serum electrolytes, glucose level

Fetal Status:

FHR pattern using auscultation or electronic monitoring as appropriate
Fetal presentation, changes in station and position
Signs of fetal distress: nonreassuring FHR patterns, passage of meconium, nonreactive NST, low BPP score, positive CST
Fetal lung maturity; gestational age

Progress of Labor:

Uterine activity: characteristics and progress of uterine contractions
Cervical changes: passage of mucous plug, ripening, effacement, and dilation
Pattern of labor progress: partogram is used
WARNING! To prevent infection, vaginal examinations to determine the progress of cervical change and fetal descent are performed only as warranted and not at a set frequency. Prevention of infection is especially important once membranes are ruptured.

F. **Health teaching and supportive interventions for women at risk for preterm birth**
1. Medication instructions
    a. Safe administration of the drug prescribed to include when and how to take it and assessments to be done before the dose
    b. Pump maintenance measures
    c. Signs of toxicity and what to do if they appear
2. Signs of labor: assessment to include how to use a home uterine activity monitor
    a. Assume a lateral recumbent position and assess for uterine contractions for 1 full hour twice a day
    b. Palpate uterine fundus with fingertips taking note of muscle tightening, *or* apply external monitor over fundus; the monitor records uterine activity and stores data for later telephone transmission

Text continued on p. 194

TABLE 7-1 Administration and Nursing Implications of Tocolytics

Tocolytic	Principles of Administration	Nursing Implications
Beta-sympathomimetics Ritodrine (Yutopar): Only drug approved by the FDA for labor suppression Used less often owing to side effects, especially with IV use	Intravenous route: Prepare ritodrine solution by mixing ritodrine in an isotonic solution; label the bag (150 mg in 500 ml of solution) Attach ritodrine solution to a controller-pump Piggyback ritodrine solution to the primary line at the port closest to the IV insertion site (port most proximal to the woman) Begin infusion, increase rate, and maintain infusion according to agency protocol, physician order, and woman's response Document the status of the maternal-fetal unit and labor at each increment on chart or flow sheet and monitor strip (see Box 7-1, p. 189) Begin oral tocolytics approximately 30 min before discontinuing the infusion Oral route (limited effectiveness from limited absorption, side effects, poor client compliance, and rapid contraction breakthrough): 5-10 mg every 4 hr; must be taken on time with food to limit GI distress Check pulse before each dose; acceptable range of 90-110 beats/min; hold if pulse is >120	Provide explanations before treatment initiation Assess status of maternal-fetal unit and labor at frequent intervals, especially during IV administration (see Box 7-1, p. 189) Position woman on her side Observe for specific side effects from administration of beta-sympathomimetics such as: Maternal-fetal tachycardia and palpitations with skipped beats Alteration in BP with widening pulse pressure progressing to hypotension Fluid volume excess progressing to pulmonary edema Transient hyperglycemia with increased insulin secretion and metabolic acidosis; transient hypokalemia Nausea and vomiting CNS irritability: tremors, nervousness, agitation, restlessness Neonatal glucose imbalance may occur during the first 24 hr after birth Observe for signs of reportable conditions that require the treatment be discontinued and physician notified:

Continued

Notify health care provider:

Drug side effects such as palpitations, pulse >120 beats/min, chest pain, dyspnea, tremors, nervousness

Signs of labor

Signs of infection

Terbutaline (Brethine)

More commonly used than ritodrine

Usually given SQ and via continuous pump infusion

Subcutaneous route:

Injection of 0.25 mg every 30 min for 2 hr, then a maximum dosage of 0.5 mg every 4-6 hr

Terbutaline pump increases contraction breakthrough time to 6 wk, thus prolonging pregnancy; it provides:

Continuous maintenance (low) dosage of 0.05-0.1 mg/hr

Bolus dosage of 0.25 mg every 4-6 hr according to woman's unique contraction pattern; hold for pulse >110 beats/min

Approximately 3 mg/24 hr are administered

Teach woman and family principles of treatment including:

Use of pump: change of syringe, rotation of site (every 3-4 days), adjustment of dosage

Site assessment for signs of infection

Self-assessment for signs of labor and side effects of terbutaline

Maternal HR >120-140 beats/min, cardiac dysrhythmias

FHR >180 beats/min

BP <90/60 mm Hg

Signs of pulmonary edema, chest pain

WARNING! Keep propranolol (Inderal) 0.5-1 mg at the bedside for emergency administration when toxic effects appear from cardiac function

Limit fluid intake to 90 ml/hr

Maintain strict asepsis to prevent infection especially if membranes are ruptured

Intervene to minimize the effects of bed rest

Assist with antiembolic stockings, range-of-motion exercises to lower extremities to prevent blood pooling

Alternate position

Cough and breathe deeply

Provide comfort measures, emotional support, relaxing diversions

Provide home care support and follow-up with telephone contact and home visitation weekly or biweekly

TABLE 7-1 Administration and Nursing Implications of Tocolytics—cont'd

Tocolytic	Principles of Administration	Nursing Implications
Magnesium Sulfate Along with terbutaline, this is a first-line drug for suppression of labor Effective with fewer side effects than the beta-sympathomimetics	Intravenous route: Prepare a loading dose of 4-6 g of magnesium sulfate in 100-250 ml of IV solution and administer via infusion pump over 15-20 min; one dose of terbutaline, 0.25 mg SQ, may be given just before the loading dose because magnesium sulfate has a slower onset than other tocolytics Continue infusion at 1 g/hr, gradually progressing to 3 g/hr; follow agency protocol and physician's order for dosage and maintenance until uterine contractions are suppressed or magnesium toxicity occurs Begin oral tocolytics or terbutaline pump before discontinuing the infusion Monitor urine output because an output <25 ml/hr increases likelihood of hypermagnesemia	Provide explanations before treatment initiation Assess maternal-fetal unit and labor status at frequent intervals (see Box 7-1, p. 189) Observe for specific findings that indicate hypermagnesemia: Transient flushing, sweating at start of treatment Depression of CNS as noted in diminished level of consciousness, and deep tendon reflexes, drowsiness Check DTR every hour Depressed cardiac and respiratory function Check respirations every hour Check for hypotension Assess chest sounds taking note of signs of pulmonary edema

GI distress: nausea and vomiting

Serum magnesium levels should be 6-8 mg/dl (4-7 mEq/L)

Hypocalcemia: paresthesia, tetany

Neonatal hypermagnesemia: especially if maternal levels rose above 8 mEq/L—noted as transient lethargy and poor feeding behavior

Observe for reportable conditions that require the treatment be discontinued and physician notified:

RR <12 breaths/min

Absence of deep tendon reflexes

Severe hypotension

Serum magnesium rising above therapeutic level

WARNING! Keep calcium gluconate (1 g of a 10% solution) at the bedside for emergency administration to reverse CNS depression and diminished respirations

Additional care interventions include comfort, emotional support, diversional activities, and minimizing the effects of bed rest

    c. Record time, frequency, duration, and perceived intensity of uterine contractions experienced

    d. Take note of any associated signs of labor

    e. Report findings during daily telephone contact with a nurse

  3. Actions to take if signs of labor are noted

  4. Interventions to prevent the onset of preterm labor and cope with required lifestyle changes

    a. Balance activity and rest, pace activities, and take frequent rest periods in the lateral recumbent position; bed rest may be required; avoid lifting

    b. Take a leave of absence from a job

    c. Avoid sexual activity, which leads to orgasm and stimulates the cervix

    d. Avoid stimulation of nipples (endogenous oxytocin)

    e. Prevent genitourinary tract infection because infection is associated with premature rupture of membranes and onset of labor

    f. Maintain nutrient and fluid balance and appropriate weight gain: small, frequent meals and adequate fluid intake (2 to 3 L/day); avoid caffeine and other stimulants

    g. Reduce stress by engaging in pleasant, distracting activities, and performing relaxation techniques

    h. Involve family in the treatment regimen; make referrals to home care agencies

III. Spontaneous rupture of the membranes before the onset of labor

  A. Types

    1. *Premature rupture of the membranes (PROM):* rupture of membranes after the completion of the 37th week of gestation, with labor usually beginning within 12 to 24 hours

    2. *Preterm premature rupture of the membranes (PPROM):* rupture of membranes before the 38th week of gestation

  B. Contributing factors

    1. Reproductive tract infections: microorganisms can weaken the amniotic membranes

    2. Increased intrauterine pressure as a result of hydramnios or multiple gestation

    3. Lifestyle habits, including poor dietary practices and smoking cigarettes

    4. Fetal anomalies and malpresentations

  C. Complications

    1. Risk for infection: membranes no longer protect uterus and fetus

    2. Fetal hypoxia from cord compression: prolapse or oligohydramnios

D. Management
1. Determine
   a. Time of rupture; gestational week
   b. Characteristics of fluid: amount, color, odor, ferning (present or absent), and nitrazine test (alkaline or acid result)
   c. Fetal lung maturity by the use of the amniotic fluid to determine the lecithin-sphingomyelin (L/S) ratio and the presence of phosphatidylglycerol (PG); rupture may enhance surfactant production
2. Watchful waiting if tear is small with minimal fluid loss, pregnancy is preterm, and signs of infection are absent; ongoing assessment and infection control interventions are critical
3. Prevent preterm labor onset and help the woman to cope with any required lifestyle changes; see discussion of preterm labor on pp. 186-189, 194.
4. Administer antenatal glucocorticoids to stimulate lung maturation if birth is inevitable and infection is not present
5. Assist to induce labor if pregnancy is at term and labor does not begin spontaneously

IV. *Prolonged/post-term pregnancy*
A. **Definition—pregnancy lasts 42 or more weeks; accounts for a significant number of perinatal deaths**
B. **Complications**
   1. Dystocia: from ineffective contraction patterns, macrosomia with large head and limited molding ability; pelvis unable to accommodate macrosomic fetus
   2. **Postmaturity/dysmaturity syndrome:** newborn exhibits evidence of the detrimental effects of placental aging
      a. Placental aging begins at 36 weeks' gestation, gradually limiting its ability to supply the fetus with oxygen and nutrients
         (1) Fetal hypoxia leads to nonreassuring FHR patterns, such as late decelerations and diminished variability, and the passage of meconium
         (2) Meconium in amniotic fluid increases the risk for intrauterine infection, drying of the cord, and meconium aspiration
         (3) Alteration in nutrition leads to weight loss; decreased subcutaneous tissue; dry, cracked, loose, peeling skin; and muscle wasting
         (4) Neonatal hypoglycemia as glucose stores are used up before birth
      b. Amniotic fluid begins to decrease after 38 weeks' gestation; oligohydramnios leads to cord compression and nonreassuring FHR patterns such as variable decelerations and diminished variability

C. **Management**
  1. Confirm gestational age and determine status of the maternal-fetal unit
  2. When the cervix is not ripe but the maternal-fetal unit is healthy: watchful waiting with close surveillance of the status of the maternal-fetal unit with the use of appropriate antepartal tests
  3. When the cervix is not ripe but the maternal-fetal unit is compromised by high-risk factors, signs of postmaturity syndrome, or both: ripen cervix and induce labor or perform a cesarean birth
  4. When the cervix is ripe: induce labor
  5. In oligohydramnios, use an *amnioinfusion,* an instillation of warm normal saline into uterine cavity to relieve cord compression

V. Stimulation of the process of labor
  A. *Augmentation of labor*
  1. Definition—enhancement of existing uterine contractions to facilitate the progress of labor
  2. Purpose: used for hypotonic dysfunctional labor, protracted active phase, and slowing of labor progress as from epidural anesthesia
  3. Methods
    a. Breast stimulation—facilitate endogenous release of oxytocin from the posterior pituitary gland by stimulation of the nipple manually or with a breast pump
    b. *Amniotomy*—an artificial rupture of the amniotic membranes, enhances prostaglandin production and allows fetal head to act as cervical dilator
      (1) It is recommended that cervix be dilated by at least 4 cm and the fetal presenting part be engaged or at station 0
      (2) Assessment and care interventions before and after amniotomy are the same as for spontaneous membrane rupture
    c. IV administration of Pitocin (Table 7-2)
  B. *Induction of labor*—stimulation of the onset of labor when a valid medical reason exists. Examples include postmaturity, intrauterine growth restriction, fetal stress, premature ruptured

TABLE 7-2   Bishop's Scale to Determine Cervical Ripeness

Cervical Factor	0	1	2	3
Dilation (cm)	Closed	1-2	3-4	5-6
Effacement (%)	0-30%	40-50%	60-70%	80%
Station (cm)	−3	−2	−1, 0	+1
Consistency	Firm	Medium	Soft	—
Cervical position	Posterior	Midline	Anterior	—

membranes **(PROM), chorioamnionitis, high-risk pregnancy, history of precipitous labor and birth.**

C. **Assessment of the readiness of the maternal-fetal unit for labor stimulation procedures**
   1. Criteria for stimulation are met
      a. Fetal lung maturity is established
      b. Fetus is capable of passage through pelvis
      c. Fetal presenting part is engaged or at station 0
      d. Uterine myometrium is capable of withstanding the demands of childbirth
   2. Current physical status of the maternal-fetal unit is determined (see Box 7-1)
   3. Cervical ripeness and readiness for a response to labor stimulation is determined by the use of Bishop's scale (Table 7-2); Bishop's scale is used to determine the score that indicates cervical ripeness
      a. Score of less than five indicates a relatively unreceptive cervix, with limited chance for successful stimulation of labor
      b. Score of five to eight has a 95% success rate
      c. Score of nine or over has little to no chance of failure
D. **Pharmacologic interventions used to ripen the cervix: assess status of the maternal-fetal unit** (see Box 7-1, p. 189) **and determine Bishop's score** (see Table 7-2) **before and after administration of ripening agent. Ensure that the criteria for stimulation of labor have been met.**
   1. Prostaglandin E_2 is used most often in the form of dinoprostone gel (Prepidil Gel) or dinoprostone insert (Cervidil)
   2. Administration of a Cervidil insert
      a. Do not use in the presence of nonreassuring FHR patterns, maternal fever or infection, vaginal bleeding, hypersensitivity, or regular progressing contractions
      b. Use with caution if woman has history of asthma, glaucoma, renal, hepatic, or cardiovascular disorder
      c. Insert into posterior fornix
      d. Assist woman to maintain a supine with lateral tilt or side-lying position for 2 hours
      e. Assess for hyperstimulation of uterus with nonreassuring FHR pattern; if this is found, remove the insert
      f. Determine cervical ripeness; when the cervix is ripe the insert is removed and induction begins if needed within 30 minutes after removal
E. **Administration of Pitocin to augment or induce labor; Table 7-3 (p. 198) describes principles of Pitocin administration during labor and nursing implications associated with its use.**

TABLE 7-3 **Administration and Nursing Implications of Induction and Augmentation of Labor Using Pitocin***

Pitocin	Principles of Administration	Nursing Implications
Synthetic form of the posterior pituitary hormone oxytocin Stimulates the uterine myometrium to contract by increasing prostaglandin production and formation of oxytocin receptors Dose can be decreased as labor progresses because sensitivity to oxytocics increases and body production of prostaglandins and oxytocin is adequate to maintain labor	Establish a primary line with an isotonic electrolyte solution to prevent water intoxication from the antidiuretic effect of Pitocin; the primary line provides a route for other IV medications that may be needed and a means to maintain access to the circulatory system if Pitocin is discontinued Add Pitocin (usually 10 U) to an isotonic solution (1 L) and label the bag; the type and amount of the IV solution as well as the amount of Pitocin added are determined by physician's orders and hospital protocol; consideration is given to the hydration status of the client Never add any other medication to the Pitocin solution Insert tubing from Pitocin solution through infusion pump-controller Piggyback Pitocin solution to the primary line at the port closest to the IV insertion site (proximal port) Turn on the piggyback at the desired rate of infusion and follow protocol for advancement of rate: Start at 0.5-2 mU/min (induction) or 0.5 mU/min (augmentation) Increase in increments of 1-2 mU/min every 15-60 min; document maternal-fetal unit and labor status before and after each increment in the chart or flow sheet and on the monitor strip	Provide explanation before procedure initiation Assess status of maternal-fetal unit and labor at intervals of at least 15 min when increasing dosage, and 30 min when maintaining or decreasing dosage (see Box 7-1, p. 189) Observe for signs of reportable conditions that require treatment be discontinued and physician notified: Uterine hyperstimulation of the uterus: Frequency: < every 2 min. Duration: >90 sec Minimal to no relaxation of uterus during resting phase and excessive intrauterine pressure during a contraction (>100 mm Hg) Nonreassuring FHR patterns Inadequate response at 20 mU/min Emergency interventions for hyperstimulation: Discontinue Pitocin infusion but maintain primary infusion Turn the woman on her side Administer oxygen via mask at 8-10 L/min Increase primary infusion rate if fluid overload is not present Prepare to administer tocolytics to reduce uterine hyperstimulation Document all assessment findings, actions taken, and results of actions

Usual maximum dosage required for induction is 20 mU/min or less, and 10 mU/min or less for augmentation

Rates >20 mU/min require physician assessment and order because side effects become more likely at the higher rates; rate should never exceed 40 mU/min

Increments continue until contractions meet these criteria:

Frequency every 2-3 min

Duration 40-90 sec

Moderate to strong intensity; 30-sec rest period with adequate resting tone

Cervical dilation of 1 cm/hr during active phase

Requirements should be met within 8-12 hr of start of induction; if not, induction is discontinued and the client is allowed to rest; induction may be resumed at a later time or a cesarean birth is performed

Once criteria for contractions are met the infusion is maintained at the rate attained until the cervix is dilated to 5-6 cm; at that point a gradual decrease in oxytocin may begin

Maintain adequate hydration: IV infusion rate of 125 ml/hr

Provide comfort measures and emotional support

Explain progress

*Protocols for Pitocin use in augmentation and induction of labor vary according to agency protocol and physician preferences. All protocols must reflect application of professional standards.

VI. *Cesarean birth*

A. Definition—transabdominal delivery of the fetus through an incision in the abdomen and uterus when a sound medical orobstetric reason exists, other interventions to secure safe delivery have failed, or the health of the maternal-fetal unit is in jeopardy

B. Incisions: abdominal transverse, suprapubic and uterine transverse into lower uterine segment

C. Types

1. Emergency: unexpected cesarean birth from changes in the status of the maternal-fetal unit such as fetal distress, failure to progress from cephalopelvic disproportion, prolapse of the umbilical cord, maternal hemorrhage from placental previa or abruptio placenta, or worsening of preeclampsia

2. Elective: planned cesarean birth from such factors as scarring of upper uterine segment associated with previous classic (vertical uterine incision) cesarean birth or uterine surgery or trauma, active genital tract infection, positive HIV status, or fetal factors such as hydrocephalus, spinal bifida, breech or shoulder presentation, or multiple gestation

D. Preoperative care interventions are similar to those for most abdominal surgeries

1. Physical interventions specific to cesarean birth
   a. Insert Foley catheter into the bladder
   b. Administer antacid such as Bicitra to neutralize GI secretions if an emergency cesarean birth is to be performed under general anesthesia
   c. Tocolytics (SQ terbutaline) if strong contractions are present

2. Psychosocial interventions; especially important if surgery is unexpected and the result of an emergency situation
   a. Explain clearly and simply the reason for cesarean birth, purpose for the preparatory interventions, and what to expect in the operating room
   b. Check for or secure a written informed consent
   c. Approach the woman and her family in a calm, assured manner
   d. Encourage a family-centered approach as much as is possible, for example, for a father in the operating room, encourage immediate interaction with newborn at birth

E. Postoperative care interventions are similar to those for most abdominal surgeries

1. Physical interventions specific to cesarean birth
   a. Assess condition of the breasts and fundus, and the characteristics of the lochia
   b. Limit IV fluid intake, with rapid progress to a regular diet within 24 hours

Box 7-2
Selected Nursing Diagnoses for the Complications of Childbirth

Maternal and Family Diagnoses

Ineffective breathing pattern related to:
  Depressant effects of magnesium sulfate
  Pulmonary edema associated with ritodrine administration
  Experience of incisional discomfort when taking deep breaths
  Decreased CO related to tachycardia associated with terbutaline administration
  Fluid volume excess related to fluid retention associated with ritodrine
    administration
Risk for infection related to:
  Premature rupture of amniotic membranes
  Alteration in skin integrity after cesarean birth
Pain related to:
  Hypertonic uterine contraction pattern
  Abdominal and uterine incision associated with cesarean birth
  Fatigue related to interruption of sleep patterns associated with prolonged labor
    process
Anxiety related to:
  Preterm onset of labor or prolonged pregnancy
  Lack of knowledge about labor induction and its effects
  Situational low self esteem related to perceived inability to secure safe passage for
    self and fetus
  Altered family processes related to limitation placed on maternal role as part of
    treatment regimen to prevent preterm birth

Fetal and Newborn Diagnoses

Impaired gas exchange related to:
  Aging of placenta associated with prolonged pregnancy; aspiration of meconium
  Hyperstimulation of uterus associated with Pitocin induction of labor
  Compression of umbilical cord associated with oligohydramnios
Risk for fetal injury related to:
  Macrosomia requiring an operative birthing intervention
  Intrauterine infection
  Precipitous birth
Alteration in nutrition (less than body requirements) related to:
  Ineffective feeding behaviors associated with high magnesium levels
  Ineffective breast feeding associated with maternal pain and fatigue after cesarean
    birth
  Risk for neonatal injury related to hypoglycemia associated with prolonged
    pregnancy

    c. Administer oxytocics to enhance contraction of uterus; Pitocin often is added to the first one or two liters of IV fluid

    d. Perineal care

2. Psychosocial interventions

    a. Encourage expression of feelings about an inability to give birth vaginally, and of the childbirth events

   b. Assist with parental attachment to the newborn, breast feeding, and newborn care; may be inhibited as a result of maternal pain, fatigue, and limited mobility
   c. Prepare the woman and family for requirements of a longer recovery period; make referrals as needed
F. **Vaginal Birth After Cesarean (VBAC)**
   1. Should be encouraged for subsequent pregnancies because low segment incisions are less likely to rupture, making labor and vaginal birth after a cesarean nearly as safe as labor and birth after a previous vaginal delivery
   2. Trial of labor (TOL): 4 to 6 hours of labor to determine how labor will progress and if VBAC is possible and safe; also used when there are questions about the adequacy of maternal pelvis

WEB Resources

http://www.csection.com
   Cesarean birth rates at hospitals in New York state and California are provided at this site along with many relevant links and references related to childbirth, cesarean birth, and VBACs.

http://www.obgyn.net
   OBGYN.net is the Universe of Women's Health. Begin by clicking on Medical Professionals Section, then click on Pregnancy and Birth in the left-hand column. Scroll down and click on archive of articles to gain access to articles related to complications of pregnancy, cervical ripening and labor induction and augmentation, and cesarean section and VBAC.

http://www.efn.org/~djz/birth/birthindex.html
   OBC-Online Birth Center. Scroll down and click on High-Risk Situations and Complications for access to information related to cesarean section, VBAC, and complications of labor and birth.

REVIEW QUESTIONS

1. Uterine dystocia may be associated with a pattern of hypotonic uterine contractions. Nurses should base actions on which of these statements?
    1. Hypotonic contractions typically occur during the active phase of the first stage of labor
    2. Nulliparous women are most likely to exhibit this type of contraction pattern
    3. Hypotonic contractions are characteristically regular, of low intensity, and occur at a frequency of 4 or less in a 10 minute period
    4. Management often involves therapeutic rest with the use of sedatives

2. When teaching a group of pregnant women about the signs of preterm labor the nurse would describe which one of these findings?
    1. Cervical ripening with some effacement and dilation
    2. Uterine contractions that occur at a frequency of four contractions in 1 hour
    3. Persistent dull, low backache
    4. Intense pain associated with uterine contractions

3. During the assessment of a pregnant woman, the nurse should realize that which of these findings is likely to contribute to the premature rupture of the membranes (PROM)?
    1. Oligohydramnios
    2. Reproductive tract infection
    3. Singleton pregnancy
    4. Intercourse in the third trimester of pregnancy

4. A nulliparous woman in labor received an epidural block during the active phase of her labor. Shortly afterward the progress of her labor slowed. Based on physician's order, the nurse could expect which of these orders to augment the progress of this woman's labor?
    1. Administer 10 U of Pitocin over a 2-minute period directly into her vein (IV push)
    2. Assist with amnioinfusion
    3. Stimulate one nipple for short periods between contractions
    4. Apply prostaglandin E_2 gel to her cervix

5. To manage a Pitocin infusion used for the induction of labor, the nurse would take which of these actions?
    1. Piggyback the Pitocin solution to the distal port (farthest from the IV insertion site) of the primary tubing
    2. Begin the infusion at a rate of 0.5 to 2 mU/min
    3. Increase the amount of Pitocin infused by 3 mU/min every 15 minutes
    4. Use 5% dextrose in water solution for both the primary and piggyback infusions

ANSWERS, RATIONALES, AND TEST-TAKING TIPS

Rationales	Test-Taking Tips

1. Correct answer: 1

Hypotonic contractions typically follow a normal latent phase in multiparous women. These contractions do not develop a regular pattern and occur at a frequency of less than three contractions in 10 minutes. Typical management involves augmentation of labor once cephalopelvic disproportion (CPD) is ruled out.

Recall that the uterus is a muscle. In multiparous women the muscle may be stretched and flabby from use and may result in hypotonic contractions. Nulliparous women tend to have stronger uterine function in relation to the strength of the contraction. Eliminate option 2. Eliminate option 3 because hypofunction of most anything typically results in irregular, not regular, function. Eliminate option 4 because sedatives may further contribute to the hypotonicity.

2. Correct answer: 3

Uterine contractions must occur at a rate of one contraction every 10 minutes or less (six or more per hour). Discomfort is often minimal, vague, and variable such as a low, dull backache. Preterm labor may be dismissed as GI upset or even go unnoticed. The nurse should emphasize signs the woman can detect herself.

Focus on what you know. The clue in the stem is "preterm labor." It is obvious that options 2 and 4, which describe contractions, are more likely to be in labor at term births. Option 1 is a change that occurs during labor, but the woman cannot determine this herself. It is assessed by the health care provider to diagnose preterm labor.

3. Correct answer: 2

Options 1, 3, and 4 have not been associated with premature membrane rupture. In addition to infection, contributing factors include hydramnios, multiple gestations, poor diet, smoking cigarettes, and fetal anomalies and malpresentations.

Use your basic knowledge that infection causes inflammation, which in turn results in irritation of the infected, inflamed site. Thus infection in the reproductive tract is a direct attack on the pregnancy site to weaken the membranes with the result of a PROM. Sexual intercourse typically results in no threat to the pregnancy.

4. Correct answer: 3

Breast stimulation results in the release of endogenous oxytocin from the pituitary gland. Endogenous oxytocin will stimulate the uterus to contract. An amnioinfusion is used for oligohydramnios to prevent cord compression. During labor, Pitocin is always mixed in an IV solution and administered with the use of a carefully controlled drip rate. Prostaglandin E_2 gel is used to ripen the cervix in preparation for induction of labor.

Look for the clues in the options. Option 1 has the clue "IV push," which is an incorrect administration method. No information in the stem states that the amount of amniotic fluid produced was too little. Option 2 introduces new information, so eliminate it. Between option 3 and 4, if you were uncertain, put option 3 into an external action and option 4 into an internal action with the use of medication. It is safest to initially do the external action before an internal treatment. Select option 3.

5. Correct answer: 2

The proximal port should be used for this piggyback. The amount of Pitocin is increased at a rate of 1 to 2 mU/min every 15 to 60 minutes; 3mU/min is too fast. Electrolyte-based solutions such as lactated Ringer's should be used to prevent water intoxication, which would occur with 5% dextrose solutions.

Use your common sense plus knowledge to eliminate options: option 1, the distal port; option 3, with a high increase at a frequent interval; and option 4, which make one solution correct for all types of infusions—the continuous or primary infusion and the intermittent or piggyback infusions.

8

The Process of Postpartum Psychosocial Adaptation and Physical Recovery with Nursing Applications

FAST FACTS

1. The fourth stage of labor is the period of stabilization immediately after the birth of the newborn, the first 1 to 2 hours.
2. **Postpartum (postnatal) period/puerperium** is the 6- to 8-week period of recovery after birth.
3. **The fourth trimester** is the 3-month period of adjustment the postpartum woman and her family undergo as a result of pregnancy, childbirth, the transition to parenthood, and changes in family processes from the impact of newborn care responsibilities.
4. Anatomic and physiologic adaptations of pregnancy are reversed from (a) the decreased hormonal levels, especially estrogen and progesterone, after placental expulsion; and (b) the decreased uterine size, with the expulsion of uterine contents.
5. The process of recovery involves two types of changes: (a) retrogressive changes: the return of body systems to a nonpregnant state; and (b) progressive changes: continued adaptation required for nurturing and care of the newborn, including lactation and transition to parenting.

6. Puerperium is a period of vulnerability for the woman and her family. She is physically at risk for hemorrhage, infection, thrombophlebitis, urinary retention and constipation, and fatigue. She also is at risk psychosocially for depression, altered family processes, disturbance in body image and self-esteem, role conflict, and altered sexuality patterns.

7. Successful recovery is a gradual process influenced by (a) the mother's physical status, including her nutritional and hygienic habits, levels of energy and comfort, and presence of health problems; (b) her emotional status regarding her reaction to and responsibility of care for the newborn; (c) the health status of the newborn; (d) care and support from the family-support system and health care providers; and (e) the adequacy of the mother's knowledge about recovery, self-care, and newborn characteristics and care.

8. All family members—parents, siblings, and grandparents—need to make adjustments as family processes, roles, and relationships change. Adjustments are influenced by their cultural beliefs and values that affect their care of the postpartum woman and newborn.

9. A potential for crisis exists during the transition and adjustment period after the birth of a baby. A crisis can be caused by (a) the perception of the event, that is, the degree to which an addition of a new family member is viewed realistically in terms of additional responsibilities, and sibling jealousy and regression; (b) the coping mechanisms of the family; and (c) the degree to which situational support groups are available and supportive.

10. Most postpartum women experience postpartum blues approximately 3 days after birth and again at approximately 1 month postpartum.

11. A holistic approach that considers the mother's physical recovery, the psychosocial adjustment of herself and her family to the reality of a newborn, and the responsibilities of care for the newborn should be used when planning care.

12. Discharge within 12 to 24 hours after an uncomplicated vaginal birth is increasing in popularity as a means to facilitate maternal recovery and family adjustment and to reduce health care costs. However, federal law requires at least a 48- to 72-hour hospital stay before discharge if desired by the mother.

13. A comprehensive, coordinated maternal-newborn health care program at the beginning of the pregnancy supports early discharge: (a) critical care pathways can facilitate health care provision in early discharge programs that avoid duplication and prevents omissions of essential care measures. (b) Innovative care delivery systems facilitate administration of care, for example, with one room—a labor, delivery, recovery, and postpartum (LDRP) room—until discharge and being cared for by a limited number of nurses; or mother-baby or couplet care that coordinates the health care of the postpartum woman and her newborn.

14. A comprehensive, coordinated maternal-newborn health care program includes: (a) prenatal education services; (b) health care agencies that provide childbirth services, which facilitate vaginal births and are family-centered and support the recovery process after the birth; (c) discharge planning, which provides essential health care and teaching about prevention, early detection, and prompt treatment of maternal and

neonatal problems; and (d) postpartum programs, which provide continuing assessment, evaluation, and care during the 6-week recovery period.

CONTENT REVIEW

I. The nursing process provides the focus for support of family efforts to incorporate the newborn into their lives

A. **Assessment**
1. Presence of factors that influence adjustment
2. Cultural influences about the care of the mother and newborn
3. Level of parental knowledge and experience
4. Effectiveness of each family member's transition to incorporate the newborn into their lives; assessed during sibling and grandparent visitation, telephone follow-up (Box 8-1, p. 210), and home visitation (Box 8-2, p. 211), especially for primiparas and high risk women and newborns
5. Family-newborn interactions and progress in parental-newborn attachment (Table 8-1, p. 210)

B. **Typical nursing diagnoses about maternal and family recovery and adjustment**
1. Ineffective individual coping related to conflicting demands of family, newborn care, and career responsibilities
2. Situational low self-esteem related to perceived difficulty in meeting the newborn's needs
3. Potential for family growth related to the birth of a healthy newborn
4. Alteration in family processes related to the addition of a new family member
5. Risk for altered parenting related to inexperience and inadequate family support

C. **Nursing support, a critical factor in maternal and family adjustment** (Boxes 8-1 and 8-2, p. 211)
1. Encourage family members to express feelings, concerns, and questions
2. Work with the mother to develop approaches that help her balance and prioritize personal, career, and family needs
3. Provide information through health teaching
4. Create opportunities for the family to interact with and practice caring for the newborn
5. Make referrals to community agencies as indicated by family needs

⚠ Warning!

Nursing interventions must be sensitive to the cultural variations determined during the assessment process.

TABLE 8-1	Behavioral Indicators of Effective and Ineffective Attachment

Effective Attachment Behaviors	Ineffective Attachment Behaviors

Use of touch:
  Caresses with fingertips or uses hands to explore newborn's body
  Cuddles newborn close to body
  Kisses newborn
  Gently handles and administers care
	Use of touch:
	  Touches limited to essential contact: feeding, changing diaper
	  Handles with carelessness, indifference
	  Shows few signs of affection

Use of visual contact:
  Gazes at newborn
  Makes eye contact
  Inspects newborn's characteristics
	Use of visual contact:
	  Looks away from the newborn
	  Avoids eye contact

Verbalization:
  Chooses name with care
  Uses name or affectionate nickname when talking to or speaking about the newborn
  Expresses pleasure about the newborn, its appearance and behavior
  Identifies the newborn's characteristics that resemble family members
	Verbalization:
	  Makes persistent negative statements about the newborn's appearance and behavior
	  Uses derogatory nicknames when talking to or speaking about the newborn
	  Expresses continued disappointment about the newborn's gender

Expressions of interest in the newborn:
  Displays eagerness to learn about proper newborn care
  Seeks feedback about care efforts
  Asks questions about the newborn and its condition
  Expresses disappointment when the newborn must return to the nursery
  Identifies and responds to the newborn's cues such as for hunger and discomfort
	Expressions of interest in the newborn:
	  Ignores or does not recognize the newborn's cues such as hunger and discomfort
	  Expresses limited interest in learning about or caring for the newborn
	  Demonstrates eagerness to send the newborn back to the nursery
	  Asks few questions about the status of the newborn

WARNING! Behavioral indicators of ineffective attachment should be evaluated carefully, over time, and in the context of situational factors such as a history of dysfunctional labor, fatigue, pain, inexperience, fear, and cultural beliefs about interaction with a newborn. Never rush to judge.

II. Process of parental and family attachment to the newborn

  A. *Attachment:* process whereby an enduring bond is established between an infant and its parents and family
    1. Attachment and bonding: development of the parent-family-newborn relationship
    2. Bonding: early stage of attachment; parents experience attraction

Box 8-1
Postpartum Telephone Follow-up

Suggested Format for Assessment of Maternal-Newborn and Family Status

Describe how you are feeling today.
What have you been doing to take care of yourself?
How does the baby seem to you?
Describe how the baby has been eating and sleeping.
What has been the greatest source of happiness for you since coming home?
What has been the greatest source of stress for you since coming home?
How have you handled this stress?
What are your concerns?
Who has been your greatest source of support since you have come home?
How has this person helped you?
How are the other members of your family (partner, other children, grandparents) doing since you and the baby came home?
What arrangements have you made for your postpartum checkup and your baby's first newborn health checkup?
How can I help to make things easier for you?

Adapted from NAACOG: Postpartum follow-up: a nursing practice guide. OGN Nursing Practice Resource. Washington, DC, 1986, Association of Women's Health, Obstetric, and Neonatal Nurses (AWHONN; formerly NAACOG).

Box 8-2
Home Visitation After Early Postpartum Discharge

Assessments:
  Maternal recovery after the pregnancy and birth
  Newborn adaptation to extrauterine life
  Family adaptation to birth and the newborn
  Environmental adequacy: cleanliness, warmth, and safety
  Knowledge of postpartum recovery and use of interventions designed to enhance the health of mother, newborn, and family
  Need for community support services
Interventions:
  Review: signs of effective and ineffective recovery for mother and infant, action to take if signs of ineffective recovery are noted, self-care and infant care measures, breast and bottle-feeding techniques, process of infant growth and development, actions to promote positive family adaptation to newborn, and family planning methods
  Discuss: feelings and concerns about the birth experience, postpartum recovery, and infant care
  Support: parenting efforts by providing guidance, positive reinforcement, and encouragement
  Utilize: community agencies by making referrals as needed to such services as WIC (Women, Infants, and Children), lactation consultants, well baby clinics, day-care centers, family planning clinics, parenting support groups
  Involve: family in the process of assessment and care

to their newborn as they make eye contact, touch and stroke, and experience the newborn's grasp and sucking

3. Attachment: reciprocal process that represents the development of feelings of loyalty and affection that grow and strengthen over time
   a. Begins during pregnancy facilitated by hearing fetal heart beat, seeing its image on ultrasonography, perceiving fetal movements and activity responses to extrauterine stimuli such as voices, music, and emotions
   b. Continues after birth enhanced by activities that encourage early, close, and frequent contact along with interaction and communication between the newborn and its family

B. **Factors influencing the process of attachment**
   1. Nature of the relationship between the parents and with their own parents; it is within these relationships that parents learn how to love and care for others, including their new baby and other children
      a. Emotional health of each person and their ability to form strong positive relationships, to give and receive affection
      b. Stability and quality of the relationships in terms of communication, mutual respect, affection, and concern for each other
      c. Supportive social network within which these relationships exist
      d. Cultural influences associated with family relationships and responsibilities
   2. Pregnancy experience: attachment is facilitated by a positive pregnancy experience and hindered by a negative pregnancy experience
   3. Childbirth events
      a. Progress of childbirth: did it meet expectations or did problems develop that required unexpected interventions and separation of family members from each other and the newborn
      b. Interventions employed by the birthing agency to facilitate the attachment process (Box 8-3)
   4. Postpartum condition of the mother and newborn allowed for close, frequent contact with the newborn
   5. Newborn characteristics
      a. Appearance: reflects expectations, resembles family members, affected by presence of external anomalies or injuries
      b. Gender: desired gender and importance the newborn's gender is to parents and family
      c. Ability to respond to parents and family: make eye contact, grasp, respond to voices and care-giving efforts in an effective manner
      d. Temperament: ability to be consoled, cuddliness, easy or difficult to arouse, irritability
      e. Presence of physical anomalies or illnesses requiring follow-up and causing concern

Box 8-3
Nursing Interventions to Facilitate Attachment

Provide time for parents to interact with their newborn as soon as possible after birth.
Create family-centered birthing practices that include birthing rooms, the presence of
  family members at the birth, and celebratory activities (champagne, photographs,
  and so on).
"Introduce" newborn to parents, showing them about newborn characteristics,
  behaviors, and sensory capabilities.
Show parents how to communicate with their newborn by using touch, eye contact,
  and speech.
Facilitate parent participation in the care of the newborn by providing:
  Classes, demonstrations, and supervised practice about infant care
  Positive feedback about skill attainment
  Mother-baby or couplet care
  Unlimited paternal visiting hours
Demonstrate how a newborn responds to parental care and communication.
Foster family interaction with newborn by encouraging sibling and grandparent
  visitation and participation in care.

6. Parental characteristics
  a. Age and maturation level
    (1) Adolescent parents may lack the maturity to cope with the
        responsibilities and frustration of newborn care; their own
        needs and that of their infants can conflict
    (2) Older parents may encounter conflict between parenting
        and career demands
  b. Experience and knowledge about newborn care and
     characteristics, including access to information, role models,
     and guidance
  c. Ability to recognize and meet the newborn's needs with
     confidence
  d. Cultural expectations and beliefs about parental role
     responsibilities and behaviors

III. Maternal psychosocial recovery and adjustment after pregnancy and birth and maternal role attainment

A. Process of recovery is reflected by progress though a set of
   stages, as described in Table 8-2, p. 214; progress through the
   stages and achievement of confidence and competence with
   maternal role are influenced by
  1. Maternal factors
    a. Degree to which the developmental tasks of pregnancy were
       accomplished; the role the mother defined for herself
    b. Events during pregnancy and childbirth; does the mother
       believe she did a "good job" and reached her expectations

TABLE 8-2 Stages of Maternal Psychosocial Recovery After Pregnancy and Birth with Implications for Nursing

Taking in, Dependent	Taking Hold, Dependent-Independent	Letting Go, Interdependent
Duration: first 1-2 days after birth	Duration: lasts 4-5 wk and follows taking-in	Duration: recovery is completed and follows taking hold
Typical behaviors and emotions: Dependency needs predominate Physical needs for rest, food, pain relief must be met Wants to be cared for Expresses a need to reflect on events and behaviors during labor and birth Reduced attention span from pain and fatigue limits learning readiness Asks questions and expresses concern about the status of self and newborn	Typical behaviors and emotions: Vacillates between her need for nurturing and her need to take charge of self and newborn Begins to focus on meeting the needs of newborn Progresses in her ability to care for self and newborn Responsive to practice and learning opportunities Fatigue occurs from recovery and care-giving demands Baby blues may occur Daily routines and patterns are established	Typical behaviors and emotions: Gives up role as pregnant woman for role as mother Reestablishes role as spouse-partner and resumes career role Views newborn as a separate being from herself More willing to involve others in care of newborn so she can take time for self Family patterns and roles are adjusted

Implications for nursing:
Nurture the mother to help her progressively nurture her baby and care for herself
Meet needs for pain relief, nutrition, and periods of uninterrupted rest
Assist with the care of newborn so the mother can rest
Encourage participation in a childbirth review, to help her analyze and accept the experience as it occurred; videotapes of the birth can be used for this review when the mother feels ready and has someone to watch it with her and discuss her concerns and questions
Provide short health teaching sessions that focus on essential information required for a safe discharge
Incorporate practice, reinforcement, review, and written materials as appropriate

Implications for nursing:
Help mother to plan realistically for tasks ahead, including time for meeting own needs
Provide opportunity for and encourage rooming in or mother-baby care; helpful for learning and "getting to know" the newborn
Identify family members and friends who will assist her with newborn care and family demands; help her to realize it is okay to ask for and accept help
Provide teaching sessions and demonstrations that include the family
Help her to learn how to prioritize: what is essential and what can wait

Implications for nursing:
Prepare mother for feelings such as sadness and guilt that she may experience when separating self from newborn to resume career role
Discuss changes that may occur in the relationship with spouse-partner including issues of sexuality, feelings of jealousy and competition with the newborn for attention
Evaluate family recovery and make referrals if signs of ineffective recovery are present and persistent

    c. Maternal health status

    d. Stability of the relationship with family members, especially the father of the baby; their reaction to her performance

    e. Level of confidence and self-esteem

    f. Maternal age

      (1) Young mothers may lack knowledge, life experience, socioeconomic resources, and family support needed to develop as a parent

      (2) Older mothers may have sufficient knowledge, life experience, and socioeconomic support required for parenting yet experience career demands and the need to be a "perfect parent"

    g. Level of stress and role conflict

  2. Newborn factors include the health status and *temperament,* which is the responsiveness to care-giving and to affection efforts of the newborn

B. Referral to community agencies that provide home visitation may be helpful in situations in which mothers are at risk as a result of:

  1. Early discharge

  2. Limited family, financial, and emotional support

  3. Lack of experience and knowledge or conflict with other demands

  4. Inadequate attachment behaviors and disinterest in caring for the newborn

C. Alterations in maternal mood and emotions

  1. Fluctuations in mood occur as a result of many interrelated factors:

    a. Changes in hormonal levels after the delivery of the placenta

    b. Presence of fatigue, pain, and discomfort

    c. Transitions in the relationships for self and family

    d. Responsibilities of newborn care, concerns about the health status of newborn, adequacy of breast feeding, and anxiety about effectiveness as a mother

    e. Role strain and conflicts as other demands compete with those of the newborn

  2. **Postpartum blues/baby blues**

    a. Most postpartum women experience the blues approximately 3 days after the birth and again at approximately 1 month postpartum

    b. Blues are a normal occurrence, mild and transient in nature, and typically last 3 days to 1 week; may progress to a mild self-limiting depression

    c. Especially vulnerable are:

      (1) Career women who wait until later in life to have their first child and have developed an idealistic view of motherhood

      (2) Adolescent mothers

(3) First-time mothers

(4) Mothers with limited support systems

d. Characteristic behaviors: irritability, moodiness, restlessness, crying spells, sleeplessness, anger, anxiety, decreased interest in surroundings

e. Effective therapeutic interventions

   (1) Preparation of woman and her family for the stressors of the postpartum period and with healthy actions to cope with stress

   (2) Involvement of the family in a therapeutic approach that includes identification of characteristic "blues" behaviors and implementation of supportive actions

   (3) Supportive actions

      (a) Provide time for the mother: "time out" to rest, sleep, and do things for self or with friends

      (b) Share the responsibilities of newborn care with family: asking for and accepting help

      (c) Provide positive reinforcement for mothering efforts

3. **Postpartum depression with or without psychotic features:** severe mood disorder that is prolonged in nature and requires professional intervention

a. Examples of professional interventions include: psychiatric referral, hospitalization, and psychotherapeutic medications

b. Characteristic behaviors

   (1) Exaggeration of behaviors associated with the blues

   (2) Hostility and inappropriate responses directed toward self, newborn, and family

   (3) Emotional lability; difficulty coping

   (4) Behavior that is psychotic (out of touch with reality: delusions, hallucinations)

   (5) Capability of doing harm to herself or her newborn

IV. Adolescent mothers

A. **Support is required for adolescent mothers as they work to attain the role of mother**

B. **Parenting efforts should be evaluated**

1. Progress of attachment

2. Progress in the development of skills that will meet the newborn's physical, emotional, and developmental needs

3. Expression of feelings about the newborn and their skills as mothers

4. Ability to evaluate their parenting skills, seek and accept help and guidance, and identify newborn cues and needs

C. **Self-esteem and confidence should be fostered**

1. Teach and demonstrate appropriate parenting skills and responses

2. Provide opportunities for supervised practice
3. Offer praise and positive reinforcement when successful

V. Paternal adjustment

A. **Paternal role behaviors are influenced by the father's role he defined as he adapted to his partner's pregnancy and by the expectations of his culture**
   1. Often take on a more active, nurturing parent role than did their own fathers
      a. View relationship with the mother as a partnership
      b. Attend parenting classes
      c. Need to be more involved owing to dual income or dual career families, which are becoming the norm
   2. Paternal role behaviors may emphasize socialization and play activities rather than care-giving behaviors
   3. Parental role responsibilities should be mutually defined by both parents and result in a satisfying experience for both
   4. Paternal participation in active care-giving should be fostered by including him in newborn care classes and providing opportunities for him to participate in the care of the newborn
B. *Engrossment:* **intense paternal interest and involvement with his newborn that is facilitated by touch, eye-to-eye contact, awareness of newborn similarities to himself, and positive newborn responses to his voice and care**
C. **Fathers are an important source of maternal support: they are often identified by the mother as her most significant support person**
   1. Assess parental relationship and their ability to support each other
   2. Provide father with information about:
      a. Maternal recovery after birth, including her physical and emotional needs
      b. Supportive and care actions he can implement to facilitate her recovery
D. **Fathers are an important source of support and guidance for their children by providing:**
   1. Care and attention needed by siblings to facilitate their adjustment to the new baby
   2. Role model for male behavior needed by their children as they determine their concept of what is male and develop relationships with men
E. **There is increasing concern about societal impact of a growing number of single-parent households, with the mother as the primary care-giver and with limited to no male influence**

VI. Sibling adjustment

A. **Siblings must deal with the:**
   1. Reality of a newborn and the impact it has on their position in the family

2. Need to share their parents' love, time, and attention
3. Increased responsibilities and loss of free time as they participate in newborn care and help with household tasks

B. Influencing factors
1. Age and level of maturation; a young child may have greater difficulty waiting for needs to be met and sharing parents, whereas an older child may resent the demands of added responsibilities
2. Preparation for the birth and the degree of their participation in pregnancy and birth
3. Security of their relationship with their parents
4. Level of self-esteem they have developed
5. Nature of previous experiences they have had with newborns
6. Characteristics of newborn and degree to which the baby meets the siblings' expectations

C. Typical siblings' reactions to the newborn's arrival
1. Enthusiastic, excited, eager to help care for newborn, express concern for newborn, use gentle touch and kisses to communicate
2. Anger and rejection directed toward newborn and even parents: "If you loved me so much why did you need another baby?"
   a. Initially anger, resentment, and impatience are expected as normal reactions
   b. Continuing anger accompanied by physical expressions against newborn and disturbances in life activities such as eating, sleeping, and school require professional evaluation
3. Relationship with the mother may undergo a transitory change
   a. Reject mother on her arrival home as they react to the feeling of abandonment when she left them to give birth
   b. Cling to mother; afraid she will leave again
4. Regression may occur in young children
   a. May be used to gain attention and same loving care as newborn
   b. May ask to be breast or bottle fed, wear diapers, or sleep in parent's room with the baby
   c. Usually are self-limiting and resolved in a few days to a few weeks; continuing regression may be an indicator of adjustment problems

D. Siblings need support in their process of attachment and adjustment to the newborn (see Box 8-4, p. 220)
1. Parents play the major role in this process assisted by grandparents, other family members, friends, and health care providers
2. Nurses should inform parents about typical sibling reactions and interventions that facilitate their adjustment
3. Family-centered activities during and after birth should be encouraged

---

Box 8-4

Parental Activities that Facilitate Sibling Adjustment to the Newborn

---

Participate in sibling visitation.

Involve the siblings in the preparations made for the homecoming of the mother and newborn.

Help the siblings to choose or make a special gift to give to the mother and newborn.

Consider the feelings of siblings on arrival home with the newborn; father should carry baby into the home to leave the mother free to interact and hug the siblings.

Provide "special gifts" to give to the other siblings on arrival home and when visitors bring gifts for the baby.

Set aside a "special time" of affection and attention just for the siblings without interruption from the new baby.

Pay attention to the activities and events occurring in the lives of the siblings.

Involve the siblings in the care of the new baby according to their ability and with recognition of their need for their own time and space.

Encourage younger siblings to take care of their doll while mommy takes care of the baby.

VII. Grandparent Adjustment

A. **Grandparents are affected by the childbirth experience of their children, often playing an integral role in family adaptation to a new baby**

1. Serve as role models for parenting skills, and informational resources regarding the care of infants and children
2. Facilitate maternal physical and emotional recovery by providing comfort, care, and emotional support in an accepting, nonjudgmental manner
3. Assist parents in helping siblings to adjust to the newborn by providing them with loving care and attention
4. Care for grandchildren while parents work or go to school

B. **Grandparents' adjustment after the birth is influenced by:**

1. Relationship established with their children
2. Attitude and views about being a grandparent and what it entails
3. Groundwork laid during pregnancy
   a. Degree of involvement in the pregnancy
   b. Their children's view of the grandparent role
   c. Ability to develop, with their children, a plan for their involvement in the care and nurturing of the grandchild
4. Willingness to accept "new approaches" to child rearing adopted by their children
5. Cultural expectations and beliefs about the role of grandparents

C. **Grandparents may be placed in a more active caregiver role when the parents are adolescents**

1. Immaturity and inexperience of an adolescent parent may compel grandparents to "take over," blurring the role boundaries between grandparent and parent: Who is the major caregiver?

2. Resumption of primary parent role by the adolescent may lead to conflict not only for the grandparent but for the child as well: "Who is my mommy?"
3. Adolescent parent role should be nurtured and supported

VIII. Assessment process during the postpartal period
A. Review prenatal history and assessment to determine
1. Obstetrical history
   a. Previous pregnancies, births, and outcomes
   b. History of postpartum complications such as hemorrhage, infection, and depression
2. Nature of prenatal care
   a. Gestational week at entry into care; consistency of visits
   b. Woman's impression of care received; important for follow-through with health care during the current postpartal period and for future pregnancies
3. Health status during pregnancy
   a. Estimated date of birth
   b. Adaptations to physical and psychosocial changes of pregnancy, including the development of pregnancy-related complications
   c. Presence of pre-gestational health problems
   d. Medical interventions, including medications, hospitalization, and bed rest
   e. Laboratory and diagnostic tests performed and the results

> ## ⚠ Warning!
>
> Blood type and Rh factor are of special importance during the postpartum period so comparison can be made with the newborn's blood type and Rh factor to determine if further testing and RhoGAM administration are required.

4. Prenatal classes attended: childbirth preparation, breast-feeding techniques, parenting skills, and sibling preparation
B. Review of parturition events
1. Onset of labor compared with EDB
2. Progress of labor: onset, duration, labor patterns established, membrane rupture (time, fluid characteristics)
3. Physical and emotional status of the mother during labor:
   a. Vital signs
   b. Fluid balance in terms of intake, output, and signs of fluid deficit or excess
   c. Elimination from bladder (spontaneous, catheterization) and bowel
   d. Blood loss
   e. Pain experience and effectiveness of relief measures, including prepared childbirth techniques

Box 8-5
The Postpartum Check

Timing: Choose a time when the mother is comfortable and you will not be interrupted; this will facilitate health teaching and discussion.

Client preparation:

Fully explain the procedure in terms the woman understands.

Instruct the woman to empty her bladder and to save her perineal pad by placing it in a paper bag.

Assist the woman into a supine position with a pillow under her head and arms at her sides.

Maintain privacy throughout the procedure by pulling the curtain, closing the door, and exposing only the part of the body being examined.

Include woman's partner if they desire.

Asepsis:

Wash your hands: if you anticipate lesions on the skin, put on clean gloves at this time.

Obtain a pair of clean gloves for use to assess the perineum and the perineal pad.

Examine by proceeding from the breasts to legs, that is, examine the cleanest area first.

Examine the breasts:

Consistency of the breasts (soft, firm, engorged) and the progress of lactation

Degree of tenderness or discomfort and its location, that is, generalized or localized, unilateral, and nipples especially during latch on

Condition of the nipple-areola: intact, cracking, bruising, blisters, or redness

Leakage (characteristics)

Breast care measures such as cleansing, use of creams (purified lanolin), type of bra worn

Examine the abdomen:

Abdominal muscles will be more relaxed and palpation easier if woman bends her knees slightly (pillows underneath knees may also help) and keeps her arms at her sides.

Fundus: consistency (firm, boggy), height (fingerbreadths or centimeter at, above, or below the umbilicus), and location (midline, deviated to the right or left); presence of afterpains.

    f. Presence of a support person or coach

    g. Woman's impression of the experience and the quality of her performance

  4. Status of the fetus: FHR patterns, signs of distress, and presentation

  5. Birth

    a. Time and method of birth: spontaneous vaginal; forceps- or vacuum-assisted; cesarean birth, emergency or planned

    b. Separation and expulsion of placenta: spontaneous or manual removal, placental condition

  6. Pharmacologic interventions

    a. Oxytocics administered: which one, when, and what were the effects experienced

    b. Analgesics, anesthetics: which ones, when, and what were the effects experienced

  7. Current status of the newborn

Box 8-5
The Postpartum Check—cont'd

Examine the abdomen—cont'd:
  Abdomen: muscle tone, distention, striae, linea nigra, bowel sounds, and bowel
    elimination patterns
  Bladder: distention; voiding patterns
Examine the perineal area:
  Perineum is more easily visualized when the woman assumes a lateral position with
    her upper leg slightly flexed forward

Put on a Clean Pair of Gloves and Loosen Pad

Examine:
  Condition of the episiotomy or laceration: REEDA—Redness, Edema, Ecchymosis,
    Drainage, Approximation of wound edges
  Presence of hemorrhoids
  Presence of perineal discomfort
  Hygienic status of the perineal area
  Effectiveness of perineal care interventions used such as washing of perineal area,
    use of a peribottle, topical preparations, and sitz baths
  Perineal pad (current pad and pad saved) for lochia: stage, odor, clots, and amount
    (see Figure 5-8, p. 158)

Remove gloves and wash hands

Examine the legs:
  Circulatory status: color, warmth, capillary refill, pedal pulses, and presence of varicosities
  Edema of feet, ankles, and calves
  Signs of thrombophlebitis: erythema, swelling, tenderness, and Homan sign
  Deep tendon reflexes (DTR) especially for women with PIH
  Return of movement and sensation after the epidural or spinal anesthesia
Throughout the postpartum checkup, you should determine the woman's level of
  knowledge about her recovery and self-care, teach her how to assess herself, describe
  her current status, and explain signs indicative of effective and ineffective healing.

C. **Assessment of recovery after the birth process**
  1. Assessment of physical and psychosocial recovery must be
     thorough, accurate, and communicated and documented.
     Discharge decisions are based on the analysis of this data.
  2. Frequency of the physical assessment is determined by the status
     of the woman, presence of risk factors, and the time elapsed since
     birth
     a. Fourth stage of labor—every 15 minutes for the first hour, and
        every 30 minutes during the second hour
     b. After the fourth stage of labor—every 4 hours for the first 24
        hours; every 8 hours after the first 24 hours
  3. **Postpartum check** (Box 8-5)
     a. Systematic approach is used for assessment of essential
        factors indicative of physical recovery after the birth
        process

Box 8-6
Assessment of Psychosocial Recovery After the Birth Process

Self-Concept

Perceptions of physical self:
  Description of current health status
  Feelings expressed about current body image and how the body feels
Perceptions of personal self:
  Evaluation of the pregnancy experience and the effectiveness of performance during childbirth
  Self-ideal about being a mother compared with reality
Behaviors indicative of progress through the stages of recovery, and knowledge level about the following:
  Self-assessment measures to determine the status of effective or ineffective recovery
  Actions to enhance healing:
    Nutritional and fluid requirements
    Appropriate activity and exercises
    Hygienic practices
    Relief measures for pain and discomfort
    Rest requirements
    Stress reduction techniques

Role Function

Current roles and potential for role conflict
Parenting role:
  Beliefs and values about the roles of mother, father, and grandparents
  Personal evaluation of effectiveness as a mother
  Role mastery behaviors exhibited
  Responses of others to mother's parenting skills

Interdependence

Progress of attachment of parents and family to newborn:
  Parental expectations about the response of siblings to the newborn, including the nature of prenatal preparation for the addition of the newborn to the family
  Activities planned to facilitate siblings' adjustment to the newborn
Status of family and support system:
  Composition and availability of woman's family and support system
  Stability of the relationships
  Degree and quality of support offered by family and support system
  Willingness of woman to ask for and accept help
Adequacy of home environment to meet newborn's needs for cleanliness, warmth, and safety
Need for referral to community agencies such as WIC (Women, Infants, and Children), well baby clinics, lactation consultants, and parenting support groups

      b. A method used to provide essential information about postpartum healing; signs of effective or ineffective healing, and measures that enhance or disrupt the healing process

      c. The postpartum check can be adapted for use as a self-assessment method by the woman after discharge

    4. Assessment of physical recovery involves identification of expected findings and warning signs of ineffective recovery; use Box 8-5 (pp. 222-223) and Table 8-3 as guides

    5. Common laboratory testing—be sure to compare current findings with those obtained prenatally

      a. CBC—check the hematocrit and hemoglobin levels, and levels of RBCs, platelets, WBCs

      b. Coombs' and Rh testing—determine if Rh sensitization has occurred when an Rh-negative woman has an Rh-positive newborn

⚠ Warning!

If the woman is a candidate to receive RhoGAM, it must be administered within 72 hours of the birth.

      c. Urinalysis—performed if indicated, for example, with a history of or signs of UTI. Use a clean-catch, midstream specimen that prevents contamination of the urine sample from lochia and other secretions.

    6. Assessment of psychosocial adjustment recovery after the birth should involve the woman and her family (Box 8-6)

IX. Nursing diagnoses related to the common problems and risks encountered by the postpartal woman

A. Risk for fluid volume deficit

B. Risk for infection

C. Altered patterns of urinary elimination

D. Constipation

E. Alteration in nutrition (more or less than body requirements)

F. Pain, altered comfort

G. Risk for alteration in parenting

H. Altered family processes

I. Parental role conflict

J. Common nursing diagnoses—A to F listed above—along with selected client outcomes, and nursing interventions are described in Table 8-4. Nursing care about parenting and family processes are discussed in this chapter and Chapter 10, p. 267.

Text continued on p. 243

TABLE 8-3 **The Maternal Recovery Process—Expected Changes, Findings, and Warning Signs**

Anatomic and Physiologic Changes	Expected Assessment Findings	Warning Signs of Ineffective Recovery
Breasts: Initiation of the lactation cycle: Decrease in estrogen and progesterone levels results in increased prolactin (lactogenic hormone) secretion; alveolar cells are stimulated to secrete milk Increased blood and lymph flow to breasts Milk ducts fill with milk Lactation cycle maintained by continued secretion of prolactin from infant sucking and emptying of breasts Bottle-feeding woman: lactation cycle is suppressed as a result of the absence of sucking and emptying of breasts; milk accumulates and negative feedback suppresses cycle **WARNING!** Pharmacologic suppression of lactation using hormones or prolactin inhibitors is no longer recommended.	Postpartum days 1-3: Essentially no change Soft, not tender Secretion of colostrum, a yellowish liquid that is the precursor to milk Postpartum day 3 or 4: Engorgement: increased blood and lymph flow with progressive distention of breasts with milk (bluish-white liquid); signs and symptoms: Swollen, firm and hard Warm, prominent venous network Tender and painful Milk leakage During period of lactation: Full, not tender Areolae: intact without bruising, blisters, cracking, redness Nipples: prominent, erectile Blocked milk duct may be palpated as a lump; disappears when duct empties Recovery to nonpregnant status is about 1 mo after the cessation of lactation	Persistent lump that does not disappear after feeding, application of warm packs, or massage Cracks, blisters, bruises, and redness on nipples and areola Inverted or flat nipples; interferes with proper latch on by infant Signs of mastitis: Chills, fever Malaise, nausea Unilateral breast tenderness with localized redness and swelling

Uterus:

Involution: return of uterus to approximate nonpregnant size; remains slightly larger

Decreased estrogen and progesterone levels lead to size decrease in myometrial cells with breakdown of excess cellular protein (*autolysis*)

Uterus contracts to decrease uterine size and compress the blood vessels to prevent hemorrhage

Regeneration of endometrium

Destruction and sloughing off of outer layer of decidua

Regeneration of inner layer of endometrium without scar formation; implantation in future pregnancies can occur

Lochia: uterine discharge composed of decidual tissue, cellular debris, blood and lymph, bacteria

Progress of endometrial regeneration is reflected in the pattern of changes in lochial characteristics: stage, amount, duration

Menstrual cycle:

Decrease in estrogen and progesterone levels reverses suppression of menstrual cycle present during pregnancy

Fundal height and position:

After expulsion of the placenta: about midway between umbilicus and symphysis pubis, midline

First 12 hr after birth: fundus rises to the level of umbilicus, or 1 cm (fingerbreadth) above, midline

24-48 hr after birth: gradual descent of fundus at 1-2 cm (fingerbreadths) or a more rapid progress in breast-feeding women or women receiving oxytocics, midline

Muscular contraction of uterus:

Firm fundal consistency on palpation

Afterpains: cramping caused by periodic relaxation and contraction of the uterus:

Most common for woman with a more enlarged uterus, breast-feeding woman

Gradually diminish in intensity over first few postpartum days

Progressive changes in lochia:

Lochia rubra: 1-3 days postpartum; red, thick, small clots, trickles from vagina

WARNING! Temporary increase or a sudden gush may be noted with a contraction, breast feeding, fundal massage, ambulation.

Subinvolution: delay in or failure of uterus and placental site to heal fully:

Persistence of lochia that does not progress as expected

Periods of heavy bleeding

Reversal of lochial stages, i.e., return to rubra after progressing to serosa

Position of fundus above umbilicus and deviated to right or left of midline; usually indicative of bladder distension

Boggy (soft) fundus: uterine atony, indicating that contractions are ineffective; danger of hemorrhage:

Fundus should become firm and remain contracted after massage and administration of oxytocic medications

Results of uterine atony:

Passage of large clots

Heavy, excessive amount of lochia; pad saturated in <1 hr (1 g weight = 1 ml blood)

Signs of uterine infection (endometritis):

Fever (often first sign), malaise

Offensive, foul lochial odor

Persistence of lochia serosa, alba

Uterine tenderness

Continued

TABLE 8-3 The Maternal Recovery Process—Expected Changes, Findings, and Warning Signs—cont'd

Anatomic and Physiologic Changes	Expected Assessment Findings	Warning Signs of Ineffective Recovery
Menstrual cycle—cont'd Function of hypothalamic-pituitary-ovarian axis gradually returns First few cycles after birth may be anovulatory but ovulation and therefore pregnancy are possible First few menstrual flows may be heavier than usual	Lochia serosa: 3-10 days postpartum; light pink to brown; thinner in consistency Lochia alba: 10-14 days postpartum but can last as long as 3 wk; yellowish-white Amount decreases as stages progress: profuse, moderate, light, scant Odor: fleshy, musty; similar to menses Resumption of menstruation with ovulation: Nonlactating women: 6-8 wk: 40-45% 12 wk: 65-75% 24 wk: 90-100% Lactating women: 6 wk: 15% 12 wk: 45% 4-8 mo for women who practice complete breast feeding (no supplementation)	**WARNING!** Inadequate knowledge about the return of ovulation and menstruation can result in pregnancy before the woman is physically and emotionally recovered or ready.
Reproductive System: Cervix, Vagina, and Perineum		
Cervix: Loose, thin, fragile, soft Gradual return to firm consistency; easily distensible for about 4-6 days after delivery Internal os closes by 2 wk	Cervix: Edematous, ecchymotic External cervical os changes from circular appearance of nulliparous woman to jagged, slitlike appearance	Cervix, vagina, and perineum: Presence of nonlochial-type bleeding may indicate unrepaired or poorly repaired lacerations of cervix, vagina, or perineum; poorly repaired episiotomy; or soft tissue trauma from difficult birth, forceps, or vacuum extractor:

Continued

Resumption of mucous secretion is slow, especially for breast-feeding women; estrogen secretion is suppressed by prolactin

Vagina:
Thin, absence of rugae; reappear in 4 wk
Regains approximate nonpregnant size in 6-8 wk
Return of secretory activity depends on resumption of ovulation and secretion of estrogen

Labia: decreased tone

Perineum:
Decreased muscle tone
Episiotomy heals in 2-3 wk
Lacerations, tearing of perineum: heal in 2-3 wk:
First degree: through skin and superficial tissues
Second degree: through perineal muscle
Third degree: additionally involves anal sphincter
Fourth degree: additionally involves anterior rectal wall

Oxygenation and Circulation

Blood volume:
Reduction to nonpregnant levels in about 3-4 wk
Average blood loss with birth vaginal: 300-400 ml, Cesarean: 600-800 ml

---

Vagina:
Flattened appearance of rugae
Dryness
Dyspareunia (painful intercourse) may occur until vaginal secretions resume

Labia: appear flabby

Perineum:
Some erythema, edema, and ecchymosis may be present for the first 1-2 days
Wound edges: approximated
No drainage
Pain present but relieved with local or systemic relief interventions

Blood pressure:
Slight decrease from analgesics, sedatives
Slight increase from the change in vascular network and blood volume, physical exertion of labor, excitement after birth, pain

---

Spurting of bright-red blood from vagina, perineum
Continuous bright-red, heavy bleeding with a firmly contracted fundus
Persistent pelvic and perineal pain, pressure, swelling, which may indicate hematoma formation

Perineum:
Signs of wound infection:
Persistent erythema and edema
Separation of wound edges
Purulent drainage
Persistent pain

Blood pressure:
Increase in diastolic with narrowing pulse pressure (early sign of hemorrhagic shock)
Continuing decrease to hypotension (worsening hemorrhagic shock)

TABLE 8-3 The Maternal Recovery Process—Expected Changes, Findings, and Warning Signs—cont'd

Anatomic and Physiologic Changes	Expected Assessment Findings	Warning Signs of Ineffective Recovery
Oxygenation and Circulation—cont'd		
Reduction in physiologic edema; extravascular water retained during pregnancy enters the circulatory system and excreted as a result of diuresis and diaphoresis	Postural hypotension, especially after spinal or epidural block anesthesia, may occur when first rising to an upright position	Steady increase especially with headache (PIH)
Increased fluid volume temporarily places stress on heart and increases risk for cardiac decompensation in first 1-2 days especially in women diagnosed with cardiac disorders	Pulse: Puerperal bradycardia: slowing of pulse (50-70 beats/min) owing to hemodynamic changes after birth	Pulse: steady increase in rate and decrease in volume (hemorrhagic shock)
Vascular network	Slight increase in pulse may occur as a result of exhaustion, pain, excitement, dehydration	
Loss of uteroplacental circulatory network	Respirations: normal baseline range, full, easy, and quiet, with return to nonpregnant pulmonary function in 6-8 wk; chest sounds clear	Respirations: signs of pulmonary edema associated with cardiac decompensation; signs of respiratory distress associated with amniotic fluid embolism
Reversal of hormonal stimulation of vasodilation		
CO remains elevated for 1-2 days then declines, returning to nonpregnant levels in 2-3 wk	Hematocrit and hemoglobin: change from baseline level during pregnancy:	Signs of thrombophlebitis as a result of venous stasis associated with limited activity and clot formation associated with hypercoagulability
Position of diaphragm and heart: nonpregnant position is regained when uterus is emptied and organs return to usual positions	Decrease days 1 and 2 from hemodilution with blood loss and reabsorption of extracellular fluid	Hematocrit and hemoglobin below expected ranges for pregnant women may be indicative of excessive or continuing blood loss
Hypercoagulability of blood: reduced over 4-5 wk	Increase days 3-7 with diuresis and diaphoresis	Leukocyte Count: increase of more than 30% within a 6-hr period is strongly suggestive of infection
Varicosities of legs, anus, vulva regress as pelvic pressure is reduced with birth	Reach nonpregnant levels in 4-6 wk	

Leukocyte count:
First 10 days: increased
Average range: 14,000-16,000/mm³ but can be as high as 20,000-25,000/mm³
Lower extremities:
Edema, especially of feet and ankles; diminishes gradually
Good circulation: warm, prompt capillary return

Nutrition, and Fluid and Electrolytes

Appetite:
Returns to normal after recovery from anesthesia and fatigue
Good appetite is essential to stimulate appropriate nutritional intake to support healing and lactation

Presence of hunger and thirst after birth
Request for large portions of food, snacks
Nausea and vomiting may be present during fourth stage of labor, especially if general anesthesia was used

Poor appetite with limited intake
Expressions of:
Excessive concern with body image and weight gained during pregnancy
Determination to regain "shape" quickly

Weight loss:
Early loss results from:
Birth of fetus and expulsion of placenta, amniotic membranes and fluid
Fluid loss with diuresis and diaphoresis
Continuing weight loss results from:
Sensible dietary modifications combined with a sensible exercise and activity program
Use of fat stores during lactation

Weight loss pattern:
11-13 lb immediately after birth with loss of uterine contents
9 lb: fluid loss with diuresis and diaphoresis
Continuing loss with return to pre-pregnant weight in 2-3 mo

Temperature of over 100.4° F (38° C) after the first 24 hr strongly suggests infection, especially if accompanied by chills, malaise, signs of infection in breasts or genitourinary tract

Dehydration: may be present, especially after a long, difficult labor with limited fluid intake to balance fluid losses
Lactation: production of milk requires energy gained through:
Increased caloric intake reflected in a nutritious diet

Signs of dehydration:
Elevated temperature up to 100.4° F (38° C) in first 24 hours
Concentrated urine
Thirst

Continued

TABLE 8-3 **The Maternal Recovery Process—Expected Changes, Findings, and Warning Signs—cont'd**

Anatomic and Physiologic Changes	Expected Assessment Findings	Warning Signs of Ineffective Recovery
Nutrition, and Fluid and Electrolytes—cont'd		
Lactation—cont'd		
Use of fat stores accumulated during pregnancy		
Physical and emotional rest		
Elimination		
Bowel:		
Flatus accumulates from an increased intestinal space after birth; peristalsis begins to increase as progesterone level decreases; flatus passed	Stronger, more frequent bowel sounds Passage of flatus	Holding back on passing feces owing to fear of pain and injury Constipation: no bowel movement by day 3-4
First bowel movement may be delayed from:	Elimination of soft, formed feces by day 2-3 postpartum	Straining with passage of feces increases pain experienced and may disrupt healing
Decreased peristalsis of intestines until progesterone effect diminishes	Hemorrhoids enlarged, edematous, sore	Excessively large or bleeding hemorrhoids
Tenderness and pain from episiotomy, lacerations, hemorrhoids and fear of further pain and "ripping stitches" with bowel movement		
Decreased abdominal muscle tone		
Decreased activity level		
Effects of labor: passage of stool and limited intake of food and fluids		

Hemorrhoids: may appear or enlarge with pressure of fetal presenting part and vigorous pushing during labor; gradually decrease in size during the puerperium

Bladder:
Reversal of renal adaptations takes 2-8 wk
By-products of metabolic and regressive changes during recovery are excreted into blood and urine
Postpartum diuresis: increased production of urine to rid body of fluid retained during pregnancy; bladder fills more rapidly
Risk for urinary retention:
Edema and decreased sensitivity of bladder and urethra from the effects of labor, birth, and regional anesthetics
Discomfort of lacerations and episiotomy
Restoration of nonpregnant bladder tone and function and usual elimination patterns occur within 1 wk

Physical Activity and Rest
Abdominal muscle tone:
Returns gradually over 6 wk, depending on pre-pregnant muscle tone, degree of stretching with pregnancy, and amount of adipose tissue
Facilitated by postpartum exercises

Voiding patterns:
Voids within 4-8 hr of birth
Amount of each voiding should be at least 100 ml
Amount increases
Absence of bladder distension
Common complaints during first few days:
Delay in initiation of stream
Slower stream
Burning when urine comes in contact with episiotomy or lacerations
Urine may contain protein (+1) from autolysis, lactose with lactation, and blood from hemorrhagic areas in bladder from labor and contamination with lochia

Abdominal muscles loose and flabby; soft and doughlike on palpation
Abdominal protrusion when upright; soft distended appearance

Signs of urinary retention and bladder distension:
Frequent voiding
Continued urgency even after voiding
Bladder palpable above symphysis pubis; manual pressure on bladder produces urgency
Dullness on percussion of bladder
Displacement of uterus upward above umbilicus and laterally to right or left; results in loss of uterine contraction (boggy fundus) leads to an increase in lochia (bright-red, fresh bleeding)
Repeated or prolonged retention and distension lead to:
UTI
Delay in return of normal bladder function and elimination patterns
Decrease in bladder tone

Expressions of excessive body image concerns; may have negative influence on nutrition and exercise during the postpartum period in an effort to rush return to pre-pregnant appearance

Continued

TABLE 8-3 The Maternal Recovery Process—Expected Changes, Findings, and Warning Signs—cont'd

Anatomic and Physiologic Changes	Expected Assessment Findings	Warning Signs of Ineffective Recovery
Physical Activity and Rest—cont'd		
Abdominal muscle tone—cont'd	Diastasis recti abdominis: separation of abdominal wall muscle that can be seen when woman is supine and rolls shoulders upward placing chin on chest—abdominal muscles will protrude through separation	Limited social support may inhibit ability to achieve a healthy balance of activity and rest
Offers limited support to abdominal contents and enlarged uterus		
Movement and activity level may be affected by:	Posture slightly bent, gait slow to reduce perineal pain when moving	
Muscle strain and soreness from muscular efforts of labor and birth	Muscle aching in arms, neck, shoulders, lower back, and pelvis from childbirth and pushing efforts	
Perineal pain aggravated by movement	Change in shoe size from a larger to a smaller size	
Loss of sensation and ability to fully move lower limbs from the use of epidural or spinal anesthesia	Return of sensation and ability to feel touch and move lower limbs after spinal or epidural block	
	Joints:	
Joints:	Full active range of motion of all joints	
Stabilize within 6-8 wk		
Joints in feet may not fully return to prepregnant position; feet remain slightly larger		

Fatigue is often present from:
Sleep disturbances during later part of pregnancy
Hormonal changes
Work of labor and excitement of birth
Altered rest-sleep patterns after birth:
Hospital environment
Pain and discomfort
Responsibilities of caring for self, newborn, and family
Continuing fatigue negatively affects healing, lactation, emotions

Integument

Postpartum diaphoresis: reversal of physiologic edema of pregnancy results in profuse sweating during first week after birth
Decrease in melanocyte-stimulating hormone
Peripheral vasodilation subsides as estrogen level decreases
Elasticity of skin is regained

Night sweats
Fading or disappearance of pigmentary changes, including:
Chloasma or melasma
Nipple-areola darkening
Linea nigra
Regression of palmar erythema and epulis; spider nevi may remain
Loss of fine hair grown during pregnancy
Resumption of fingernail strength and consistency; firmer and stronger
Fading of striae gravidarum from bright reddish-pink to silvery white

TABLE 8-4	Common Nursing Diagnoses, Expected Outcomes, and Interventions for the Postpartum Period

Nursing Diagnoses, Expected Outcomes	Nursing Interventions

Risk for fluid volume deficit related to blood loss associated with process of childbirth and recovery
 	
Woman will:
Heal without excessive blood loss
Identify signs indicative of effective healing of the reproductive tract after the birth
Identify measures to enhance healing
Incorporate measures to enhance healing into her living patterns after discharge
	Assess progress of involution by checking vital signs, fundus, characteristics of lochia, episiotomy, laceration
	Massage fundus if boggy or flaccid by supporting the lower uterus, grasping the fundus through the abdominal wall, and massaging it until firm (see Fig. 5-7)
	Administer oxytocics as ordered:
	  Pitocin 10-20 U in 1 L IV fluid
	  Methergine (IM or PO), 0.2 mg, assessing BP before and 5-10 min after administration; hold dose if BP 140/90 mm Hg or higher
	Encourage woman to void every 2 hr to prevent bladder distention that can interfere with uterine contraction
	Teach and demonstrate:
	  Fundal check and massage
	  Stages of lochia and its expected characteristics (see Fig. 5-8)
	Discuss actions to enhance healing:
	  Get out of bed and begin ambulation slowly
	  Follow activity restrictions such as lifting heavy objects over 5 lb, climbing stairs
	  Do acceptable activities and postpartum exercises that enhance circulation and prevent thrombophlebitis
	  Take frequent rest periods
	  Have good nutrition that includes a balance of nutrients especially protein, vitamins, and iron
	  Use actions to prevent constipation
	  Use birth control interventions to facilitate the spacing of pregnancies; at least a 2-yr interval between pregnancies is recommended

Risk for infection related to the effects of vaginal birth

Woman will:

Heal without infection

Identify signs and symptoms indicative of infection

Identify actions that will prevent infection

Use appropriate actions to prevent infection

WARNING! Barrier methods are recommended until breast feeding is well-established. A diaphragm must be refitted after healing is complete.

WARNING! Use aseptic principles, scrupulous hand washing, and standard precautions to prevent infection while caring for the woman and her newborn.

Assess woman for infection by checking temperature, pulse, heart rate, breasts, fundus, characteristics of lochia, episiotomy or laceration, urination patterns, and urine characteristics

Teach woman the signs and symptoms of infection and how to check temperature, breasts, episiotomy or laceration, lochia, and urine for their presence

Teach and demonstrate:

Breast care (see Box 8-7, p. 241)

Perineal care (see Box 8-8, p. 242)

Teach actions to prevent bladder infection:

Practice frequent perineal care

Increase fluid intake to 3 L/day, including fluids that increase acidity of urine such as cranberry juice or take vitamin C

Empty bladder every 2 hr to prevent stasis of urine

Teach actions to enhance healing and maintain a resistance to infection:

Good nutrition: protein, fluids, vitamins

Balance of rest and activity

Stress reduction measures

Avoid intercourse until healing has taken place; use principles of safer sex

Good general hygiene

Altered patterns of urinary elimination, retention, related to effects of pregnancy and childbirth on the renal system

Woman will:

Void within 4-6 hr of birth

Empty bladder at each voiding without difficulty

Use actions to facilitate voiding:

Assist woman into an upright position to void, sitting forward so urine does not touch episiotomy

Provide privacy

Stimulate urination by running water, placing woman's hands in warm water, blowing bubbles in a glass of water using a straw, having the woman use a sitz bath

Measure first few voidings: assess amount and characteristics

Palpate abdomen, above symphysis pubis, to check for a distended bladder

Continued

TABLE 8-4	**Common Nursing Diagnoses, Expected Outcomes, and Interventions for the Postpartum Period—cont'd**

Nursing Diagnoses, Expected Outcomes	**Nursing Interventions**

Void every 2-3 hr
Not exhibit bladder distension
	Encourage fluid intake of 3 L/day
	Perform straight catheterization (requires physician order) if bladder is distended and woman is unable to void spontaneously:
	  Explain what you are going to do
	  Perform perineal care to remove lochia
	  Use good lighting because edema may make urethra difficult to visualize
	  Use gentle approach because the area is very tender

Constipation related to painful hemorrhoids, laceration or episiotomy, and decreased intestinal motility associated with pregnancy
Woman will:
Have soft, formed bowel movement by third postpartum day
Use appropriate actions to facilitate bowel elimination
	Assess woman for bowel sounds, passage of flatus, usual elimination patterns
	Use appropriate actions to facilitate bowel elimination
	Teach woman measures that are effective in safely stimulating bowel elimination:
	  Fluid intake of 3 L/day
	  Roughage and bulk in diet, including raw fruit and vegetables, bran cereals, whole wheat bread or muffins
	  Periods of activity such as ambulation, postpartum exercises
	Administer, as ordered, a stool softer [docusate sodium (Colace)], a stool softener and laxative (docusate sodium and casanthranol (Peri-Colace)], or a rectal suppository [bisacodyl (Dulcolax)]
	Administer sodium biphosphate (Fleet Enema) as ordered if above measures are ineffective; contraindicated if a 3rd to 4th degree laceration is present
	Use local pain relief interventions and proper cleansing after a bowel movement such as perineal care, sitz bath, topical applications

Alteration in nutrition (less than body requirements) related to knowledge deficit about postpartum nutrient requirements and weight loss patterns

Woman will:

State nutrient requirements of postpartum period

Maintain a nutrient intake reflective of nutrient requirements of postpartum period

Participate in an exercise program appropriate for postpartum women

Lose weight gained during pregnancy at a rate of 0.5-1 lb/wk

Weigh woman

Discuss expected progress of weight loss during the postpartum period

Explain the importance of an approach to weight loss that combines good nutrition and appropriate exercise

Teach woman components of a postpartum diet that support healing and lactation: the diet and prenatal vitamins recommended for pregnancy can be continued for the 6-wk postpartum period (see Table 3-4, pp. 64-65):

Calories supply nutrient and energy requirements for healing and lactation

Proteins are crucial for healing

Fluid intake of 3 L/day is required, with an additional 1-2 L if breast feeding

Complex carbohydrates (fruits, vegetables, whole grains) are excellent sources of nutrients and roughage

Iron-rich foods, or iron supplements or both are required, especially if hematocrit and hemoglobin levels are low

Avoid use of alcohol, tobacco, caffeine especially if breast feeding

Teach postpartum exercises that facilitate weight loss and restoration of abdominal muscle tone

Pain related to effects of vaginal birth

Woman will:

Request medication as needed for pain relief

Experience a reduction of pain after use of the pain relief interventions

Use appropriate pain relief interventions

Determine source, intensity, and duration of pain

Provide relief measures appropriate to the source and intensity of the pain

Provide local relief measures such as:

Breast care (see Box 8-7, p. 241)

Perineal care (see Box 8-8, p. 242)

Sims position for perineal pain

Squeeze buttocks together before sitting down

Continued

TABLE 8-4	Common Nursing Diagnoses, Expected Outcomes, and Interventions for the Postpartum Period—cont'd
Nursing Diagnoses, Expected Outcomes	**Nursing Interventions**

Pain related to effects of vaginal birth
 	
Woman will:
Request medication as needed for pain relief
Experience a reduction of pain after use of the pain relief interventions
Use appropriate pain relief interventions
	Instruct to request analgesic before pain becomes severe
	Provide analgesics as ordered such as:
	  Acetaminophen (Tylenol) with or without codeine
	  Ibuprofen (Motrin); especially effective for afterpains
	  Propoxyphene hydrochloride (Darvon), hydrocodone bitartrate (Lortab), oxycodone hydrochloride and acetaminophen (Tylox)
	  WARNING! Always check the components of combination analgesics to ensure both are safe for lactation and maternal allergy is not present.
	Encourage use of relaxation and breathing techniques taught in childbirth classes
	Provide comfort measures to enhance relaxation and rest along with effectiveness of pain relief measures
	Explain to woman the importance and safety of pain relief measures even for breast feeding mothers
	Assess effectiveness of pain relief measures

Box 8-7
Instructions for Breast Care During the Postpartum Period

Instructions for the Woman Who is Bottle Feeding

Hygiene: Wash breasts at least once a day as the first part of the shower or bath, use a mild soap, and rinse well.

Support: Wear a clean bra that fully supports the entire breast until breasts have returned to their nonpregnant status in about 1 month.

Care of engorged breasts:
Wear snug supportive bra or breast binder.
Avoid exposure of breasts to hot water during the shower; have water run over shoulders, not over breasts.
Apply cold packs to breasts to reduce tenderness.
Never express milk from breasts because more milk will be produced.
Change frequently the absorbent pads that are used to collect leakage.
Avoid the use of plastic liners because keeping moisture against the nipples-areolas leads to excoriation, cracking, and infection.

Instructions for the Woman Who is Breast Feeding

Hygiene: Wash nipple and areola of each breast with a clean cloth and warm water as the first part of the shower or bath, and before and after each breast-feeding session if needed; allow to air dry thoroughly; and avoid soap because it may dry and irritate the nipple-areola, leading to cracking and infection.

Support: Wear a clean bra that fully supports the entire breast until breast feeding is discontinued and breasts return to their nonpregnant status about 1 month after breast feeding is stopped.

Care of nipples-areola:
Use correct breast-feeding techniques for latch on, removal from, and position at breast.
Apply colostrum or milk after breast feeding as a safe and effective intervention to maintain suppleness and integrity of the nipples-areola.
If recommended by health care provider, use purified lanolin sparingly and apply after breast feeding to nipple-areola that have been cleansed and dried; lanolin may be removed with warm water before breast feeding.
Change absorbent pads used to collect leakage frequently.
Avoid the use of plastic liners because keeping moisture against nipples-areolas leads to excoriation, cracking, and infection.

Care of engorged breasts:
Empty the breasts frequently using good breast-feeding technique to prevent or limit the extent of engorgement.
Apply warmth (warm packs, shower) to breasts, massage breasts, express some milk to soften the breasts and nipples; this practice facilitates latch on and stimulates the let down reflex.
Apply cold packs to breasts after feeding to reduce tenderness and decrease swelling.
Wear a supportive bra.

Care of sore nipples-areola:
Initiate feeding on breast that is not sore or is least sore.
Limit the duration of sucking on the sore breast.

Continued

Box 8-7
Instructions for Breast Care During the Postpartum Period—cont'd

Instructions for the Woman Who is Breast Feeding—cont'd

Care of sore nipples-areola—cont'd:
   Stimulate the let down reflex using breast massage, before newborn latches on to the sore breast.
   Keep nipple-areola dry.
      Expose to air after feeding.
      Use breast milk to soothe.
      Use nipple shells to allow for circulation of air and to prevent further irritation from rubbing of nipple-areola against bra. Nipple shells can also be used to enhance eversion, especially when nipples are flat or inverted.

Box 8-8
Instructions for Perineal Care During the Postpartum Period

Hygiene:
   Wash perineal area from front to back using a clean washcloth, soap and water at least twice a day (morning and at night) and after a bowel movement.
   Use a different part of the cloth for each stroke, and do not separate labia while washing.
   Rinse with a peribottle filled with warm water by directing the flow backward; never direct the flow upward into the vagina.
   Pat dry.
   Use a peribottle, filled with warm water, to cleanse the perineum after each urination and pad change.
   Change peripads at least every 2 to 3 hours, putting them on and taking them off from front to back; avoid touching the side of the pad that comes in contact with the vulva and perineum.
Application of topical preparations for pain relief:
   Apply ice packs intermittently (on for 20 to 30 minutes and off for 60 minutes) during the first 12 to 24 hours after the birth.
   Use topical preparations (anesthetics and antiseptics) sparingly, no more than 4 times a day.
   Apply directly to the episiotomy or laceration after the perineum has been cleansed, and avoid application to the peripad because doing so hinders its function and minimizes absorption into the skin.
   Use preparations only as needed for discomfort.
Use of the sitz bath:
   Perform perineal care before a sitz bath is used.
   Use a sitz bath—sitting in warm water—at least twice a day to enhance healing and comfort and to facilitate cleansing.
   Use of cool to cold water may be effective to reduce discomfort.
   Use warm water and continue the bath for approximately 15 to 20 minutes.
   Wash the sitz bath basin with soap and water after each use.
WARNING!   Wear clean gloves when assisting the woman with perineal care or the sitz bath to protect yourself and prevent infection to the mother.

WEB Resources

http://www.babycenter.com
This website is created by parents with physician and expert panel support. Click on Pregnancy to access information related to the postpartum period.

http://www.parenthoodweb.com
This website covers all aspects of pregnancy including the postpartum period. Click on pregnancy to access the postpartum-related information.

http://www.fatherhood.org
This is the website for the National Fatherhood Initiative. It provides information and support designed to help men become loving, committed, and responsible fathers.

http://members.xoom.com/_XMCM/fobb
This website provides support and information for fathers of breastfed babies. It also lists many relevant links to sites on the Breastfeeding Web Ring.

http://www.promom.org
This is the website for Pro Mom—Promotion of Mother's Milk, Inc. It includes articles, essays, and a breastfeeding gallery of fine art, photography, and clip art depicting breastfeeding mothers and infants.

http://www.women.com/pregnancy
This website covers all aspects of pregnancy, birth, and parenting an infant. Scroll down to Choose a Topic and click on postpartum for access to information related to recovery and adjustment after birth.

http://www.plannedparenthood.org
Planned Parenthood Federation of America, Inc.

REVIEW QUESTIONS

1. The onset of the lactation cycle is initially dependent on which of these occurrences?
   1. Increased secretion of prolactin
   2. Increased circulation to the breasts
   3. Sucking of the newborn, which empties the breasts
   4. Decreased levels of estrogen and progesterone with the expulsion of the placenta

2. Which of these women is least likely to experience afterpains?
   1. Primiparous woman who is bottle feeding and delivered a 7-lb baby at 40 weeks' gestation
   2. Multiparous woman who delivered twin boys at 27 weeks' gestation
   3. Primiparous woman who is breast feeding and delivered an 8-lb baby at 42 weeks' gestation
   4. Multiparous woman with gestational diabetes who delivered an 11-lb macrosomic baby at 38 weeks' gestation

3. When assessing a multiparous woman on her first day postpartum, the nurse would expect which of these findings?
   1. Fundus two to three fingerbreadths below the umbilicus, and firm
   2. Lochia serosa, moderate, no clots or foul odor
   3. Full, tender breasts
   4. Painful, intact episiotomy with some erythema, edema, and bruising

4. A primiparous woman, 1-day postpartum, calls the nurse into her room. The woman anxiously tells the nurse that while breast feeding, she experienced uterine cramps and a heavy gush of flow that soaked through her peripad to her bed. The nurse should initially do which action?
   1. Palpate the woman's fundus
   2. Tell the woman that this often happens when breast feeding for the first few days after birth
   3. Administer the methylergonovine maleate (Methergine) that was ordered PRN
   4. Assist the woman with pericare and with changing her pad

5. Dyspareunia during the postpartum period is most likely the result of which change associated with pregnancy and birth?
   1. Inadequate secretion of vaginal mucous
   2. Flattened vaginal rugae
   3. Tenderness of the cervix
   4. Pressure on uterus

6. Which of these families is most likely to experience a maturational crisis related to the birth of a new baby?
   1. Father wishes to participate in the physical care of the baby while the mother has expressed the belief that baby care is woman's work
   2. Parents have planned special activities that are designed to give attention to their older children without the new baby present
   3. First-time parents have enrolled in parenting classes designed for new parents even though they also have the help and support from their extended family
   4. Before discharge from the hospital, first-time parents have asked the nurse for the name of a lactation consultant and the location of a La Leche group because the mother does not feel confident with breast feeding

7. The nurse should understand that the parent-newborn attachment process has which criteria?
   1. Begins after the baby is born
   2. Requires that parents and newborn interact with each other immediately after birth
   3. Is enhanced by early, close, frequent contact and interaction of parents with newborn
   4. Is affected by the health status of the mother during the postpartum period but not during pregnancy

8. Which of these women is least likely to exhibit postpartum blues?
   1. Multiparous woman whose husband took his 2-week vacation from work to help care for the older children while she takes care of the new baby
   2. Primiparous woman who gave birth to a healthy full-term baby boy whom she will be breast feeding
   3. Adolescent primipara, whose family is embarrassed by her pregnancy, will be living in her parents' home with the new baby until she graduates from high school in 1 year
   4. Primiparous woman, aged 39, who plans to continue her career as a lawyer and take care of her new baby girl

9. Paternal role behaviors and the degree of involvement in infant care have which characteristic?
   1. Should be determined by the mother as the primary care-giver
   2. Is fostered by encouraging the father to participate in newborn care classes
   3. Should be limited to the areas of discipline, play, and modeling of the male role
   4. Are primarily influenced by the father's culture

10. Parents should realize that which of these sibling behaviors, related to adjustment to a new baby, would require evaluation by a health care professional?
    1. Impatience and sometimes anger when the newborn's needs take precedence over their own
    2. Rejection of their mother when she arrives home with the new baby
    3. Asking to be bottle-fed or to sleep in the parent's bedroom along with the new baby
    4. Altered living patterns such as sleeping, eating, and refusal to go to school

11. The physician has ordered the administration of RhoGAM to an Rh-negative postpartum woman. The nurse should administer the RhoGAM no later than how many hours after birth?
    1. 12
    2. 24
    3. 48
    4. 72

12. A woman who is breast feeding would demonstrate the need for additional instruction about breast feeding and care if she has which action?
    1. Washes the nipple and areola of each breast with warm water but avoids the use of soap
    2. Applies a small amount purified lanolin to her nipples and areola after each feeding
    3. Feeds her baby every 4 hours
    4. Positions her baby by bringing him up to her breast

13. The breasts of a woman who is bottle feeding her baby are engorged. The nurse should tell her to use which of these relief measures?
    1. Wear a snug, supportive bra
    2. Allow warm water to soothe the breasts during a shower
    3. Express milk from breasts occasionally to relieve discomfort
    4. Place absorbent pad with a plastic liner into her bra to absorb leakage and prevent staining of clothing

14. Perineal care is an important infection control measure. When evaluating a postpartum woman's perineal care technique, the nurse would recognize the need for further instruction if the woman performs which of these actions?
    1. Uses soap and warm water to wash the vulva and perineum
    2. Washes the vulva and perineum from the symphysis pubis back to the episiotomy site, then over the episiotomy site to the anus
    3. Changes her perineal pad every 2 to 3 hours
    4. Uses the peribottle to rinse upward into her vagina

15. The bladder of a postpartum woman is distended, and she is having difficulty voiding. Before inserting a catheter, as ordered by the physician on an as-needed basis, the nurse should try which of these actions to stimulate spontaneous urination?

1. Place the woman's hands in cold water
2. Blow bubbles into a glass of water
3. Play soothing music
4. Tell woman that she must urinate to avoid being catheterized

ANSWERS, RATIONALES, AND TEST-TAKING TIPS

Rationale	Test-Taking Tips

1. Correct answer: 4

Options 1, 2, and 3 are important in the process of lactation, especially in the continuation of the cycle. However, estrogen and progesterone levels must decrease to remove the suppression on prolactin activity and allow the lactation process to begin.

The clue in the stem is the word "initially." This guides you to think as you read the options to put them in a sequence of possible events. The first event is option 4. The clue also lets you know that all of the options are correct and possible answers. Avoid looking for three incorrect and one correct option.

2. Correct answer: 1

Afterpains are most common when the uterus is overstretched as in a multiparous woman, a large fetus, and multiple gestation. In addition, breast feeding stimulates the release of oxytocin, which causes the uterus to contract.

First establish that the uterine stretch is least in a primiparous woman. Next note that the weight of the neonate is not excessive and thus the uterus would not be overly stretched. Think less stretch, less afterpains. Be aware that the question asks for the least likely person to experience afterpains. Eliminate options 2 and 4 with the multiparous women who would have greater stretch and more afterpains. With options 1 and 3 remaining, take an educated guess that the breast-feeding mother would have the release of more hormones to contract the uterus than a mother who bottle feeds her baby. The critical element to get this question correct is to keep in mind the question of "least likely." For these types of questions, after you have made a selection take the extra time and effort to read together the question and option you have selected one last time.

3. Correct answer: 4

Episiotomies often exhibit the findings described as a result of the pressure of birth, local anesthesia, and the

Option 1 would be 2 or 3 days after the birth. The uterus descends at a rate of 1 to 2 cm/day. *Lochia serosa,* a light pink to brown

inflammatory process essential for healing. The fundus should be one finger below and midline. *Lochia ruba,* 1 to 3 days postpartum, should be red, thick, moderate, with no large clots or foul odor; small clots or trickles from the vagina are expected. Breasts should be soft and should not be tender.

drainage with a thinner consistency, occurs 3 to 10 days postpartum. The final drainage, *lochia alba,* a yellowish white, can last as long as 3 weeks. Full, tender breasts may indicate mastitis, especially if found unilaterally.

4. Correct answer: 1

Although this is an expected finding with breast feeding, fundal massage, or ambulation, the nurse should still make sure that the fundus is firm. If firm, the nurse can then implement options 2 and 4. If the uterus is boggy, it should be massaged. If the uterus does not remain contracted after massage, then Methergine is administered and the physician is notified.

A basic rule for postpartum is when women have complaints that are associated with bleeding, check the fundus first. The nursing process could be used as a guide to the correct answer. When the client has a complaint do further assessment to collect more information about the complaint.

5. Correct answer: 1

Until resumption of ovulation and the secretion of estrogen, vaginal dryness will be present related to limited production of lubricating mucous. Rugae do not affect intercourse. Options 3 and 4, while possible, are unlikely to be problematic once intercourse resumes a few weeks after birth.

Think about your general knowledge of dyspareunia, abnormal pain during sexual intercourse. A common cause is dry vaginal mucosa, especially in older women with hormonal changes of menopause. Then associate the changes in hormonal production in the postpartum period. Make an educated guess to select option 1.

6. Correct answer: 1

In option 1 the parents have not developed mutually acceptable parental role responsibilities. Options 2, 3, and 4 reflect a realistic view of postpartum stressors and appropriate coping mechanisms to deal with the stressors.

You can cluster the options 2, 3, and 4 under the theme "working as a team." In option 1, each parent has a different view, which can contribute to a maturational crisis.

Rationales   **Test-Taking Tips**

7. Correct answer: 3

Attachment begins during pregnancy as the fetal heatbeat is heard, the fetal image is viewed in a sonogram, and the mother perceives fetal movement. Events and well-being during all stages of pregnancy affect attachment, which is progressive and ongoing. Therefore failure to have immediate contact between the parents and neonate because of maternal or newborn health problems will not have serious long-term effects. However, opportunities for close and frequent contact need to be provided.

Read the options carefully to identify the clues associated with timeframes: in option 1, the timeframe of "after" the baby is born; in option 2, "immediately after" birth; in option 3, a more general time of "early"; and in option 4 "during postpartum. . . not pregnancy." Then look at the verbs: begins, requires, enhanced, and affected. Of these verbs matched with the timeframes, the less restrictive timeframe and the positive verb make option 3 the best answer. Note that the question is of a more general nature so the option with the more general focus usually is the best answer.

8. Correct answer: 1

Option 1 reflects past experience and support, both of which help reduce the incidence of the blues. Options 2, 3, and 4 describe women who have one or more risk factors associated with the blues and depression. These are adolescent mothers with limited support, older mothers with a career, and women who are primiparous.

Read the question carefully, then look for the mother with least risk. Avoid looking for the mother with the most risk. Another approach if you had no idea of a correct answer is to cluster the options 2, 3, and 4 because these options include first-time mothers. Select the odd one, option 1. Last, note that with a support system and repeated experience, less emotional reaction take places with most events. Compare first semester nursing students' emotional reactions to the course and clinical assignments during school with the reactions of the students in the third semester. The emotional reactions are minimized in the third semester because students have experience and established support systems.

9. Correct answer: 2

Both parents should determine paternal behaviors and degree of involvement in infant care to their mutual satisfaction. Paternal role responsibilities are unlimited, especially today, as many fathers want to play a more active role in childcare. Many factors, in addition to culture, influence the father's role such as the relationship with their own father, education, lifestyle, and friends.

Did you find the clues of the restrictive words in options 1, 3, and 4? In option 1 "determined by the mother" is too one-sided. In option 3, "should be limited to" is too narrow of an approach to childcare. In option 4, "primarily influenced by. . . culture" is too narrow of a base to establish roles in infant care.

10. Correct answer: 4

Options, 1, 2, and 3 all are typical sibling reactions, especially in young children who have more difficulty understanding the impact of a new baby. Disturbances in life activities, especially if persistent, reflect a problem with adjustment that necessitates the care of a health care provider before more serious difficulties develop.

If you have no idea of a correct answer, look for the theme clue. Each option is focused on a specific situation or more general actions. Options 1, 2, and 3 present specific events. Option 4 is a more global option with the words "living patterns." Select the odd option, option 4.

11. Correct answer: 4

Although often given shortly after birth, 72 hours is the latest that RhoGAM can be given effectively.

Use the 48-to-72-hour rule if you had no idea of the correct answer. This means that many events cluster around the 48-to-72-hour timeframe: bowel sounds return after surgery, the action of warfarin (Coumadin) becomes effective, the time for physiologic jaundice in neonates, and the time to read a TB skin test. See if you can add to this list. Take 48 to 72 seconds to brainstorm for other events.

12. Correct answer: 3

Options 1, 2, and 3 are correct techniques. If lanolin is used, it is best applied after feeding

Avoid narrow thinking by focusing only on the baby. Think of the mother's need to empty her breasts

Rationales	Test-Taking Tips

once the breasts have been cleansed with warm water and air-dried. Colostrum or milk also can be used. A breast-fed baby should be fed every 2 to 3 hours to provide for food and fluids and to prevent overdistended breasts.

of milk. The baby may be able to go 4 hours between feedings. However the mother will have discomfort.

13. Correct answer: 1

Cold packs reduce tenderness, whereas warmth increases circulation and thereby increases discomfort. Expressing milk results in continued milk production and a rebound type of event, resulting in engorgement. Plastic liners keep nipples-areola moist, which leads to excoriation and cracking.

Avoid the temptation to select option 1 and not read the other options. This type of action and bad habit can cause you to miss many easy questions. When you are tempted to do this, go immediately to option 4 to start a reverse order of reading: options 4, 3, 2, and 1. Using this process will clear your mind and make you more alert to the information given.

14. Correct answer: 4

Options 1, 2, and 3 are appropriate measures. The peribottle should be used in a backward direction. The flow should never be directed upward into the vagina.

If you missed this question you probably read too quickly over option 4, which has two parts. Avoid the error of reading the second part of an option too quickly by simply first identifying that the option has two parts. Then read the second part of the option first, and the first part second. In this situation you would read "into the vagina use the peribottle to rinse upward."

15. Correct answer: 2

The sound of bubbles often stimulates the urge to void and successful voiding. Another effective approach is to place the woman's hands in warm water—not cold—or run warm

It is obvious that option 4 is not therapeutic. Auditory prompts are important to stimulate voiding and must be associated with a component of water movement. Thus, eliminate option 3. Of the

water over her hands, and let her listen to the sound of running water. Option 3 might relax her or divert her attention with no enhancement for her to void. Option 4 would increase her anxiety to further inhibit urination. A sitz bath of warm water or pouring water over the vulva also is helpful.

remaining options, option 2 fits the criteria for the stimulation to void better than does option 1.

9

Complications in Postpartum Recovery

FAST FACTS

1. Major complications from ineffective postpartum recovery are hemorrhage, infection, thrombophlebitis, and postpartum depression (see Chapter 8, p. 216).
2. Complications are more common among women whose (a) pregnancy was high risk; (b) labor was dysfunctional, requiring medical or surgical intervention; and (c) postpartum lifestyle is inadequate in terms of rest, nutrition, hygiene, finances, and social support.
3. Postpartum complications are a major cause of **maternal mortality,** which is the number of maternal deaths from complications of pregnancy, birth, and the puerperium per 100,000 live births.
4. Hemorrhage is a major cause of maternal mortality. Postpartum hemorrhage is the most common type of excessive blood loss associated with pregnancy.
5. Early discharge after birth requires that women be instructed about interventions related to the (a) prevention of complications by self-care measures related to hygiene, nutrition, rest, activity, and social support; (b) early detection of signs and symptoms that indicate an ineffective recovery and the development of complications; and (c) prompt treatment when signs of complications are detected, for example, massage the fundus and call the health care provider.
6. Complications interfere with maternal attachment to the newborn and the development of parenting skills.
7. Nursing actions to help with maternal attachment to the newborn, family coping and parenting skills are as follows: (a) providing short periods, within the tolerance level of the woman, for interaction with her newborn, giving her a chance to see, touch, and gradually care for the newborn; (b) encouraging expression of feelings by the mother and other family members; (c) providing opportunities for family members to be together; and

(4) discussing strategies that may be helpful in constructively readjusting the family processes: involvement of the grandparents, other family members, and friends in care of other children, the use of homemaker services.

CONTENT REVIEW

I. Postpartum hemorrhage

A. **Definition—Blood loss of more than 500 ml after a vaginal birth or more than 1000 ml after a cesarean birth, a 10% change in hematocrit since admission for childbirth, or a need for erythrocyte transfusion. The hypervolemic state of pregnancy provides initial protection and delays the onset of shock.**

B. *Early* **postpartum hemorrhage occurs within the first 24 hours after birth with these major causes:**
   1. **Uterine atony:** uterine hypotonia noted as a boggy or soft fundus
   2. Lacerations of the labia, perineum, vagina, and cervix
   3. **Hematoma:** accumulation of blood within the connective tissue of the pelvis or genitalia—the labia, vagina, vulva, and perineum—from bleeding of a blood vessel damaged during the childbirth process. The use of forceps or vacuum extraction and pressure from the presenting part are common causes for this damage.
   4. Clotting disorders
      a. *Disseminated intravascular coagulation (DIC)*—abnormal, diffuse clotting pattern that depletes clotting factors and results in massive bleeding
      b. Decreased platelets associated with severe preeclampsia and the HELLP syndrome (hemolysis, elevated liver enzymes, and low platelet count occurring in association with preeclampsia)
   5. Inversion of the uterus

C. *Late* **postpartum hemorrhage occurs from the second postpartum day (24 hours after birth) until the 28th postpartum day and most often during the first week or two. Major causes are** *subinvolution*—**the delayed return of the uterus to nonpregnant state—retained placental fragments, and infection**

D. **Risk factors associated with postpartum hemorrhage:**
   1. Dystocia
      a. Prolonged or precipitous labor patterns
      b. Interventions: external version, forceps, vacuum extraction, or cesarean birth
      c. Stimulation of labor with oxytocin (Pitocin)
   2. Overstretching of the uterus: inhibits the ability of the uterus to contract, and leads to atony. Examples include macrosomia, hydramnios, multiple gestation, and grand multiparity.
   3. Placental abnormalities: abruptio placenta, placenta previa, placental adherence that require manual removal, and retention of fragments that limits the ability of uterus to contract

4. Magnesium sulfate: used to treat preterm labor or severe preeclampsia. Magnesium relaxes the smooth muscle of the uterus.
5. Uterine infection (chorioamnionitis)

E. **Selected nursing diagnoses and major assessment findings related to hemorrhage. The goal is early detection and prompt intervention to prevent hemorrhagic shock with major life-threatening complications**
   1. Fluid volume deficit related to blood loss; assess the amount, character, and source of blood loss
      a. Uterine: profuse, bright-red blood with clots and a boggy fundus
      b. Laceration, episiotomy: bright-red blood in a steady stream or trickle, with a firm fundus
      c. Hematoma: blood accumulates in tissue resulting in increased pelvic pain and pressure, vaginal fullness, the urge to defecate, tissue swelling, and a firm fundus
      d. Alteration in vital signs reflecting fluid deficit (hypovolemia)
         (1) BP
            (a) Initially a narrowing of the pulse pressure: a decrease in the systolic pressure with a compensatory increase in the diastolic pressure associated with peripheral vasoconstriction
            (b) Progresses to hypotension
         (2) Pulse: rapid, strong and regular, usually with a sustained increase of at least 20 beats per minute over the client's baseline, with progression to being thready, weak, and irregular
         (3) Respirations: rapid; deep, progressing to shallow; and irregular
   2. Alteration in renal tissue perfusion related to hypovolemia associated with hemorrhage; decreasing urine formation progressing from oliguria (less than 25 ml/hr) to anuria
   3. Alteration in peripheral tissue perfusion and integument related to compensatory vasoconstriction: pallor; cool, progressing to cold; dry, progressing to moist and clammy; and delayed capillary refill of more than 3 to 5 seconds after blanching of the nail bed base
   4. Alteration in cerebral tissue perfusion related to hypovolemia: restlessness, anxiety, lightheadedness, faintness, dizziness, vertigo, diminishing level of consciousness and responsiveness, and mental confusion

F. **Interventions related to the source and degree of blood loss**
   1. Reduce blood loss
      a. Uterine atony: stimulate uterine contraction
         (1) Massage uterus until firm
         (2) Stimulate nipples manually or with breast feeding (endogenous oxytocin)
         (3) Administer **oxytocics** (listed in order of use)
            (a) Pitocin infusion, adding 10 to 40 U to 1000 ml of an

isotonic solution; administer at a recommended rate of 125 to 200 mU/min; observe for nausea and vomiting and signs of water intoxication

(b) Methylergonovine maleate (Methergine), 0.2 mg IM, every 2 to 4 hours up to 5 doses; watch for hypertension and headache

> ### ⚠ **Warning!**
>
> Assess BP before and 5 to 10 minutes after administration of oxytocics because hypertension is a dangerous side effect; hold dose if BP is 140/90 mm Hg or higher.

    (c) Prostaglandin $F_{2\alpha}$ (carboprost tromethamine; Hemabate), 0.25 mg, IM or intramyometrially; used if uterine atony is unresponsive to other drugs; repeated every 15 to 90 minutes for up to eight doses; watch for nausea and vomiting, fever, and headache

    (4) Insert Foley catheter into bladder: prevent bladder distension to allow uterus to contract; monitor renal perfusion by notation of the hourly urine output

  b. Surgical intervention to evacuate a hematoma, remove placental fragments, or repair lacerations or episiotomy

2. Replace fluid losses
   a. Carefully monitor response to replacement by measuring input and output and assessing for signs of fluid volume excess or deficit
   b. Use crystalloid or colloid solutions and packed RBCs

3. Enhance the circulation to the heart and lungs and facilitate venous return by
   a. Positioning the woman with a small pillow under her head and with legs elevated from the hips to an angle of 20 degrees
   b. Alternating the position frequently
   c. Encouraging coughing and deep breathing

4. Strict asepsis for care measures: an increased risk for infection occurs with hemorrhage

5. Reduce fear and anxiety to enhance rest
   a. Provide explanations to keep the woman and family informed
   b. Consolidate care to provide periods of uninterrupted rest
   c. Provide comfort measures to enhance relaxation

II. Postpartum infection

  A. **Major sites for infection during the postpartum period**

    1. The reproductive tract

      a. **Endometritis**—uterine infection, usually at the placental site, that can spread to the fallopian tubes and peritoneum. It is a major threat to fertility and life.

      b. Cervix, vagina, perineum, or vulva

2. The urinary tract: bladder and kidney
3. Wounds: episiotomy, laceration, abdominal incision of cesarean birth
4. **Mastitis:** breast infection that usually is unilateral but can be bilateral

B. **Risk factors associated with postpartum infection**
　1. Dystocia
　　a. Prolonged labor process: duration of more than 24 hours
　　b. Multiple invasive procedures
　　　(1) Repeated vaginal examinations
　　　(2) Urinary catheterizations
　　　(3) Interventions such as forceps, vacuum extraction, and cesarean birth
　　　(4) Internal fetal monitoring
　　c. Prolonged rupture of membranes: more than 24 hours before birth
　　d. Retained placental fragments
　2. Inadequate hygienic practices
　3. Health problems, for example, repeated genitourinary infections, diabetes, anemia, and poor nutrition
　4. Postpartum hemorrhage
　5. Ineffective breast-feeding techniques lead to cracking and breakdown of nipples and areola; increased risk with nulliparous woman

C. **Postpartum infection—major assessment findings and nursing diagnoses. The goal is early detection, which leads to prompt intervention and prevention of complications that can permanently affect reproductive functions.**
　1. General assessment findings related to infection
　　a. Alteration in body temperature related to infectious processes
　　　(1) Body temperature over 100.4 F (38° C) or higher; fever is often the first sign of infection
　　　(2) Present on two consecutive days after the first 24 hours of birth
　　　(3) Accompanied by tachycardia and tachypnea
　　b. Risk for fluid volume deficit related to diaphoresis, anorexia, nausea, and vomiting
　　c. Altered comfort related to malaise, fatigue, lethargy, chills, and headache
　　d. Elevation in WBC count from the previous baseline
　2. Specific assessment findings related to a site of infection
　　a. Reproductive tract: foul-smelling lochia, altered comfort from uterine tenderness, low backache, pelvic pain, and dysuria
　　b. Incisional infection: erythema, edema, purulent drainage with foul odor, separation of wound edges, incisional pain, and tenderness of surrounding tissue
　　c. Urinary tract: frequency, urgency, dysuria, cloudy urine, odor, and hematuria

    d. Breasts—findings are usually unilateral
       (1) Infected fissure or crack in nipple or areola
       (2) Edema and engorgement as infection spreads to breast tissue
       (3) Hard, red, and tender over the mass or an abscess

D. Interventions relate to the severity of the infection and the site of involvement

 Warning!

Consideration of standard precautions and aseptic principles is critical to prevent the spread of infection to other sites and persons.

  1. Interventions related to alteration in body temperature
    a. Monitor temperature, vital signs, and fluid balance
    b. Administer antibiotics to destroy causative organism
       (1) Obtain specimen of body substance such as wound drainage or urine for culture before initiation of antibiotic treatment
       (2) Administer antibiotic IV (piggyback) or orally, which are the most commonly used routes
       (3) Use appropriate principles to obtain maximum antibiotic effect
    c. Remove causative organism by incision and drainage of abscesses
    d. Administer antipyretics when fever is elevated over 102° F and is accompanied by discomfort such as headache and joint pain
    e. Encourage nutrient and fluid intake to prevent dehydration and energy depletion: small, frequent meals of easily digested foods with fluid intake of at least 3 L/day
    f. Administer IV fluids if oral intake is insufficient to balance fluid loss and energy depletion
    g. Use appropriate interventions to cool the body and cleanse the skin
  2. Interventions related to alteration in comfort
    a. Apply heat or cold locally using packs, pads, or sitz bath as ordered. Take into consideration the woman's preferences if possible.
    b. Keep breasts empty and preserve the lactation process by pumping breasts and discarding milk until the infection is resolved and antibiotics are discontinued
    c. Cleanse skin and mucous membranes of irritating, foul-smelling drainage
  3. Interventions related to fatigue and anxiety
    a. Organize care to provide uninterrupted rest periods
    b. Provide explanations, keeping the woman and family informed of progress because fear about future reproduction and the ability to continue breast feeding may be present

III. Thromboembolic disease: clot (thrombosis) formation in a blood vessel from inflammation (*thrombophlebitis*) or partial obstruction of a vessel. Pregnancy increases the risk for thrombosis formation from hypercoagulability of blood, venous stasis associated with the pressure of an enlarged uterus, and the decreased activity level of the woman.

A. **Types**
 1. Superficial venous thrombosis: most common form of postpartum thrombosis
 2. Deep vein thrombosis (DVT): major complication is pulmonary embolism

B. **Nursing diagnoses and major clinical manifestations related to thrombosis formation**
 1. Altered comfort from venous inflammation and blockage of the circulation
   a. Superficial venous thrombosis: pain and tenderness at site, warmth, erythema; vein is enlarged and hard over the thrombosis
   b. DVT: pain and calf tenderness in one leg or thigh, edema, erythema and warmth, and positive Homan sign. Some women may have no apparent signs or symptoms.
 2. Ineffective breathing pattern related to the blockage of a pulmonary vessel associated with pulmonary embolism: sudden dyspnea, tachypnea, cough, hemoptysis, tachycardia, and chest pain
 3. Anxiety related to an unexpected change in physical status after birth

C. **Interventions related to the type of thromboembolic problem**
 1. Administration of anticoagulants (primarily with DVT)
   a. Heparin: IV or SQ administration for several days
   b. Coumadin (Warfarin): oral administration after initial Heparin treatment. The oral medication is started while the client is still on heparin. An overlap of IV and PO medication is common for 48 to 72 hours to allow for the attainment of therapeutic prothrombin levels from the Coumadin. The oral medication may continue for several months after the initial therapy.
 2. Comfort interventions
   a. Limit activity; bed rest with DVT
   b. Elevate leg; change positions frequently if on bed rest
   c. Apply warm, moist heat to the site
   d. Administer analgesics *without aspirin* because aspirin potentiates the anticoagulation action of the oral medication
   e. Apply elastic support stockings after the acute phase
 3. Support measures
   a. Explain the basis of the health problem
   b. Inform the woman that breast feeding can continue

c. Teach about the
(1) Purpose of the specific treatments
(2) Use of anticoagulants; importance of follow-up appointments, which usually are weekly then biweekly throughout therapy
(3) Measures to prevent bleeding and injury while taking anticoagulants
(4) Importance to avoid pregnancy until warfarin sodium (Coumadin) is discontinued because it is teratogenic
(5) Need to maintain a normal intake of foods high in vitamin K. If these foods are increased in intake, the Coumadin may have decreased effectiveness.

WEB Resources

http://members.aol.com//KPPDK/index.html
Postpartum Stress Center provides information and support related to postpartum depression and other mental health problems associated with pregnancy.

http://www.psycom.net
This website is devoted to mental health. Click on Depression Central and then scroll down and finally click on Postpartum Depression to access information and links related to mood disorders during pregnancy and the postpartum period.

http://www.epregnancy.com
This website provides articles, interactive features, forums, and resources for women and families from before conception to after birth. Use the Search Feature and type in postpartum to access information related to concerns and care during recovery and adjustment after pregnancy and birth.

REVIEW QUESTIONS

1. Early postpartum hemorrhage—hemorrhage that occurs within the first 24 hours after birth—is least likely to occur as a result of which physiology?
   1. Subinvolution of the uterus, especially the placental site
   2. Uterine atony
   3. Lacerations of the labia, perineum, vagina, or cervix
   4. Hematoma formation within the tissue of the pelvis and genitalia

2. A postpartum woman gave birth 12 hours ago and is still receiving IV magnesium sulfate for preeclampsia. She has begun to experience excessive uterine bleeding. The nurse would expect to administer which medication?
   1. Cervidil
   2. Pitocin
   3. Methergine
   4. Fentanyl

3. Which of these factors presents the lowest risk for postpartum infection?
   1. A labor of 14 hours followed by a spontaneous vaginal birth
   2. Membranes ruptured for 28 hours before birth
   3. Vacuum extractor used to assist with internal rotation and birth of the fetal head
   4. Internal monitors applied to assess FHR patterns and intrauterine pressure

4. A woman diagnosed with mastitis and receiving antibiotics should perform which of the following actions?
   1. Feed her baby from the uninfected breast only
   2. Discontinue breast feeding
   3. Continue to breast feed as usual
   4. Maintain lactation by pumping both breasts and discarding the milk

5. When caring for a postpartum woman with a uterine infection, the nurse should take which action?
   1. Isolate the woman from her newborn to prevent transmission of infection
   2. Provide at least 2000 ml/day of fluid
   3. Obtain appropriate specimens for cultures before the initiation of antibiotic treatment
   4. Reassure the woman that future reproduction will not be affected

ANSWERS, RATIONALES, AND TEST-TAKING TIPS

Rationale	Test-Taking Tips

1. Correct answer: 1

Subinvolution is most closely associated with late postpartum hemorrhage—the second day until the 28th day—along with retained placental fragments, infection, or both. For subinvolution think of slow involution.

Think logically. Hemorrhage with lacerations occurs then hematoma formation. Eliminate options 3 and 4. Recall that atony means loss of muscle tone of an organ, which could be the bladder, uterus, or intestine. This situation with a uterus leads to a boggy uterus, with risk of hemorrhage. Eliminate option 2. Select option 1, then reread the question to ensure you have read it correctly to ask for the least likely occurrence.

2. Correct answer: 2

Pitocin is used for uterine contractions, which this client needs. The magnesium sulfate would have a tendency to minimize uterine contractions to increase the risk of bleeding. Cervidil is used to ripen the cervix, not contract the uterus. Methergine should not be used for women who have hypertensive problems because it can further elevate the BP. Fentanyl is a narcotic analgesic.

With uncertainty of which actions all of these medications have, focus on the medication for which you know the action, Pitocin. Avoid wrong answers by second-guessing yourself by selecting something you do not know. Note the clue of "preeclampsia" indicates hypertension problems.

3. Correct answer: 1

Of the four options listed, option 1 represents the lowest risk. Fourteen hours is an average duration for labor and spontaneous birth, without the use of forceps or vacuum extractor. Option 2 is a risk factor because the rate of infection increases dramatically if the membranes have been ruptured for more than 24 hours.

Careful reading is required to select the lowest risk for infection. If you are tired or tense, the tendency is to miss these key words. Did you notice that this is the second question to ask what is the "lowest" or the "least likely" in the middle of the question? Be prepared to switch gears in thinking and to avoid question hangover from prior questions.

Options 3 and 4 increase infection risk because they are invasive procedures.

4. Correct answer: 4

Infants usually do not receive breast milk as long as antibiotic therapy is being administered to the mother. Lactation should be maintained because breast feeding may be resumed once the problem is resolved. The mother will have to pump the breasts at regular intervals and discard the milk. Breast feeding usually should not resume until 24 to 48 hours after the final antibiotic dose. Mastitis usually is unilateral but also can be bilateral.

Option 1 is not a comprehensive answer because it does not state what to do with the milk from the infected breast. Option 2 is partially true, that is, to stop breast feeding, but does not give enough information to be the best answer. Option 3 is incorrect information. Option 4 is the most comprehensive answer and therefore more likely to be the correct answer.

5. Correct answer: 3

There is no basis for isolation of the woman from her newborn as long as standard precautions are maintained. At least 3 L/day of fluid are required for postpartum women. There is no way to be sure that reproduction will not be affected. False assurance should not be given. The nurse should explain treatments and the progression of healing.

Keep focused on the given situation and basic protocol for antibiotic therapy. The location of the infection is the uterus, which is of no risk to the infant. Option 3, the correct answer, is the golden rule with antibiotic therapy.

10

Nursing Process Applications in the Physiologic Adaptation of the Neonate to Extrauterine Life

FAST FACTS

1. **Neonatal period,** the first 28 days of life, is a period of rapid growth and development.
2. Deviations from the norm, if left undetected and untreated, may result in irreversible damage to the newborn and its well-being. For example, oxygen deprivation associated with ineffective breathing patterns may adversely affect the neurologic system.
3. A healthy term newborn requires close and ongoing observation to distinguish expected assessment findings and variations from warning signs of ineffective adaptation and deviations from the norm that require intervention by a health care provider.
4. The newborn's parents must receive support, guidance, and instruction in the observation and care of their new baby. Parents must be informed about normal and abnormal findings, how to assess newborn, and when to call the health care provider.
5. Early discharge programs must ensure a follow-up plan for the newborn and its parents by competent health care providers.

6. A full-term healthy neonate typically has less mature function of its body systems than an adult, resulting in (a) limited reserves in times of stress, for example, the stress of a common cold in a newborn can compromise the respiratory system and deplete glucose stores; and (b) risk for infection, hypothermia or hyperthermia, fluid imbalances, injury, and hyperbilirubinemia.

7. Newborn health assessment and care are based on understanding that (a) the origin of many adult health problems are found early in life and influenced by parental habits and knowledge and care of the infant; (b) infancy is most hazardous year of life until the age of 65; (c) the highest mortality rate occurs during the neonatal period, the first 28 days of life; (d) gross inequities exist in health care systems for the care of infants: the poor, the uninsured, the homeless, minorities, and those living in rural areas are not afforded the same opportunities for quality health care as are other population groups.

8. Predictors of infant morbidity and mortality are classified into maternal and infant predictors.

9. The maternal predictors are (a) under 20 years of age or over 35 years; (b) member of a minority group; (c) unmarried, with a limited support system; (d) inadequate education and health care; and (e) exposure to teratogens, including the use of tobacco, alcohol, and drugs before and during pregnancy.

10. The major infant predictor is **low birth weight** (LBW); weight at birth of less than 2500 g from intrauterine growth restriction (IUGR), preterm birth, or both.

11. Infant mortality statistics show that the United States ranks 23rd among industrialized nations in infant mortality.

12. Infant mortality statistics also show that **infant mortality rates,** that is, the number of deaths in first year of life per 1000 live births, are as follows: 7.2 for all infants, 13.7 for black infants, and 6.0 for white infants.

13. Avoid the prone position (on abdomen) for neonates and infants because it may interfere with breathing and has been associated with Sudden Infant Death Syndrome (SIDS).

14. Use a rear-facing, safety-approved car seat at all times when traveling with a newborn. Follow the directions for its use. The car seat can be turned to face forward once the infant weighs more than 20 lb.

15. Never use honey on a nipple or in a newborn's food because a dangerous botulism infection may occur.

CONTENT REVIEW

I. Mortality rates
A. **Neonatal mortality rate: number of infant deaths in the first 28 days of life per 1000 live births**
   1. Closely associated with intrauterine events and LBW
   2. Rates: 4.8 for all infants, 9.2 for black infants, and 4.0 for white infants

B. **Postneonatal mortality rate: number of infant deaths after the first 28 days of life per 1000 live births**
1. Closely associated with inadequate social and environmental conditions, resulting from poverty; unsafe and unsanitary housing; and limited resources to provide for infant needs in terms of health care, nutrition, and development
2. Rates: 2.4 for all infants, 4.5 for black infants, and 2.1 for white infants
C. **Leading causes of infant mortality**
1. Congenital anomalies
2. LBW
3. SIDS
4. Respiratory distress syndrome
5. Newborns affected by maternal complications of pregnancy
D. **Interventions identified as effective in reducing infant mortality and in improving infant health**
1. Preparation for pregnancy and parenthood
   a. Parenting classes before becoming pregnant, prenatally, and after birth
   b. Family planning classes and services
   c. Preconception care
2. Counseling to prevent congenital anomalies
3. Comprehensive, ongoing prenatal care beginning early in pregnancy
4. Parental health habits and lifestyle that focus on health promotion and disease prevention
   a. Maintenance of ideal weight with a balance between good nutrition and adequate exercise
   b. Measures to prevent infection, with good hygiene and safer sex practices
   c. Healthy stress management, with a balance of the activities of sleep, rest and relaxation, activity and work, and recreation
   d. Avoidance of alcohol, tobacco, and drug use before, during, and after pregnancy

II. Physical assessment of the newborn
A. **Guidelines**
1. Use Table 10-1 (p. 269) as an assessment guide to determine newborn health status, adequacy of growth in utero, and success in adapting to extrauterine life

⚠ Warning!

Perform physical assessments frequently immediately after birth and during the transition period of adaptation to extrauterine life, carefully documenting all observations and immediately reporting any deviations from the norm that could indicate neonatal distress.

Text continued on p. 293

TABLE 10-1 Anatomic and Physiologic Adaptations to Extrauterine Life, Expected Findings, and Warning Signs of the Full-Term Neonate

Anatomic and Physiologic Adaptations	Expected Assessment Findings and Variations	Warning Signs of Ineffective Adaptation
I. Oxygenation Effective function of respiratory and circulatory systems is critical for newborn survival; both systems function interdependently **A. Respiration** First breath stimulated by: Brief period of hypoxia at birth; carbon dioxide is retained and the respiratory center is stimulated Recoil of the chest after compression during passage through birth canal Exposure to environmental stimuli: light, cool air, touch Lungs expand easily as a result of: Surfactant: reduces surface tension of alveoli; facilitates alveolar expansion and contraction with breathing Fluid fills lungs while in utero; lungs are maintained in partial expansion Fetal breathing movements occur in utero. Lung fluid must be removed to facilitate newborn respiration:	First breath occurs immediately at birth; progresses to lusty, rhythmic cry Respirations reflect these characteristics: Rate: average of 40 breaths/min; range, 30-60 breaths/min Quiet, effortless without retraction or nasal flaring Rate, depth, rhythm vary according to activity level Brief periods of apnea without evidence of respiratory distress or cyanosis Diaphragmatic in nature; abdomen moves more noticeably with breathing than does chest Auscultation of lungs: Generally clear without presence of adventitious sounds	Persistent: Bradypnea (15 breaths/min or less) Tachypnea (60 breaths/min or more) Crackles with findings of respiratory distress Episodes of apnea 15 sec or longer accompanied by cyanosis and signs of respiratory distress Signs of respiratory distress: Nasal flaring Expiratory grunting Persistent sternal, intercostal retractions even at rest Chin tug Persistent and copious watery drainage from nose Bulging or malformations of chest

One third is squeezed out with chest compression during passage through birth canal

Remaining fluid is reabsorbed into circulatory and lymphatic systems within 12 hr of birth

WARNING! Crackles may be noted until lung fluid clears; respiratory distress is absent.

Nose:
Symmetric, intact, broad nose; midline placement
Patent: small amount of mucous
Sneezes to clear nasal passages
No flaring of nares with breathing
WARNING! Nasal patency must be maintained because newborns are nasal breathers.

Chest:
Circular, barrel-shaped
Expands and contracts symmetrically with breathing
Chest and abdomen move in synchrony with breathing
Crying: strong, lusty, moderate tone and pitch

Asymmetric chest expansion
Seesaw respirations: asynchronous movement of chest and abdomen with breathing
Crying: high-pitched or shrill, weak, or absent

B. Circulation

Circulation changes from a fetal to adult pattern:
Loss of placental circulatory network with the cutting of the cord
Decreased venous return leads to decreased pressure in right side of heart
Increased arterial flow with increase in systemic vascular resistance leads to increased pressure in left side of heart

Blood pressure:
Average 75/42 mm Hg at birth
Range of 60-80/40-50 mm Hg
About the same in upper and lower extremities

Apical pulse:
Located on left side, 4th intercostal space; pulsations may be visible and palpable

Hypotension or hypertension
Systolic pressure in lower extremities 6-8 mm Hg less than upper extremities
Apical beat auscultated on right side of chest
Persistent:
Tachycardia: greater than 160 beats/min
Bradycardia: less than 110 beats/min or resting rate <80-100 beats/min

Continued

TABLE 10-1 Anatomic and Physiologic Adaptations to Extrauterine Life, Expected Findings, and Warning Signs of the Full-Term Neonate—cont'd

Anatomic and Physiologic Adaptations	Expected Assessment Findings and Variations	Warning Signs of Ineffective Adaptation
Foramen ovale (fetal shunt between right and left atria) closes	Rate 110-160 beats/min varies with newborn's activity level:	Dysrythmias
Ductus venosus (liver bypass shunt) closes	Sleep: as low as 100 beats/min	Murmurs
Lungs fill with air with the first breath	Activity-crying episode: as high as 160 beat/min with transient irregularity	Femoral pulses: weak, absent, or asymmetric
Decreased pulmonary vascular resistance	Transient tachycardia after birth as high as 180 beats/min	Temperature of extremities: asymmetric with one side warmer or cooler than the other
Decreased pressure in right side of heart		
Increased pulmonary circulation leads to increased blood return to left side of heart and increased pressure on left side of heart	Regular, strong, sharp, and clear heart sounds	
	Transient, minor murmurs may be auscultated until shunts fully heal over	
Ductus arteriosus (fetal lung bypass shunts) closes to allow full pulmonary circulation and blood gas exchange	Femoral pulses: equal and strong bilaterally Temperature of extremities: warm bilaterally, with cooler hands and feet especially on exposure	
WARNING! Ineffective respiratory patterns can lead to hypoxia with reopening of ductus arteriosus; permanent closure of the foramen ovale and the ductus arteriosus does not occur until infancy.		
Color of newborn is influenced by: Adequacy of respiratory and circulatory functioning	Pink color with ruddy (deep red color) appearance after activity and crying episodes	Cyanosis: circumoral, generalized Pallor, grayness Plethora: very dark red color

Continued

Sluggish peripheral circulation results in color variations related to position and environmental temperature

Elevated RBC count

Blood vessels are closer to body surface from limited amount of subcutaneous fat

Fetus produces a large number of RBCs to ensure adequate oxygen transport during intrauterine life

Hyperbilirubinemia (elevated bilirubin levels primarily from unconjugated bilirubin) can occur:

Neonatal breathing supplies sufficient oxygen

Excessive RBCs are destroyed causing bilirubin level increase

Breakdown and excretion of bilirubin are limited by:

Immaturity of the liver and its ability to breakdown bilirubin

Limited milk intake, which inhibits subsequent stool and reduces excretion of bilirubin leading to bilirubin reabsorption into the circulatory system

Acrocyanosis: bluish tinge to hands and feet especially when exposed; hands and feet also feel cooler to the touch

Mottling (cutis marmorata): marbled, irregular coloration of skin when exposed to decreased environmental temperature

Harlequin sign: difference in color of skin from the position of the newborn, e.g., when lying on side, lower half of body becomes pinker while upper half of body becomes pale pink

Hemoglobin: 14-29 gm/dl, with a mean of 17

Hematocrit: 43-69%, with a mean of 55%

RBC count: $4.7\text{-}5.8/mm^3$

Physiologic jaundice:

Develops after first 24 hr of life and resolves by the 9th–10th day

Serum (unconjugated, indirect) bilirubin levels do not exceed 12 mg/dl nor is there an increase of >5 mg/day

Conjugated, direct bilirubin levels do not exceed 1-1.5 mg/dl

Jaundice tends to progress in a cephalocaudal and proximodistal direction; the extent is exhibited in dermal zones to approximate the bilirubin level, e.g.:

Face: 5 mg/dl

Chest: 7 mg/dl

Abdomen: 10 mg/dl

Thighs: 12 mg/dl

Knees to ankles, elbows to wrists: 15 mg/dl

Hemoglobin or hematocrit levels are less or greater than expected

Pathologic jaundice appears in the first 24 hr or does not meet the criteria listed for physiologic jaundice

TABLE 10-1	**Anatomic and Physiologic Adaptations to Extrauterine Life, Expected Findings, and Warning Signs of the Full-Term Neonate—cont'd**		
Anatomic and Physiologic Adaptations	**Expected Assessment Findings and Variations**	**Warning Signs of Ineffective Adaptation**	
Postnatal bleeding tendency occurs as a result of: Inability to synthesize vitamin K until intestinal flora develops as part of digestion process Immaturity of liver in terms of production of prothrombin and other clotting factors Hemorrhagic areas occur from pressure and trauma of birth process	Petechiae: red pinpoint hemorrhagic areas usually on the presenting part Hemorrhagic area noted in sclera or conjunctiva Ecchymosis (bruising): Facial from pressure of forceps' use Occipital from pressure of vacuum extractor Buttocks, sacrum with a breech birth	Petechiae and ecchymosis: generalized or over areas of body unrelated to pressure of birth, especially if persistent in nature	
II. Nutrition, Fluid and Electrolytes Adequacy of intrauterine nutrition and fetal growth is reflected in: Neonatal body size and weight Presence of subcutaneous fat (adipose) tissue **WARNING!** Limited oral intake coupled with fluid loss through bowel and bladder elimination, during the first few days of life, results in a loss of weight and a tendency toward dehydration.	Measurements: Fall within the 10th–90th percentile and are appropriate for estimated gestational age Are consistent: fall in the same percentile Comparisons should be made with parental body builds and size of their other newborns Weight: Average range of 2500-4000 g (5 lb, 8 oz–8 lb, 13 oz) Appropriate for gestational age (AGA) Expected weight loss of 5-10% of birth weight during the first week of life; regained within 2 wk	Measurements: <10th or >90th percentile Inconsistent: fall in different percentiles Weight: <2500 g, or 5lb, 8 oz: considered **low birth weight** as a result of: Intrauterine growth restriction: small for gestational age (SGA) Preterm birth >4000 g, or 8 lb, 13 oz: considered macrosomia or large for gestational age (LGA) Weight loss of >10% during the 1st wk or a delay in the return to birth weight may reflect inadequate nutritional intake	

Head circumference:
  Average range of 32-37 cm (12.5-14.5 inches)
  Usually 2-3 cm (1 inch) larger than chest circumference
  Molding may alter circumference for the first few days
Chest circumference: ranges from 30-33 cm (12-13 inches)
Length: 45-55 cm (18-22 inches)
Fat deposits present:
  Sucking pads: fat deposits in cheeks; rounded, full appearance
  Integument: full with few wrinkles
  Buttocks: rounded and full
Hydration status:
  Weight gain or loss follows expected patterns
  Turgor: resilient, hydrated integument; determined by pinching skin over abdomen or thigh; skin returns to original state immediately on release
  Anterior fontanel flat
  Temperature, normal range, stable
  Voiding: 6-10 times/day of pale yellow urine
  Moist mucous membranes

Head circumference:
  <32 cm
  Is 4 cm or more larger than chest
Fat deposits are limited:
  Loose, baggy, wrinkled skin
  Prominent clavicles and ribs
  Small, absent sucking pads
Hydration status indicators of dehydration and inadequate nutrient intake:
  Weight loss
  Decreased urination
  Poor turgor
  Depressed anterior fontanel
  Temperature elevation may occur
  Dry mucous membranes

Continued

TABLE 10-1	Anatomic and Physiologic Adaptations to Extrauterine Life, Expected Findings, and Warning Signs of the Full-Term Neonate—cont'd		
Anatomic and Physiologic Adaptations	**Expected Assessment Findings and Variations**	**Warning Signs of Ineffective Adaptation**
Digestion and utilization of nutrients: Adequate for protein and simple carbohydrates	Liver: palpable in the upper right quadrant about 2 cm below costal margin—sharp edge	Liver: enlarged with rounded edge Glucose level fails to stabilize within the expected range
Limited with regard to complex carbohydrates and fats	Hyperbilirubinemia with resultant physiologic jaundice after the first 24 hours of life	Signs of hypoglycemia are exhibited: Irritability, jitteriness
Liver functions on an immature level with limited ability to:	Slight peripheral edema at birth, especially at body areas that had pressure during birth process	Tremors Lethargy Poor feeding behavior
Conjugate bilirubin, including that formed as a by-product of RBC breakdown	Postnatal bleeding tendency	Cyanosis
Produce plasma proteins, prothrombin, other coagulation factors	Increased tendency for hypoglycemia—glucose levels:	
Store glycogen	Decrease after birth as a result of limited stores and utilization of glucose for energy	
	Should be at least 45 mg/dl	
	Stabilize at 50-60 mg/dl during transition period after birth	

Effective feeding behaviors must be present to supply the required fluids and nutrients for optimum growth, development, and well-being

Stomach:

Filled with mucous and amniotic fluid during intrauterine life; removed after birth via vomiting and regurgitation; feeding and digestion are facilitated once contents are removed

Capacity is limited to approximately 90 ml; emptying time: 2-4 hr

Cardiac sphincter at entrance into stomach from esophagus is immature; regurgitation is possible, especially with rapid and/or overfeeding, which leads to risk for aspiration

Gastric acidity is reduced after 1st wk of life; formation of gas increases and colic or gas pain develop

Feeding reflexes are necessary for adequate intake:

Rooting reflex:

Stimulus: before feeding, stroke side of cheek, lips, mouth with finger or nipple

Response: turns head toward stimulus, opens mouth, takes hold, and starts to suck

Sucking reflex: strong and rhythmic

Swallow: coordinates with suck

Exhibits hunger every 3-4 hr by eagerness to feed, as demonstrated by sucking movements of mouth, active rooting, crying

Exhibits satisfaction after feeding by sleeping several hours

Gains about 5-7 oz/wk

Mother and newborn demonstrate satisfaction and comfort with chosen feeding method

Regurgitation of small amounts of milk after or during feedings

Weak or absent or asymmetric rooting reflex

Weak suck: need for continued encouragement to continue to suck and swallow

Swallow is not coordinated with suck, which leads to:

Excessive regurgitation while feeding

Gagging, coughing, vomiting

Projectile vomiting

Sleepy and lethargic behavior, slow to rouse, needs to be awakened to feed

Continued

TABLE 10-1	Anatomic and Physiologic Adaptations to Extrauterine Life, Expected Findings, and Warning Signs of the Full-Term Neonate—cont'd		
Anatomic and Physiologic Adaptations	**Expected Assessment Findings and Variations**	**Warning Signs of Ineffective Adaptation**	

III. Temperature Regulation

Anatomic and Physiologic Adaptations	Expected Assessment Findings and Variations	Warning Signs of Ineffective Adaptation
Temperature regulation is immature and places the newborn at risk for hyperthermia and hypothermia	Axillary temperature: 36.5-37° C (97.7-98.6° F)	Temperature does not stabilize by 10 hr after birth
Limited subcutaneous fat to insulate body, bringing blood vessels closer to surface of body; blood influenced by environmental conditions	Temperature stabilizes within about 8-10 hr of birth	Hypothermia (subnormal temperature) or hyperthermia (elevated temperature) may occur as a result of:
Larger body surface (heat loss) compared with body mass (heat production)	Transitory dehydration fever can occur at about 2-4 days after birth until fluid intake balances losses; easily reversed by increasing fluid intake	Environment that is too cold or too hot
Sweat glands ineffective for the first month of life; unable to sweat to dissipate heat		Over- or underdressed
Inability to change body posture to reduce body surface area exposed to cool temperatures		Infection
Inability to shiver for heat production		Dehydration
Brown fat: specialized fat located in several areas of newborn's body (i.e., nape of neck, between scapula, around kidneys, etc.) is capable of a high metabolic rate that produces heat; blood is warmed as it circulates through this fat		Cold stress that results from exposure to cold temperatures or inadequate warming measures or both, resulting in:
		Increased activity with crying, restlessness, muscular movement lead to increased basal metabolic rate (BMR), which leads to heat production
		Increased RR to meet increased oxygen demand leads to stress on respiratory system and respiratory depression
		Depletion of glucose stores to meet energy demands of increased BMR leads to increased risk of hypoglycemia
		Increased activity level leads to fatigue
		WARNING! Hyperthermia can result in dehydration, leading to cerebral damage.

IV. Elimination

A. Bowel:

Abdominal muscles are not fully developed, leading to limited ability to fully support abdominal contents

Intestinal capacity is small, leading to more frequent bowel movements or gastrocolic reflex (bowel movement during or just after a feeding as a result of its stimulation of peristalsis)

Fecal characteristics are influenced by the nature of the oral intake

Abdomen: rounded, symmetric, protuberant, dome-shaped; prominence increases after feeding

Bowel sounds present within 1-2 hr of birth: intermittent, soft, tinkling sounds every 10-20 sec

Anus is patent (open), with active wink reflex: anus contracts when touched

Bowel movements:

First bowel movement within 24-36 hr of birth is influenced by the timing of the first feeding

Frequency of stools:

Approximately 5-6/day during first 2 wk

Individual elimination pattern develops that varies from a BM every other day to 3-6/day

Type of stools:

Meconium: dark, greenish-black, sticky, stool composed of amniotic fluid, intestinal secretions, bilirubin, cells, blood, all passed during the first few bowel movements:

Transitional stool: thin, slimy, greenish-brown to yellow

Milk stool:

Breast-fed newborn: loose, golden-yellow, nonirritating, sour milk odor

Bottle-fed newborn: soft, pale yellow to light brown, more offensive odor

Abdomen:

Flat or flabby

Hard, distended

Asymmetric

Bowel sounds: absent or hyperactive with visible peristaltic waves

Anus: imperforate

Bowel movements:

No stool by 36 hr or more

Meconium has strong, foul odor

Passage of hard, formed constipated-type stool

Passage of green, watery, diarrhea-type stool

Newborns receiving phototherapy for hyperbilirubinemia exhibit frequent, loose, green stool

Presence of blood or mucous in stool

Continued

TABLE 10-1 Anatomic and Physiologic Adaptations to Extrauterine Life, Expected Findings, and Warning Signs of the Full-Term Neonate—cont'd

Anatomic and Physiologic Adaptations	Expected Assessment Findings and Variations	Warning Signs of Ineffective Adaptation
B. Bladder: Kidneys must take over elimination and filtration functions of the placenta Renal system functions at an immature level with limited ability to: Concentrate urine Maintain fluid, electrolyte, and acid-base balance especially in times of stress, e.g., vomiting, diarrhea, infection, improper dilution of formula Bladder capacity is about 40 ml	Voiding: First urination is within 24 hr of birth Frequency is approximately: 2-6 times for the first 2 days then up to 20 times/day 6-10 times/day after the first week of life Stream of urine: full Urine: Pale yellow, dilute, nearly odorless Rust-stained diaper as a result of uric acid crystals in the urine Specific gravity of 1.005-1.015 once fluid intake is established	Failure to void by 24 hr after birth Distended bladder Weak, hesitant stream
V. Neurologic Function Nervous system: Lacks complete integration and function Is characterized by primitive reflex activity Stimuli are used to elicit a variety of reflexes as part of the assessment of neurologic function integrity	Common newborn reflexes **Moro reflex:** Stimulus: hold in semi-sitting position and allow head and trunk to fall backward to an angle of 30°, or place in a supine position on a flat surface then strike surface or clap hand above newborn; any sudden, intense stimulus should elicit the response	Reflex responses to stimuli exhibit: Asymmetry with one side of body responding in a different manner or with less strength Absent or weak response despite application of a strong stimulus and newborn not in a deep sleep state

Continued

When testing reflexes:

Responses should be bilateral, strong, and symmetric

Accuracy is facilitated when newborn is in a quiet, alert state

Repeated stimulation of a reflex will result in a diminished response as a result of the newborn's ability to shut out environmental stimuli (*habituation*)

Stimulation may be ineffective in eliciting reflexes when newborn is in a deep sleep state

Reflexes disappear during infancy and are replaced by purposeful activity

Neurologic development follows a predictable sequence:

Cephalocaudal: from head to foot; able to support head before sitting, able to sit before standing and walking

Proximodistal: from midline to peripheral; able to control shoulder movement before movement of hands and fingers, masters gross movement before fine movement, e.g., able to walk before able to write

Response: immediate extension and abduction of arms with fingers fanning out as thumb and forefinger form a C; followed by adduction and flexion of arms into an embrace type position; the legs may move into similar positions as the arms

Grasp (palmar-plantar) reflex:

Stimulus: place finger in palm of hand; place finger at base of toes

Response: fingers curl firmly around the finger (palmar) and toes curl downward (plantar). This response can facilitate the formation of parent-infant attachment.

Tonic neck (fencing) reflex:

Stimulus: place in a supine position then turn head to one side; repeat stimulus to other side; may occur spontaneously

Response: extends arm and leg on side to which head is turned while opposite arm and leg flex

Step-walk (dance) reflex:

Stimulus: hold in an upright position and allow feet to touch flat surface

Response: flexes and extends knees making steplike movements

Crawling reflex:

Stimulus: place in a prone position (on abdomen)

Response: crawling movements are made with arms and legs

Persistence of reflex response beyond expected time of disappearance

TABLE 10-1 Anatomic and Physiologic Adaptations to Extrauterine Life, Expected Findings, and Warning Signs of the Full-Term Neonate—cont'd

Anatomic and Physiologic Adaptations	Expected Assessment Findings and Variations	Warning Signs of Ineffective Adaptation
V. Neurologic Function—cont'd		
Skull bones are slightly separated to allow for expansion of skull during brain growth	**Babinski reflex:** Stimulus: stroke sole of foot upward beginning at heel along lateral aspect of sole then move across ball of foot to big toe Response: toes hyperextend (fan out) and big toe dorsiflexes (positive) **Magnet reflex:** Stimulus: partially flex both legs applying pressure to soles Response: both legs extend against pressure Head is symmetric and round once molding subsides: Palpate sutures and fontanelles when infant is quiet: Sutures: space between skull bones; slightly separated; transient overlap of skull bones related to molding Fontanelles: spaces in skull where suture lines meet: Flat, some bulging (intermittent) when crying or stooling Flat when upright and quiet Anterior fontanelle: diamond-shaped Posterior fontanelle: triangular-shaped	Head: persistent asymmetry or irregularity in shape; depressions or fractures Sutures, fontanelles: Widely spaced, enlarged or closed, fused sutures or fontanelles Sunken-depressed fontanelles Persistent/bulging fontanelles at rest; may indicate increased intracranial pressure

Caput succedaneum: edema over the presenting part of the head as a result of pressure during birth

Cephalhematoma: development of a hematoma between periosteum and skull bone as a result of trauma or pressure during birth

VI. Muscular Activity and Rest

Posture: after birth the newborn tends to assume its intrauterine posture

Upper and lower extremities: appearance and function are influenced by both the maturity and development of the neuromuscular system and intrauterine position

Posture is general flexion:
Extremities moderately flexed and adducted
Fists clenched
Slight tremors with movement and crying; occasional spontaneous startles
Temporary positional variations gradually subside:
Facial asymmetry as a result of intrauterine pressure from shoulder or arm; legs in extension and stiff as a result of a breech presentation

Face:
Symmetric appearance at rest and when crying and feeding
Bilateral symmetry in the movement of facial features

Neck:
Short, thick with skin folds, flexible
Limited ability to support head in upright position, except for short periods

Posture:
Hypotonia with relaxed, extended extremities and floppy, lethargic posture
Hypertonia, jitteriness, irritability
Face: persistent asymmetric appearance or movement

Neck:
Webbing
Masses, enlarged lymph nodes or thyroid, distended veins
Limited or absent range of motion of neck; head held at an angle
Fracture of clavicle: crepitation, asymmetric movement of arms with limited movement on fractured side

Spine:
Presence of pilonidal cyst, sinus or dimple, tuft of hair along spine
Limited movement
Asymmetry, lateral curvature

Continued

TABLE 10-1	Anatomic and Physiologic Adaptations to Extrauterine Life, Expected Findings, and Warning Signs of the Full-Term Neonate—cont'd		
Anatomic and Physiologic Adaptations	**Expected Assessment Findings and Variations**	**Warning Signs of Ineffective Adaptation**	
VI. Muscular Activity and Rest—cont'd	Ability to lift head (momentarily) and turn it to side when in the prone position	Spina bifida: congenital neural tube defect that results in lack of union between the laminae of the vertebrae, primarily in the lumbar area; spinal cord, membranes, and fluid may herniate through the opening to back	
	Full range of motion of shoulders and neck		
	Clavicles intact		
	Spine: midline, straight, flexible, intact		
	Extremities are bilaterally symmetric as to size and movement:	Extremities:	
	10 fingers and 10 toes, with full range of motion and strong grasp	Asymmetry of extremities as to appearance, size, movement	
	Creases on palms of hands; intact nails to fingertips (sharp)	Fingers and toes: missing or too many digits; webbing between digits	
	Creases on ⅔ of soles; plantar fat pad creates a flat-footed appearance	Simian crease on palms of hands suggests Down syndrome	
	Arms slightly longer than legs	Club foot: foot positioned downward and inward	
	Legs may appear to be bowed, with feet turning in slightly	Limitation, lack of movement of an extremity	
	Strong muscle tone of arms and legs; offers resistance to extension by examiner	Hip displacement as exhibited by:	
	Full range of motion of all joints but movement is asynchronous; arms and legs move fully but not in same way at the same time	Asymmetric gluteal folds	
		Presence of a click or slipping of femur when performing Ortolani's maneuver	

Transitional period after birth, about the first 6-8 hr of life, is characterized by instability and occurrence of **periods of reactivity.** The newborn's behavioral states and physiologic function fluctuate widely.

Observation of neonatal behaviors during these periods provides important data related to its health and well-being

Newborns develop individualized patterns of sleep and activity states

Hips and femur are intact as exhibited by:
Symmetric gluteal folds
Absence of a click with Ortolani's maneuver

First period of reactivity: first 15-30 min after birth:
Tachycardia (160-180 beats/min)
Irregular, rapid respirations (60-80 breaths/min), with brief periods of apnea
Transient rales and crackles, grunting, nasal flaring, chest retractions
Alert, cries, sucks, displays interest in environment, makes eye contact
Transient tremors, spontaneous startles
Able to begin feeding and interact with parents

Period of inactivity and rest for next 2-4 hr (some authorities say 60-90 min):
HR slows to 100-120 beats/min
RR slows to 50-60 breaths/min; becomes easy and quiet
Activity level decreases, infant becomes drowsy and enters a deep sleep state; level of responsiveness decreases, difficult to arouse
Bowel sounds can be auscultated

Second period of reactivity that lasts 10 min to several hours (some authorities say 4-6 hr): HR and RR fluctuate with transitory periods of tachycardia, tachypnea, and brief periods of apnea

Newborn's behaviors do not meet expectations with regard to periods of reactivity, stability of body systems, or sleep-activity patterns

Continued

| TABLE 10-1 | Anatomic and Physiologic Adaptations to Extrauterine Life, Expected Findings, and Warning Signs of the Full-Term Neonate—cont'd |

Anatomic and Physiologic Adaptations	Expected Assessment Findings and Variations	Warning Signs of Ineffective Adaptation
VI. Muscular Activity and Rest—cont'd	Awakens from sleep, becomes alert and responsive to feeding and environment; activity alternates with periods of sleep Gastric and respiratory secretions increase; gagging and regurgitation can occur Bowel sounds increase; passes meconium Voids After this period the newborn begins to exhibit stability of body systems Sleep-wake states: infant develops individual pattern of deep sleep, light sleep, drowsy, quiet alert, active alert, and crying states	
VII. Endocrine and Reproductive Function Influence of maternal hormones, primarily estrogen, affect appearance of breasts and genitalia of male and female newborns Pressure during a breech birth may result in bruising and increased edema of the genitalia	Breasts: Symmetric with 3-10 mm of tissue Slight swelling and secretion of milky substance called witch's milk Nipples prominent, formed; areola may be pigmented Female genitalia: Labia majora: edematous, pigmented, meet at midline and cover labia minora	Breasts: Malpositioned or widely spaced Erythema and firmness around nipples Supernumerary nipples: extra nipples along nipple line; often associated with renal anomalies Ambiguous genitalia: genitalia do not exhibit characteristics typical of either sex, i.e., not clearly male or female

Continued

Clitoris: edematous and prominent
Urinary meatus: located below clitoris
Vernix caseosa found between labia and at groin
Pseudomenstruation: odorless, mucoid blood-tinged vaginal discharge
Male genitalia:
Scrotum: edematous, pigmented, pendulous and covered with rugae
Testes bilaterally descended and palpable in scrotum
Penis; slender; erection may occur when genitalia are touched
Urinary meatus: slitlike opening at tip of penis
Prepuce (foreskin) membrane that covers glans penis; not easily retracted; removed at circumcision
Smegma: white cheesy substance found under foreskin
Cremasteric reflex: retraction of testes when chilled

Female genitalia:
Enlarged clitoris with meatus at the tip
Fused labia
Absence of vaginal opening
Fecal discharge from vagina
Inflammation of urethra
Foul-smelling discharge
Male genitalia:
Absence of rugae
Testes undescended
Hydrocele: accumulation of fluid in scrotal sac
Adherent, tight prepuce
Urinary meatus not at tip of penis
Epispadias: urinary meatus is on the dorsum (upper side) of penis; sphincter is defective
Hypospadias: urinary meatus is on the underside of the penis; sphincter intact
Inguinal hernia in either of the lower abdominal quadrants

Eyes:
Size, shape symmetric
Position: distance between inner aspects of eyes equals length of eye
Eyebrows: distinct

Eyes:
Size, shape, structures asymmetric
Closely/widely set eyes
Opacities/cataracts or ulcerations of cornea/lenses

VIII. Sensory Function

Fairly well developed at birth providing newborn with ability to interact with environment and people in it; attachment is enhanced by newborn's ability to make eye contact, attend to voices, respond to touch

TABLE 10-1	Anatomic and Physiologic Adaptations to Extrauterine Life, Expected Findings, and Warning Signs of the Full-Term Neonate—cont'd	
Anatomic and Physiologic Adaptations	Expected Assessment Findings and Variations	Warning Signs of Ineffective Adaptation
VIII. Sensory Function—cont'd	Eyelids: equal, freely moveable, open adequately; slightly edematous from the pressure at birth; erythema may be present as a reaction to ophthalmic ointment used after birth to prevent infection	Pink color of iris
		Purulent discharge; persistent erythema
		Epicanthal fold
	Eyeballs: round and firm	Asymmetry of pupil size; limited/absent (fixed dilation or constriction) reaction to light
	Pupils: round, equal, reactive to light	
	Iris: intact; blue-gray or brown	
	Sclera: clear, bluish-white (slightly yellow in dark skinned races); hemorrhagic area(s) may be present related to pressure at birth	Blue-yellow sclera
		Persistent strabismus
		Unable to follow to midline or fixate on objects
	Cornea and lenses: clear, intact	
	Conjunctiva: pink, moist; clear drainage and erythema may be present as a result of medication used after birth	
	Tears: scant or absent because tear glands begin to function at 2-4 wk of age	
	Eye movement:	
	Random, somewhat jerky movements	
	Follows objects (about 8 inches away) to midline; fixates momentarily on objects	

Makes eye contact and gazes intently

Pseudostrabismus: transient occurrence of a cross-eyed appearance until eye muscles are fully developed at about four months of age

Doll's eye phenomenon: as head is turned eye movement lags behind first 10 days of life

Blink/Glabellar reflex:

Stimulus: tap forehead at bridge of nose with finger

Response: both eyes blink simultaneously with first 4 to 5 taps

Ears:

Symmetric appearance and placement with upper part of pinna slightly above outer canthus of eye

Well formed with curved pinna and firm resilient cartilage

Infant responds to sounds:

Moves head in direction of sound

Loud, sudden noise: Moro or startle reflex, cries

Low pitched sound: quiets, soothes

High-pitched sound: alerts

Smell: responds to various odors in different ways

Turns away from strong or foul odors

Turns toward pleasant or familiar odors such as mothers scent and her milk

Ears:

Placement below outer canthus of eye

Asymmetric placement or appearance

Overly prominent or protruding ears

Limited amount of cartilage

Presence of skin tags, sinuses

Limited or absent response to sounds

Continued

TABLE 10-1	Anatomic and Physiologic Adaptations to Extrauterine Life, Expected Findings, and Warning Signs of the Full-Term Neonate—cont'd		

Anatomic and Physiologic Adaptations	Expected Assessment Findings and Variations	Warning Signs of Ineffective Adaptation
VIII. Sensory Function—cont'd	Taste: responsive to different tastes Tasteless: no response Sweet-pleasant taste: eager sucking, satisfaction Sour-bitter taste: puckering, anger, grimace, cry Touch: responsive to touch: Gentle patting, rubbing, cuddling; soothes, calms Painful stimulus: cries, anger, increased activity	
IX. Integument Delicate and easily damaged Sensitive to handling and exposure to environment and substances, including clothing, linens, diapers, lotions and soaps, urine, feces Breaks in the integrity: umbilical cord, circumcision, rashes, abrasions, cracks increase risk of infection	Skin: Color: generally pink with deepening pigmentation related to ethnic-racial origin begins after birth Transient hyperpigmentation may occur from the maternal hormones: areola, genitalia, linea nigra Soft, smooth, full with few wrinkles Resilient (turgor), well hydrated with dryness, cracking at ankles, feet, wrists	Skin: Characteristics present associated with a preterm newborn: Deep, ruddy color Edema: hands, feet, labia Thin, smooth Abundant lanugo and vernix caseosa Characteristics present associated with a postmature newborn: Thick, dry skin

Integument is protected in utero by **vernix caseosa** (white cheesy substance) and **lanugo** (hairy growth) that cover the surface of the body. Both begin to wear away as term approaches. Sweat and sebaceous glands do not begin to function until the second month of life.

Reddened, irritated areas may occur where skin comes in contact with environmental substances

Vernix caseosa: white, odorless, cheesy substance; removed with first bath though some may remain in creases and folds (groin, axilla, labia)

Lanugo: fine downy hair found on shoulders, back, pinna of ears, forehead

Milia: plugged sebaceous glands that look like pimples (white heads) and found on face especially on chin and nose; disappear spontaneously

Erythema toxicum: newborn rash characterized by round, erythematous areas with small, raised, yellowish centers; often a response to the environment; resolves spontaneously

Mongolian spots: hyperpigmented, ecchymotic-like areas usually over buttocks and sacrum; commonly occur among dark-skinned newborns; fade gradually

Telangiectatic nevi (stork bite marks): flat, pink, *easily blanched* localized areas of dilated blood vessels found on the eyelids, bridge of nose, occiput, and nape of neck; deepen in color with crying; fade gradually over 1-2 yr

Desquamation (peeling)
Absence of lanugo and vernix caseosa
Presence of pustules, blisters, rashes, lacerations, excoriations, ecchymoses (bruises)
Cafe-au-lait spots: light-brown spots over body: presence of more than 6 is considered abnormal
Vernix caseosa: yellow-green reflects intrauterine passage of meconium; odor may indicate infection
Hemangioma: birth marks associated with capillary formations:
Strawberry mark (nevus vasculosus): raised, sharply demarcated, bright or dark red, rough-surfaced lesion that resembles a strawberry
Port-wine stain (nevus flammeus): nonraised, red-purple lesion that varies as to size, shape, location (most frequently the face); does not blanch or fade with pressure

Hair:
Coarse, brittle
Fine, wooly (preterm)
Unusual growing patterns
Mouth, oral cavity:
Thrush (candidiasis): white, adherent patches or plaques on tongue, palate, and buccal membranes; bleed when touched

Continued

TABLE 10-1 **Anatomic and Physiologic Adaptations to Extrauterine Life, Expected Findings, and Warning Signs of the Full-Term Neonate—cont'd**

Anatomic and Physiologic Adaptations	Expected Assessment Findings and Variations	Warning Signs of Ineffective Adaptation
IX. Integument—cont'd	Hair: silky, single strands; lies flat, growing toward face and neck	Cleft lip, palate
	Mouth, oral cavity:	Large, protruding tongue; limitation in movement
	Mucous membranes: pink, moist, intact, with no white patches	Profuse salivation or drooling
	Epstein's pearls: whitish, hard epithelial cysts on hard palate and gums	Umbilical cord:
	Soft/hard palate intact	Bleeding, oozing around cord
	Lips: symmetric, midline, intact, sucking blisters	Yellow-green discoloration or odor
	Tongue: nonprotruding, freely moveable, symmetric	One artery may indicate internal anomalies such as renal
	Saliva: scant to none	Umbilical hernia: outpouching or protrusion of abdominal contents into the area of the cord
	Umbilical cord:	Signs of infection, inadequate healing
	Gelatinous, full at birth	
	Whitish gray color	
	Odorless	
	Two arteries and one vein	
	Progressive drying with no signs of infection present	
	Falls off after about 1 wk; slight bleeding (a few drops) can occur at that time	

2. Adjust the environment: warm, draft-free, and well lighted
3. Avoid chilling the newborn: perform the assessment efficiently with all equipment available, exposing only areas being examined; a radiant heat warmer can be used to maintain body temperature during the examination
4. Employ the principles of asepsis throughout the examination
   a. Progress from head to toe
   b. Use good hand-washing technique before and after the examination, and during the examination if contaminated
   c. Use equipment appropriately
      (1) Use alcohol swabs to clean equipment, such as earpieces and diaphragm of the stethoscope
      (2) Use disposable, paper tape for measurement
      (3) Place a clean scale paper on the scale for each newborn
5. Make use of the newborn's activity level when making observations
   a. Checking when infant is at rest: vital signs, posture, color, and fontanels
   b. Checking when infant is active: musculoskeletal activity, reflexes, and color changes
6. Use techniques that facilitates accuracy and safety
   a. Vital signs
      (1) Accuracy is essential
      (2) Count apical rate and RR for 1 full minute
      (3) Assess temperature using axillary or tympanic route; rectal route can perforate the rectum
   b. Measurements
      (1) Weight
         (a) Weigh every day at same time, preferably in the morning *before a feeding*
         (b) Remove all clothing
         (c) Place clean scale paper on the scale
         (d) Balance the scale
         (e) Place the newborn on the scale, keep hand over the newborn, and keep full attention on the newborn during the entire procedure

 Warning!

Never turn away or leave the newborn unattended.

      (2) Measure the head, chest, abdomen, and length using a nonstretchable, disposable, paper tape
         (a) Measure head circumference at the greatest diameter of the head, that is, across the forehead at the level of the ears over the occiput
         (b) Measure the chest circumference at the nipple line

(c) Measure the abdominal circumference just below umbilicus

(d) Measure length from the top of the head to the buttocks then stretch the legs and measure to the heels

7. Involve parents and family members as a means of facilitating attachment and getting to know their baby; especially important with early discharge because parents must learn how to monitor their newborn's condition

B. **Methods for data collection and assessment of the newborn**

1. Review antepartal and parturition records to determine quality of fetal-newborn responses to pregnancy, labor, and birth

   a. Physical status of the mother and responses of the mother and family to the pregnancy

   b. Antepartal testing performed and results

   c. Gestational age of the pregnancy and duration of labor

   d. Medications and anesthetics administered to the mother during labor and birth

   e. Method of birth (vaginal or cesarean), birth presentation, and use of instruments

   f. Fetal monitoring used during childbirth and results

2. Apgar score performed at 1 and 5 minutes after birth

3. Full physical assessment of health status (see Table 10-1, pp. 270-272)

4. Gestational age assessment and determination of adequacy of intrauterine growth

   a. Assess gestational age within 12 hours after birth by observation of the signs that indicate the degree of neuromuscular and physical maturity; compute the score to determine gestational age (Figure 10-1)

   b. Weigh the newborn and measure the head and length; plot on graphs to determine adequacy of intrauterine growth (see Figure 10-1)

   c. Describe infant as

      (1) **Small for gestational age** (SGA): weight is below growth expectations for gestational age: below the 10th percentile or 2 standard deviations below the mean for gestational age

      (2) **Appropriate for gestational age** (AGA): weight meets the growth expectations for gestational age: between the 10th and 90th percentiles or within 2 standard deviations of the mean for gestational age

      (3) **Large for gestational age** (LGA): weight exceeds the growth expectations for gestational age: above the 90th percentile or 2 standard deviations above the mean for gestational age

5. Laboratory testing

   a. Source of specimens for testing

      (1) Cord blood at the time of birth

      (2) Lateral heel stick to obtain capillary blood for testing

NEUROMUSCULAR MATURITY

	-1	0	1	2	3	4	5
Posture							
Square Window (wrist)	> 90°	90°	60°	45°	30°	0°	
Arm Recoil		180°	140°-180°	110° 140°	90°-110°	< 90°	
Popliteal Angle	180°	160°	140°	120°	100°	90°	< 90°
Scarf Sign							
Heel to Ear							

A

PHYSICAL MATURITY

MATURITY RATING

Skin	sticky friable transparent	gelatinous red, translucent	smooth pink, visible veins	superficial peeling or rash, few veins	cracking pale areas rare veins	parchment deep cracking no vessels	leathery cracked wrinkled
Lanugo	none	sparse	abundant	thinning	bald areas	mostly bald	
Plantar Surface	heel-toe 40-50 mm: -1 <40 mm: -2	>50 mm no crease	faint red marks	anterior transverse crease only	creases ant. 2/3	creases over entire sole	
Breast	imperceptible	barely perceptible	flat areola no bud	stippled areola 1-2 mm bud	raised areola 3-4 mm bud	full areola 5-10 mm bud	
Eye/Ear	lids fused loosely: -1 tightly: -2	lids open pinna flat stays folded	sl. curved pinna; soft; slow recoil	well-curved pinna; soft but ready recoil	formed & firm instant recoil	thick cartilage ear stiff	
Genitals (male)	scrotum flat, smooth	scrotum empty faint rugae	testes in upper canal rare rugae	testes descending few rugae	testes down good rugae	testes pendulous deep rugae	
Genitals (female)	clitoris prominent labia flat	prominent clitoris small labia minora	prominent clitoris enlarging minora	majora & minora equally prominent	majora large minora small	majora cover clitoris & minora	

score	weeks
-10	20
-5	22
0	24
5	26
10	28
15	30
20	32
25	34
30	36
35	38
40	40
45	42
50	44

Figure 10-1 Estimation of gestational age. **A,** New Ballard Scale for newborn maturity rating. Expanded scale includes extremely premature infants and has been refined to improve accuracy in more mature infants. (Part A is from Ballard J, et al. New Ballard Score, expanded to include extremely premature infants. *J Pediatr* 1991, 119(3):417.)   *Continued*

        (3) Venipuncture to obtain venous blood to recheck or confirm abnormal values

        (4) Urine using a collection bag

        (5) Body secretions and drainage for culture

    b. Common laboratory tests performed

        (1) Direct Coombs' test to determine if antibodies against Rh-positive blood have been formed by an Rh-negative mother and transferred to her fetus by way of the placenta; negative

CLASSIFICATION OF NEWBORNS—
BASED ON MATURITY AND INTRAUTERINE GROWTH
Symbols: X - 1st Examination   O - 2nd Examination

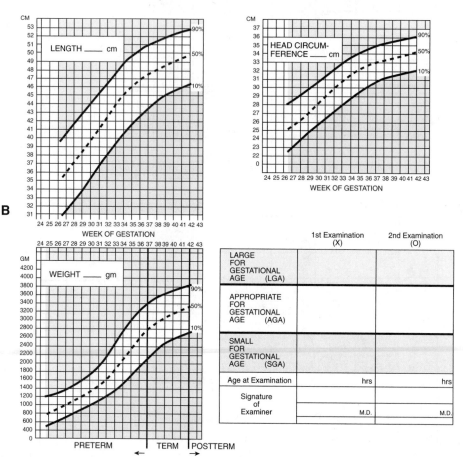

Figure 10-1, cont'd   B, Newborn classification based on maturity and intrauterine growth. (Part *B* is modified from Lubchenco L, Hansman C, and Boyd E. Intrauterine growth in length and head circumference as estimated from live births at gestational ages from 26 to 42 weeks. *J Pediatr* 1966, 37(3):403; and Battalgia F, and Lubchenco L. A practical classification of newborn infants by weight and gestational age. *J Pediatr* 1967, 71(2): 159.)

(no antibodies); positive (antibodies present that can destroy Rh-positive blood cells)
(2) Rapid plasma reagin (RPR) test and Venereal Disease Research Laboratory (VDRL) test to determine if intrauterine exposure to syphilis occurred; nonreactive (no exposure); reactive (exposure)
(3) CBC: WBC, 18,000/mm^3; hemoglobin, 14 to 29 g/dl; and hematocrit, 43% to 69%

(4) Dextrostix to determine blood glucose level
   (a) Performed frequently during the first 4 to 6 hr after birth as determined by hospital policy
   (b) Should be above 45 mg/dl stabilizing at 50 to 60 mg/dl
(5) Bilirubin levels (direct or indirect) to confirm the presence of hyperbilirubinemia when jaundice is observed
(6) Screening for metabolic disorders that require immediate treatment to prevent permanent damage such as mental and growth retardation; testing is often required by state law; if not performed before discharge, parents must be informed of the importance of bringing their newborn in for testing
   (a) PKU test within 72 hours of initial feeding to detect phenylketonuria, an inborn error of protein metabolism
   (b) Thyroid (T_4) testing to detect presence of hypothyroidism
   (c) Additional testing for other inborn errors of metabolism (branched-chain ketonuria, galactosemia) and sickle cell trait and disease may be required
(7) HIV testing to determine if the newborn's blood contains the HIV antibody. The mother's blood may be tested instead of or in addition to the newborn. Many states require testing of the newborn, mother, or both.

III. Psychosocial assessment of the newborn and family
A. **Essential components**
1. Quality of attachment of the newborn with parents and parents with newborn
2. Reaction of family members to the newborn
3. Stability of parental and family relationships
4. Level of parental knowledge and skill about the newborn's characteristics and care; availability of resource persons such as grandparents, friends, and health care providers
5. Safety and adequacy of the home environment
6. Ability to provide for the health care of the newborn
   a. Knowledge about the importance and frequency of regular health assessments during infancy and signs that require an emergency visit or call
   b. Arrangements made for health care (private pediatrician, clinic) and availability of health insurance
   c. Knowledge about the importance of immunizations
B. **Methods to use for assessment**
1. Observe parents and family as they care for and interact with the newborn
2. Review antepartal history
3. Interview parents before discharge
4. Follow-up phone calls and home visits after discharge

Box 10-1
Safety Tips for Parents of Newborns and Young Infants

Hold the newborn securely by supporting the head, neck, and spine.

Never leave the newborn unattended on a flat surface without side rails, such as a changing table, countertop, or bed because even newborns can roll off.

Assemble all equipment you will need ahead of time and place within easy reach.

Place hand securely on infant, if you must turn away.

Keep a bassinet or crib nearby in which to place the newborn in case you are suddenly called away.

Place the newborn in a crib and playpen that meets the standards of the U.S. Consumer Products Safety Commission (CPSC):

  Position the crib and playpen away from draperies, blinds, or shades that have long cords.

  Avoid the use of cribs that have special carvings, knobs, and indentations.

  Ensure that side-rail slats are no more than 2-⅜ inches apart.

  Make sure that the side rails can be raised and secured in place.

  Use a firm mattress that fits securely and snugly in the crib; never use a water mattress; make sure matting in the playpen is secured so the infant cannot get under or twisted in it.

  Fasten all bed linen securely so it cannot twist around the newborn.

  Avoid placing objects, especially ones that are soft, in the crib.

Position the newborn to ensure good breathing and prevent choking:

  Use a side-lying position with a secure back support after feeding.

  Use a supine (on back) position for sleeping.

  Avoid the prone position (on the abdomen) because it may interfere with breathing and has been associated with SIDS.

Learn infant CPR and first-aid measures.

Use interventions to prevent choking:

  Use only approved pacifiers.

  Keep small and sharp objects such as pins, scissors, and buttons out of the reach of a newborn.

  Do not tie anything around the newborn's neck, including bibs. Use bibs that have snaps.

Put the child in a rear-facing, safety-approved car seat at all times when traveling in the car. Follow directions for its use. The car seat can be turned to face forward once the infant weighs more than 20 lb.

Use safety straps in high chairs.

Instruct other children about newborn safety.

Keep emergency phone numbers next to the telephone, i.e., your health care provider, poison hot line, local hospital, and so on.

IV. Nursing diagnoses and interventions during the neonatal period

A. Nursing diagnoses for the healthy full-term newborn are primarily related to the newborn's risk for developing health problems as a result of:

1. Physiologic systems that are not fully mature and have limited reserve capacity in times of stress
2. Parents who may be inexperienced or lack the resources to ensure the newborn's well-being

B. Nursing interventions

1. Focus on early detection and prompt treatment to prevent more serious problems or even permanent damage or death
   a. Assessment of vital signs to detect early indicators of respiratory distress and cold stress
   b. Strict adherence to asepsis and standard precautions to prevent infection
   c. Administration of vitamin K using correct injection technique for newborns to enhance the clotting ability of the newborn for prevention of excessive bleeding from the cord or circumcision
2. Emphasize the education of parents about these topics
   a. Characteristics of newborn, including what to expect and what indicates a developing problem that requires prompt attention from a health care provider
   b. Newborn requirements for health care
   c. Interventions to ensure effective breathing, stable body temperature within normal limits, and adequate nutrient and fluid intake
   d. Infection control measures
   e. Instruction on how to keep the environment safe and secure to prevent accidental injury (Box 10-1)
   f. Instruction on how to stimulate growth and development
3. Teaching methodologies
   a. Group and one-on-one classes and demonstrations; a good time to teach is during the newborn's bath or when a physical assessment is being performed
   b. Videos and written materials that can be used as references after discharge
   c. Postpartum parenting classes and support groups
   d. Follow-up phone calls and home visits

C. Common nursing diagnoses with selected client outcomes, nursing interventions, and evaluation criteria encountered during the neonatal period are described in Table 10-2 (p. 300)

Text continued on p. 309

TABLE 10-2	**Common Nursing Diagnoses, Outcomes, and Interventions for the Neonatal Period**

Nursing Diagnoses, Expected Outcomes	**Nursing Interventions**
Risk for impaired gas exchange related to immature status of neonatal respiratory system and presence of mucous in respiratory tract	Assess adequacy of oxygenation including respiratory patterns and circulatory status
	Maintain airway patency:
Newborn will exhibit:	Gently suction oro-nasopharynx as needed; breathing and cry sound congested; use:
Easy, full, quiet respirations at 30-60 breaths/min	bulb syringe
	Suction mouth before nose
Clear chest sounds after first few hours following the birth	Compress bulb before insertion
	Insert along side of mouth not over tongue; into each nostril separately
Regular, strong apical beat at 120-140 beats/min	Release bulb slowly while removing
	Mechanical suction (more copious and tenacious secretions) set at low suction, <80 mm Hg
Pink color of conjunctiva and oral mucous membranes	Lubricate sterile catheter with sterile water
	Insert catheter gently with suction off
Parents of newborn will identify:	Apply suction with removal of catheter
Characteristics of effective breathing in the newborn	Suction for 5 sec/insertion or less, with rest periods in between, oxygenate if needed
	Suction until cry and breathing sound clear
Measures that facilitate newborn breathing and maintain airway patency	Report suspicious secretions; may require testing for infection
	Position newborn to facilitate drainage of mucous, prevent aspiration, and enhance breathing:
	Side-lying position with a secure back support
	Reclining position at a 30-45° angle or side-lying position after feeding
	Avoid prone position: may interfere with expansion of chest; has been associated with SIDS
	Burp infant well after feeding; avoid overfeeding

Avoid feeding newborn for about 2 hours before circumcision to prevent vomiting and aspiration (see Box 10-4, p. 308)

Reduce factors that place stress on respiratory system:

Hypoglycemia: facilitate feeding

Cold stress, hyperthermia: use interventions to maintain stable temperature within normal limits

Infection; asepsis, standard precautions

Teach parents:

Signs indicative of respiratory health

Use of bulb syringe

Emergency care for infant who is choking, not breathing, or needs CPR

Actions to prevent respiratory tract infection and injury:

Stop smoking, especially in proximity to newborn

Avoid contact with persons who have a respiratory tract infection

Use correct feeding techniques (Boxes 10-2 and 10-3, pp. 306-307)

Create a safe environment (see Box 10-1, p. 298)

Avoid use of talc powder; use cornstarch by applying it into hand then on to baby; never sprinkle on the baby

Ineffective thermoregulation related to immaturity of the newborn's thermoregulatory function

Newborn's temperature will stabilize between 97.7° F and 99° F within 8-10 hr of birth

Newborn will not exhibit signs of cold stress or hyperthermia

Parents will:

Demonstrate correct technique for taking newborn's temperature using axillary or tympanic method

Assess newborn's temperature every hour until stable and periodically thereafter; check immediately after circumcision

Use radiant heat warmer and thermistor probe during transition period while temperature stabilizes

Place thermistor probe over skin on upper right quadrant of abdomen, below ribs

Cover probe with reflective material to avoid false readings

Attach thermistor to control panel and set to desired temperature; alarm will ring when temperature is reached so newborn is not overheated

Advance to axillary or tympanic method once stabilized

Continued

TABLE 10-2   Common Nursing Diagnoses, Outcomes, and Interventions for the Neonatal Period—cont'd

Nursing Diagnoses, Expected Outcomes	Nursing Interventions

Ineffective thermoregulation related to immaturity of the newborn's thermoregulatory function—cont'd
 	
Parents will:
Identify interventions effective to maintain the newborn's body temperature within the normal range
	Teach parents to:
	  Avoid use of rectal method:
	    Danger of perforating rectum
	    Remains elevated until severe cold stress is present
	  Assess for signs of cold stress or hyperthermia
	Employ actions that are effective to maintain a stable body temperature and teach applicable measures to parents
	  Place undressed newborn under prewarmed radiant warmer or in a prewarmed incubator until temperature is stabilized
	  Adjust environment: 75° F, draft-free
	  Keep newborn and clothing dry
	    Wipe dry of amniotic fluid immediately after birth
	    Change wet clothing and bedding promptly
	    Perform first bath only after temperature has been stable at 97.8° F or higher for at least 1 hr
	    Use warm water (98-99°F) for bath and a warm, draft-free room
	    Wash head first before unwrapping, then rest of body; expose only part to be washed
	    Dry body parts immediately during bath
	  Avoid placing crib near heaters or windows (drafts, sunlight)
	  Use self as guide when dressing newborn; do not over- or underdress
	  Wrap newborn in blanket to keep limbs close to the torso:
	    Decreases heat loss by reducing the amount of body surface area exposed to air
	    Provides a sense of comfort and security
	  Use cap to decrease heat loss

Risk for infection related to immaturity of newborn's immunologic system

Newborn will not exhibit signs of infection

Newborn's cord or circumcision will heal without development of infection

Parents will:

Demonstrate correct care interventions for newborn's integument, cord, and circumcision

Employ infection control interventions in their home

Identify signs indicative of newborn infection

Assess newborn for signs indicative of infection:
Temperature instability; varies >1° C or 1.8° F from one reading to another
Subnormal temperatures
Lethargy, restlessness, irritability
Poor feeding behavior, vomiting
Diarrhea: green, watery stools
Decreased urine output
Respiratory distress
Lesions, rashes, pallor, jaundice
Erythema, edema, warmth, purulent drainage at sites where skin integrity is interrupted such as cord, circumcision, abrasions and cuts
Employ actions that are effective to prevent infection and teach applicable measures to parents:
Wash hands as per hospital policy, before and after care
Limit contact of newborn with those who have infections, including hospital personnel, crowds
Provide newborn with its own supplies and equipment and keep all items clean including toys and pacifiers
Support breast-feeding efforts
Prepare and store formulas correctly
Skin care:
Cleanse skin with warm water, using mild soap only for very dirty areas, e.g., buttocks after a bowel movement; make sure to rinse well
Bathe every other day, except for essential areas of scalp, face, creases in neck, genitalia, buttocks
Change diapers promptly and cleanse area:
Expose buttocks to air
Apply thin layer of Vaseline, K-Y jelly, or A and D Ointment
Avoid use of powders
Avoid rubbing of skin
Wash clothes and bedding separately, using hot water, mild detergent, and double rinse

Continued

TABLE 10-2	Common Nursing Diagnoses, Outcomes, and Interventions for the Neonatal Period—cont'd
Nursing Diagnoses, Expected Outcomes	**Nursing Interventions**
Risk for infection related to immaturity of newborn's immunologic system—cont'd	Umbilical cord care: Use alcohol or triple dye to enhance drying and prevent infection Expose to air; fold diaper and shirt away from cord Sponge bathe until cord falls off and site heals Eye care: Apply erythromycin ointment within 1 hr of birth Wash eyes at beginning of bath with clean cloth and water, from inner to outer canthus; use separate part of cloth for each eye Nails: cut straight across when newborn is asleep, using blunt-ended scissors Circumcision care (Box 10-4, p. 308) Administer hepatitis B vaccine IM as ordered by physician Teach parents importance of immunizations and make referrals as needed

Risk for alteration in nutrition (less than body requirements) related to parental lack of knowledge and experience regarding newborn nutrition and feeding technique

Newborn will:

Lose no more than 5-10% of birth weight in 1st wk of life

Gain approximately 1 oz/day

Consume approximately 80-100 ml/kg of fluid and 100 cal/kg/day for first 3 mo of life

Exhibit signs of hunger about every 3 hr

Exhibit satiety after feeding by resting quietly, sleeping

Parents will:

Demonstrate skill with their chosen feeding method

Identify signs of adequate nutrition and hydration in newborn

Recognize behaviors indicative of hunger and satiety in newborn

Assess nutritional status, and feeding behaviors and patterns:

Strength and coordination of rooting, suck, swallow; frequency of feeding

Patterns of weight gain and loss

Signs of hydration status

Feeding technique and skill of parents

Parental, newborn satisfaction with feeding method chosen

Determine if daily requirements for calories and fluid are being met

Calories: 100 kcal/kg (breast milk and formula contain 20 kcal/oz)

Fluid: 80-100 ml/kg; includes milk; may need to be increased in hot weather

Teach parents:

Expected frequency of feeding and amounts

Feeding readiness cues: hand-to-mouth or hand-to-hand movements, sucking motions, mouthing, rooting

Signs of satiety after feeding; stops sucking, turns away

Signs of adequate hydration and nutrition in terms of voiding patterns, expected weight gain, resiliency of integument, condition of anterior fontanel

Assist parents with feeding method of choice (Boxes 10-2 and 10-3, pp. 306-307)

Box 10-2
Guide for Successful Breast Feeding

Recommended Breast-Feeding Technique

Initiate feeding when the newborn is awake, alert, and exhibiting feeding cues; every 1.5 to 3 hours.

Assume a position of comfort in a relaxing environment. Relax the newborn during feeding by making eye contact, talking, and singing.

Alternate the newborn's breast-feeding position with each feeding: football, traditional (cradle), cross-over (modified cradle), and side-lying.

Alternate the starting breast. Place safety pin on bra to remember.

Initiate effective latch on:
  Support the breast with four fingers on bottom and thumb on top.
  Bring newborn to breast (not breast to newborn) and stimulate the **rooting reflex.**
  Guide the nipple and areola into newborn's open mouth; the newborn's mouth should cover the nipple and most of the areola.
  Observe for correct latch-on: sucking is rhythmic, with occasional brief rest periods and audible swallowing.

Remove newborn from the breast when the breast is empty or the newborn is finished (about 10 minutes) by releasing suction: insert finger into side of mouth.

Burp the newborn before changing breasts and at the end of the breast-feeding session.

Continue this process on the other breast.

Do not let the newborn continue to suck after the breast is empty.

Cleanse the nipples and areolas with warm water as needed. Air dry.

Apply a small amount of milk or purified lanolin on nipples-areola and air-dry. Use nipple shells as needed to facilitate drying, protect nipples from irritation and enhance the eversion of flat or inverted nipples.

Begin supplementation, as needed, once lactation and feeding patterns have been established in about 3 to 4 weeks. Breast milk can be collected and stored for this purpose. Use clean bottles and store in the freezer or refrigerator.

Use gentle massage to stimulate the let down reflex, keep milk flowing during breast feeding, and prepare breasts for expression of milk manually or with a pump.

Box 10-3
Guide for Successful Bottle Feeding

Recommended Bottle-Feeding Technique

Initiate feeding when newborn is awake, alert, and exhibiting feeding readiness cues; every 2.5 to 3 hours.

Assume a position of comfort in a relaxing environment. Relax the newborn during feeding by making eye contact, talking, and singing.

Hold the newborn closely (once nipple is in the mouth) in an en-face position. Change holding position with each feeding: football and traditional holds and using different arms.

Position the bottle so the milk fills the nipple and top of the bottle, thereby preventing entrance of air into the newborn's stomach.

Use nipples that allow dripping of milk. The nipple hole should not be so large that milk streams out nor so small that the newborn must struggle during sucking.

Stimulate the rooting reflex, then place the nipple into the open mouth.

Burp the newborn after every half to one ounce of formula and at the end of the feeding.

Never prop up the bottle for feeding because it increases the danger of choking, may block the airway, and decreases interaction with the newborn.

Stop feeding when the newborn signals satiety (stops sucking, turns away) not when the entire bottle is empty. Discard any formula remaining in the bottle.

Monitor the amount of formula taken at each feeding, then determine the amount taken daily.

Formula Preparation

Use the formula that is best for you: ready-to-use in bottles (most expensive) or prepared formulas using powder or concentrate.

Never use honey because a very dangerous botulism infection can occur in the newborn.

Follow directions exactly with regard to preparation. Never over- or underdilute because serious health problems will occur, including fluid and electrolyte imbalances.

Wash hands, the can opener, and the tops of cans and containers before opening. Use clean bottles, nipples, and equipment that have been thoroughly washed in hot water and soap and then fully rinsed.

Store formulas properly: ready-to-use and concentrates at room temperature until opened; reconstituted formulas and opened containers and cans in the refrigerator.

Feed newborn formula that is at room temperature or that has been warmed by placing the bottle in a container of hot water. Test the heated formula on your wrist before feeding the newborn.

Never use a microwave oven to the warm formula, because overheating can easily occur.

Box 10-4
Circumcision Care Guidelines

Nursing Interventions Before Circumcision

Ensure that informed consent from one parent has been obtained; discuss the procedure and available options.

Do not feed the newborn for approximately 2 hours before the procedure to reduce the possibility of vomiting and the risk of aspiration. *Note.* Check with the physician and agency policy because holding the feeding before circumcision may not be required.

Prepare equipment for a surgical aseptic procedure: sterile instruments, gloves, gowns, Vaseline gauze, anesthetics, and syringes (if used).

Advocate the use of anesthesia to reduce pain experienced by the newborn.

Assess vital signs.

Restrain the newborn.

Nursing Interventions after the Circumcision

Apply Vaseline (gauze, jelly) or A and D ointment to the site. Diaper the newborn. Cloth diapers may be recommended for the first day or so. *Note.* If the Plastibell is used, Vaseline or A and D ointment is not applied. The plastic rim remains in place for about 1 week while healing occurs, and then it falls off.

Assess vital signs.

Wrap the newborn and take to mother for feeding and comfort.

Assess site for bleeding every hour for 12 hours. If active bleeding occurs, apply gentle pressure with sterile gauze to the site of bleeding and notify the physician.

Change diaper promptly and cleanse thoroughly with water after elimination. Reapply Vaseline or A and D ointment to the site if Plastibell was not used.

Note time of first voiding after the procedure. Urination may be inhibited by edema around urethra.

Discuss the expected appearance of the circumcision site and care measures:

Glans will appear reddened and will become covered with a yellowish, protective exudate after the first 24 hours. The exudate will disappear in 2 to 3 days and should not be removed.

The plastic rim should fall off within 8 days.

Apply gentle pressure to the site if active bleeding occurs and notify the physician.

Signs of infection include continued erythema, edema, and purulent, malodorous drainage.

Change diaper promptly, cleanse site with warm water, and apply ointment as appropriate. Avoid the use of soap or baby wipes (they contain alcohol) until the site is fully healed.

Position the neonate on his side to keep pressure off of the penis.

WEB Resources

http://www.brightfutures.org

Bright Futures is a practical developmental approach to providing health supervision for children of all ages from birth through adolescence. The website is sponsored by the National Center for Education in Maternal and Child Health (NCEMCH) and the Health Resources and Services Administration.

http://www.abcparenting.com

The following is a comprehensive website that focuses not only on parenting and childcare issues but also provides access to information on pregnancy.

http://www.parentsoup.com

This website is part of the i Village.com network. It provides information and support for parents and prospective parents from the pre-pregnancy period through parenting of teenagers.

http://www.bflrc.com

Bright Future Lactation Resource Center. This website is designed to support people who support breast feeding.

http://www.lalecheleague.com

La Leche League International. This website is designed to provide mother-to-mother support, education, and encouragement regarding breast feeding.

REVIEW QUESTIONS

1. The parents of a newborn become concerned when they notice that their baby seems to stop breathing or hold its breath for a few seconds. After a confirmation of the parent's findings by observing that the newborn has occasional periods of apnea lasting 2 to 3 seconds, the nurse should take which action?
   1. Notify the physician
   2. Assess newborn for additional signs of respiratory distress
   3. Explain to the parents that this is the expected pattern of breathing for a newborn
   4. Tell the parents not to worry because their newborn is healthy

2. When assessing the apical HR of a newborn, the nurse should recognize which of these characteristics as expected?
   1. Resting rate may be as low as 80 beats/min
   2. Rate immediately after birth may exhibit transient tachycardia with a rate as high as 200 beats/min
   3. Rate after a crying episode may be as high as 160 beats/min, with transient irregularity
   4. Baseline rate range is 110 to 170 beat/min

3. An 18-hour-old newborn exhibits each of these variations in skin color. Which one would be a warning sign of ineffective adaptation to extrauterine life?
   1. Jaundice
   2. Acrocyanosis
   3. Mottling
   4. Petechiae on forehead

4. The birth weight of a breast-fed newborn was 8 lb, 4 oz. On the third day the newborn's weight was 7 lb, 12 oz. Based on this finding the nurse should take which action?
   1. Encourage the mother to continue breast feeding because it is effective in meeting the newborn's nutrient and fluid needs
   2. Suggest that the mother switch to bottle feeding because breast feeding has been ineffective in meeting the newborn's needs for fluid and nutrients
   3. Notify the physician because the newborn is being poorly nourished
   4. Refer the mother to a lactation consultant to improve her breastfeeding technique

5. An assessment finding indicative of effective newborn feeding behavior would be which of these?
   1. Exhibits signs of hunger and eagerness to feed at least every 3 to 4 hr
   2. Sleeps for 1 hour after a feeding

3. Gains approximately 2 to 4 oz weekly
4. Sleeps through the night by 2 weeks of age

6. Biostatistical data provide health care professionals with information about the health status of a population. Which of these is a correct interpretation of current trends in infant mortality in the United States?
   1. Neonatal and postneonatal mortality rates are approximately the same
   2. The infant mortality rate for black infants is nearly double that of white infants
   3. SIDS is the leading cause of neonatal mortality
   4. The major cause of infant mortality is respiratory distress syndrome

7. Weight at birth is an important factor in terms of a newborn's ability to adjust to extrauterine life. Which of these statements is accurate?
   1. A weight of less than 3500 gm at birth is considered to be LBW
   2. Preterm newborns are considered to be SGA
   3. The weight of a newborn considered to be LGA is at or above the 80th percentile
   4. A newborn whose weight falls within the 10th and 90th percentiles is described as being AGA

8. When weighing a newborn, the nurse should follow which guideline?
   1. Leave its diaper on for comfort
   2. Place a sterile scale paper on the scale for infection control
   3. Keep hand on the newborn's abdomen for safety
   4. Weigh the newborn at the same time each day for accuracy

9. A newborn female, 41 weeks' gestation, would exhibit which characteristic?
   1. Creases over entire plantar surface of feet
   2. Prominent clitoris and labia minora
   3. Her leg can be extended so that her heel touches her ear
   4. Flat areola

10. After the circumcision of a newborn, the nurse provides instructions to its parents about postcircumcision care. The nurse should tell the parents to follow which of the following care guidelines?
    1. Remove the Plastibell rim after 24 hr
    2. Do not remove the yellowish exudate that will cover the glans after the first 24 hours
    3. Change the diaper every 2 hr, and cleanse the site with soap and water or baby wipes
    4. Apply firm squeezing pressure with the fingers to the site if bleeding occurs, and call the physician

ANSWERS, RATIONALES, AND TEST-TAKING TIPS

Rationale	Test-Taking Tips

1. Correct answer: 3

Newborns typically exhibit irregular respirations with periods of apnea. Periods of apnea should be less than 15 seconds and cyanosis should not occur. Because this newborn exhibits a normal breathing pattern options 1 and 2 are not required. Option 4 does not give parents enough information about typical newborn breathing characteristics.

Option 1 is incorrect because no information in the stem warrants an alert to the physician. Option 2 has the clue "additional signs of respiratory distress," which is an incorrect statement because the findings in the stem are not respiratory distress. Option 4 has a phrase that typically makes an option incorrect—not to worry.

2. Correct answer: 3

Resting apical rate can be as low as 100 beats per minute. Transient tachycardia can be as high as 180 beats per minute, not 200. The average baseline apical rate range is 110 to 160 beats per minute, with rate and regularity influenced by activity level. This is the range for a fetus, a newborn, or an infant up to 1 year of age.

Associate that the normal HR range for adults is 60 to 100 beats per minute, with the HR of the newborn or infant starting at 100 at the lowest and 160 at the highest. Remember that 100 plus 60—an adult's highest and lowest rates, respectively—equal 160 for the fetus, newborn, and infant up to 1 year of age.

3. Correct answer: 1

Options 2, 3, and 4 are expected normal variations for an 18-hour-old newborn. Jaundice in the first 24 hours of life is pathologic rather than physiologic jaundice. It may reflect a problem related to excessive hemolysis by antibodies formed when the mother and newborn are incompatible as to Rh factor or blood type.

Avoid misreading the question as asking about an effective adaptation. To prevent this testing error, once you have selected your answer read the question and your option together. If you have misread or missed some clues, they will become evident at this last reading of both items together.

4. Correct answer: 1

A weight loss of 8 oz falls within the 5% to 10% expected weight loss during the first few days of life. For this newborn it would be 6.6 to 13.2 oz. Breast feeding is obviously effective. Options 2, 3, and 4 are inappropriate at this time.

If you have no idea of a correct answer, simply read the options for clues. You will note that three of them are negative, and state that a problem exists. Only option 1 suggests a positive result without a problem at this time. Select this option that is different. The others are too similar to be correct answers.

5. Correct answer: 1

A newborn should sleep at least 2 hours after a feeding and gain 5 to 7 oz/wk. The newborn is not expected to sleep through the night.

Associate the maximum weight gain with the days in a week—7 days and a maximum of 7 oz. Note the important term in the question "effective newborn feeding behavior." Then make an educated guess based on what you know: that babies are fed every 3 to 4 hr in the hospital, and this schedule is typically continued at home.

6. Correct answer: 2

The neonatal morbidity rate is nearly twice as high as the postneonatal mortality rate. The leading cause of neonatal mortality is intrauterine events and LBW. The major cause of infant mortality is congenital anomalies.

If you have no idea of a correct answer, match the clue in the stem, "infant mortality" with the same words in the stem to narrow the options to either 2 or 4. Reread the question and then eliminate option 4 because the focus is the cause and the question asks about a current trend. Option 2 is stated in terms more aligned with trends.

7. Correct answer: 4

Low birth weight is less than 2500 g. Preterm newborns may be SGA, AGA, or LGA, depending on their gestational age and weight. The weight of a newborn classified as LGA is above the 90th percentile or 2 standard deviations above the mean for gestational age.

If you have no idea of a correct answer, look for clues in the options. Options 1, 2, and 3 focus on abnormal findings. Option 4 focuses on what is appropriate. Therefore, an educated guess is to select the statement with normal information.

| Rationales | Test-Taking Tips |

8. Correct answer: 4

Weigh baby undressed for accuracy, with a hand above, not on, the abdomen for safety. Clean scale paper is used.

Caution. Read the options slowly for each clue. The words "sterile" in option 2 and "hand on" in option 3 make them incorrect. Option 1 can be eliminated by the use of common sense. Apply the general principles to obtain a client's weight: weigh the infant at same time of day, using the same technique, while the infant is wearing the same clothes or no clothes at all.

9. Correct answer: 1

Option 1 is the only expected finding for a full term newborn female. Options 2, 3, and 4 are signs noted in the preterm newborn.

A first action is for you to note the number of weeks as within the normal range of weeks for pregnancy. Then as you read the options, keep the focus of "normal" in mind, rather than abnormal. Option 1 is the only normal finding for a full term newborn.

10. Correct answer: 2

The Plastibell rim should fall off spontaneously within 8 days. The diapers are changed frequently, and the site is cleansed with warm water only. Gentle pressure, not squeezing pressure, should be applied to the site of bleeding if it should occur. A sterile gauze square should be used with application of gentle pressure rather than with the bare fingers.

As you read attempt to recall what you know about the healing process—it occurs with most wounds in 5 to 10 days. Thus, eliminate option 1 because the Plastibell is applied for protection and would be needed for more than 24 hr. Note the clue in option 3, soap or baby wipes. Either of these may result in irritation of the fresh surgical site. With the options narrowed between 2 and 4, option 2 is a better choice because it presents a more common finding in a healing wound than option 4, which focuses on bleeding. Bleeding is more often a complication. Select option 2, which is the expected normal finding

11

Ineffective Adaptation of the Neonate to Extrauterine Life

FAST FACTS

1. Newborns may experience difficulty adapting to extrauterine life from the effects of an unhealthy intrauterine environment that exposes them to stressors such as teratogens, insufficient uteroplacental circulation, and inadequate nutrition.
2. Exposure to intrauterine stressors may result in intrauterine growth restriction, LBW, congenital anomalies, and preterm birth.
3. Intrauterine growth restriction may result in the birth of a small for gestational age (SGA) newborn, a newborn whose measurements and weight do not meet growth expectations for gestational age.
4. SGA refers to size, not gestational age. These newborns can be preterm, full-term (see Figure 11-1, p. 316), or post-term.
5. SGA newborns have difficulty adapting to extrauterine life from a hypoxic state during pregnancy, hypoxia during labor and birth, and ineffective nutrition.
6. A hypoxic state during pregnancy stimulates the formation of more RBCs than expected, increasing the risk for neonatal polycythemia and hyperbilirubinemia.
7. Hypoxia may be the result of a small placenta that limits gas exchange, especially during the intense and frequent contractions of active labor. Hypoxia can lead to the passage of meconium to increase the risk for meconium aspiration.
8. Ineffective nutrition limits the formation of nutrient stores and subcutaneous fat to increase the risk for neonatal hypoglycemia and cold stress.

9. For gavage feedings, measure the length of the gastric tube from the tip of the nose to the lobe of ear, to midpoint between zyphoid process and umbilicus; mark the tube (see Figure 11-2, p. 323).
10. The mouth is preferred for gastric tube insertion with intermittent feedings because newborns are nasal breathers and because the tube stimulates sucking.
11. Include the gastric content aspirated as part of fluid used for a feeding, unless it contains blood or mucous or is more than one quarter of the previous feeding, which reflects too much residual milk in the stomach from that feeding.

CONTENT REVIEW

I. The preterm newborn experiences difficulty adapting to extrauterine life because of gestational age and an immature body system. Figure 11-1 illustrates some of the differences that can be seen when comparing a full-term and a preterm newborn.

   A. Major problems encountered by preterm newborns include:
   1. **Respiratory distress syndrome (RDS)**
      a. Definition—ineffective respiratory function primarily from the lack of pulmonary **surfactant,** a substance that coats the lining of the alveoli to facilitate alveolar expansion and contraction during respiration. Inadequate surfactant causes the alveoli to become stiff and difficult to expand, limiting gas exchange.
      b. Weak, poorly developed respiratory muscles also contribute to breathing difficulty
   2. Circulatory problems: cardiovascular immaturity and limited oxygen lead to persistent fetal circulation with continued patency of the ductus arteriosus and foramen ovale
   3. Risk for infection from
      a. Immaturity of the immunologic system
      b. Increased number of invasive procedures
      c. Delicate, easily traumatized integument
   4. Hyperbilirubinemia associated with immature hepatic function
   5. Hypothermia related to limited brown fat, glucose stores, subcutaneous fat, and muscular activity, including the ability to assume and maintain a flexed posture
   6. Renal immaturity, which increases the risk for fluid, electrolyte, and acid-base imbalances
   7. Immaturity of brain development coupled with treatment interventions such as mechanical ventilation, which increase the risk for intracranial hemorrhage
   8. Nutritional deficits such as hypoglycemia and hypocalcemia from:
      a. Limited gestational time to form nutrient stores and stressors encountered, which rapidly deplete limited stores

CLINICAL EVALUATION

PRETERM	TERM

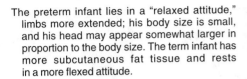

The preterm infant lies in a "relaxed attitude," limbs more extended; his body size is small, and his head may appear somewhat larger in proportion to the body size. The term infant has more subcutaneous fat tissue and rests in a more flexed attitude.

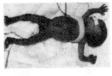 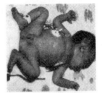

The preterm infant's ear cartilages are poorly developed, and the ear may fold easily; the hair is fine and feathery, and lanugo may cover the back and face. The mature infant's ear cartilages are well formed, and the hair is more likely to form firm separate strands

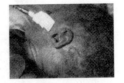 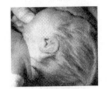

The sole of the foot of the preterm infant appears more turgid and may have only fine wrinkles. The mature infant's sole (foot) is well and deeply creased.

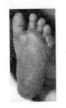 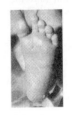

The preterm female infant's clitoris is prominent, and labia majora are poorly developed and gaping. The mature female infant's labia majora are fully developed, and the clitoris is not as prominent.

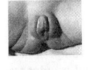 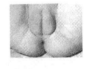

The preterm male infant's scrotum is undeveloped and not pendulous; minimal rugae are present, and the testes may be in the inguinal canals or in the abdominal cavity. The term male infant's scrotum is well developed, pendulous, and rugated, and the testes are well down in the scrotal sac.

Scarf sign—The preterm infant's elbow may be easily brought across the chest with little or no resistance. The mature infant's elbow may be brought to the midline of the chest, resisting attempts to bring the elbow past the midline.

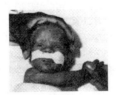 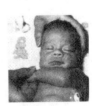

Figure 11-1 Clinical and neurologic examinations comparing preterm and full-term infants. (From Wong DL, et al: *Whaley and Wong's Nursing care of infants and children,* ed 6, St. Louis, 1999, Mosby. Data from Pierog SH, Ferrara A: *Medical care of the sick newborn,* ed 2, St. Louis, 1976, Mosby.)

Continued

NEUROLOGIC EVALUATION

PRETERM	TERM

Grasp reflex—The preterm infant's grasp is weak; the term infant's grasp is strong, allowing the infant to be lifted up from the mattress.

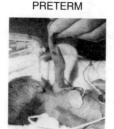
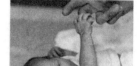

Heel-to-ear maneuver—The preterm infant's heel is easily brought to the ear, meeting with no resistance. This maneuver is not possible in the term infant, since there is considerable resistance at the knee.

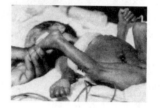
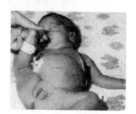

Figure 11-1, cont'd Clinical and neurologic examinations comparing preterm and full-term infants. (From Wong DL, et al: *Whaley and Wong's Nursing care of infants and children,* ed 6, St. Louis, 1999, Mosby. Data from Pierog SH, Ferrara A: *Medical care of the sick newborn,* ed 2, St. Louis, 1976, Mosby.)

  b. Limited ability to supply nutrients during extrauterine life from weak and immature GI functions that interfere with nutrient digestion and absorption

B. Close observation of high-risk newborns is essential to ensure early detection and prompt treatment for a problem before permanent damage and possibly death occur

C. Care management of the high-risk newborn should emphasize
1. Support of respiration
2. Prevention of cold stress
3. Facilitation of adequate nutritional intake and fluid, electrolyte, and acid-base balance
4. Detection and reduction of elevated bilirubin levels
5. Prevention of infection
6. Promotion of attachment and reduction of stressors for the newborn and the newborn's family

II. Respiratory distress

A. High-risk newborns may have respiratory distress as they adapt to extrauterine life and may require assistance to maintain airway patency, breathe, and obtain adequate oxygen

B. Clinical manifestations of respiratory distress
1. Tachypnea: more than 60 breaths per minute, progressing to 80 to 120 breaths per minute; more frequent periods of apnea
2. Nasal faring and expiratory grunting

3. Retractions (sternal, costal), reflecting increased work of breathing
4. Crackles bilaterally over the lung fields progressing to pulmonary edema; diminishing breath sounds
5. Central cyanosis
6. Hypercapnia and respiratory acidosis
7. Hypotonia with diminished responsiveness to stimuli

C. **Treatment interventions must be instituted immediately**
   1. Reduce stress on the respiratory system by maintaining:
      a. A **thermoneutral environment** to prevent cold stress and hyperthermia
      b. Nutrient and fluid, electrolyte, and acid-base balance to prevent hypoglycemia, dehydration or fluid excess, electrolyte imbalance, and alkalosis or acidosis
   2. Provide oxygen and breathing assistance with signs of respiratory distress and partial pressure of oxygen in arterial blood (PaO_2) of less than 60 mm Hg or oxygen saturation of less than 92%
      a. Oxygen should be warmed and humidified
      b. Oxygen concentration, volume, temperature, and humidity must be carefully controlled
      c. The method used depends on the response to treatment and the degree of difficulty experienced
         (1) Plastic hood placed over the newborn's head to supply humidified and warmed oxygen for infants who do not need mechanical ventilation
         (2) Nasal cannula for infants who require low-flow amounts
         (3) Continuous positive airway pressure (CPAP) provides a continuous infusion of oxygen under pressure by means of nasal prongs, face mask, or endotracheal tube for newborns who do not respond favorably to the hood or nasal cannula
         (4) Mechanical ventilation breathes for the newborn and supplies oxygen when the hood, cannula, or CPAP are ineffective to maintain oxygenation and support respiration
      d. Observe newborn responses to oxygen treatment every 1 to 2 hours
         (1) Physical assessment noting reversal or worsening of respiratory distress
         (2) Monitor blood gas levels and use pulse oximetry (95% to 100%)
   3. Surfactant administration to prevent and treat RDS by administering surfactant by way of an endotracheal tube into the lungs
   4. Maintain airway patency
      a. Note that respiratory secretions can become tenacious, thick, and copious
      b. Observe the newborn and auscultate the lungs before and after airway clearance measures
      c. Use percussion and vibration to loosen secretions
      d. Suction only after validating the need to because damage to delicate respiratory structures can occur with frequent suctioning

5. Change position frequently using supported side-lying or supine position, with slight neck extension
6. Provide oral and skin care to prevent breakdown—intact skin is a barrier to infection

III. Thermoregulatory instability

A. **Thermoregulation is immature in all newborns but cold stress is more likely to occur in high-risk newborns, especially if LBW. Cold stress is likely to be more hazardous in high-risk newborns because compensatory mechanisms and body functions are less effective.**

B. Cold stress, **or hypothermia, can rapidly lead to other problems:**
   1. Respiratory distress and hypoxia
   2. Metabolic acidosis
   3. Hypoglycemia

C. **Interventions to support thermoregulatory stability**
   1. Create a **thermoneutral environment:** environment that assists the newborn to maintain a stable body temperature between 97.7° F and 99.5° F (36.5° C to 37.2° C) with minimal expenditure of oxygen and nutrients
      a. A radiant warmer or incubator
      b. Close bundling in blankets, covering head and feet when the newborn is taken out of the warmer or incubator to be fed, held, and cuddled by the family
   2. Keep the newborn under a radiant warmer or in an incubator until the newborn is capable of maintaining a stable body temperature without assistance; assess axillary temperature periodically to double-check the temperature recorded on the warmer control panel
   3. Use a radiant warmer or an incubator to assess the newborn and perform treatments and procedures, because the newborn is undressed except for a cap and sometimes foot coverings
   4. Warm and humidify oxygen and air—reduces heat loss through evaporation
   5. Warm all surfaces (scale, examination table, treatment table), and objects (blankets, instruments, hands) that come into contact with the newborn to reduce heat loss through conduction—use of a heated water pad under the infant may assist with conservation of heat and preservation of skin integrity
   6. Bathe the newborn judiciously
   7. Assist the newborn in assuming and maintaining a flexed posture

IV. Alteration in nutrition (less than body requirements)

A. **Hypoglycemia: low serum glucose levels**
   1. Glucose levels—should be determined more frequently for high-risk newborns
   2. Use glucose monitor (dextrostix)—confirm low readings with laboratory testing

3. Glucose level—reflective of hypoglycemia
   a. Dextrostix—blood glucose is less than 45 mg/dl
   b. Blood glucose—laboratory testing
      (1) Less than 35 mg/dl in first 72 hours
      (2) Less than 45 mg/dl after first 72 hours
      (3) Less than 25 mg/dl in LBW newborn
4. Findings include
   a. Jitteriness, tremors, and twitching, progressing to convulsions and coma
   b. Poor feeding behavior
   c. Lethargy
   d. Cyanosis and respiratory distress
   e. Weak, high-pitched cry
5. Prevent by beginning feedings early and reducing stressors that can deplete glucose stores
6. Treatment
   a. Increase frequency of oral feedings to at least every 2 to 3 hours, with careful assessment of blood glucose levels on regular basis after each feeding
   b. Administer IV glucose
B. **Interventions to ensure adequate nutrient and fluid intake**
1. Oral feedings are preferred
   a. Assess strength and coordination of suck and swallow along with the gag and rooting reflexes by an initial feeding of sterile water
   b. Observe the newborn's behavior during feeding, tolerance for oral feeding, and amount of fluid retained
      (1) In high-risk newborns, feeding should take less than 30 minutes
      (2) Feeding smaller amounts more frequently may be helpful for the newborn that tires easily
   c. Attempt bottle or breast feeding using the correct technique with the newborn wrapped securely during feeding to prevent cold stress; supplemental oxygen may be needed
2. **Gavage feeding**
   a. Definition—feeding by way of a gastric tube inserted through the newborn's nose or mouth and into the stomach
   b. Required by newborns who are unable to obtain sufficient nutrients and fluids orally
      (1) Tires during feeding; takes longer than 30 minutes to complete feeding
      (2) Suck and swallow are weak and uncoordinated; the gag reflex is weak
      (3) Respiratory distress occurs during feeding
      (4) Weight loss of more than 15% of birth weight, or more than 2% in a 24-hour period

c. Methods
  (1) Intermittent feeding
    (a) Most commonly used method
    (b) Helpful for newborns who have some ability to suck yet become tired or cyanotic during feeding
    (c) Gavage and oral feedings can be alternated
  (2) Continuous drip using an infusion pump
d. Technique
  (1) Choose appropriate GI tube (15-inch #5 or #8 F)
  (2) Measure tube length from the tip of the newborn's nose to the earlobe, to midpoint between zyphoid process and the umbilicus; mark the tube (Fig. 11-2)
  (3) Lubricate the tube with sterile water
  (4) Insert the tube through the nose or mouth to the mark; the mouth is preferred for intermittent feedings because newborns are nasal breathers and sucking will be stimulated
  (5) Tape the tube to the newborn's cheek
  (6) Aspirate gastric contents and measure the amount
    (a) Is a method to determine tube placement; another method to check placement is to inject 1- to 3-ml of air and auscultate for gurgling at epigastric area
    (b) Evaluates tolerance for the amount of milk used by indicating residual milk in the stomach (should be less than one quarter of the previous feeding)
  (7) Include aspirated gastric content as part of fluid used for the feeding, unless it is more than one quarter of the previous feeding or contains blood or mucous
  (8) Use formula, breast milk, or other fluid
  (9) Instill fluid by gravity flow at rate of 1 ml/min
  (10) Enhance tolerance for feeding and prepare for oral feeding by:
    (a) Allowing the newborn to suck on a pacifier during feeding—helps associate sucking with satiety
    (b) Holding and cuddling the newborn—provides pleasurable physical contact that becomes associated with feeding
  (11) Assess tolerance for feeding by noting:
    (a) Amount taken and retained
    (b) Occurrence of vomiting and regurgitation and amount
    (c) Degree of abdominal distension
    (d) Bowel and bladder elimination
    (e) Weight gain or loss; hydration status
    (f) Blood glucose levels
3. Other feeding methods that may be used
  a. Gastrostomy feeding for infants with congenital anomalies
  b. Total parenteral nutrition (TPN) when enteral feedings are ineffective

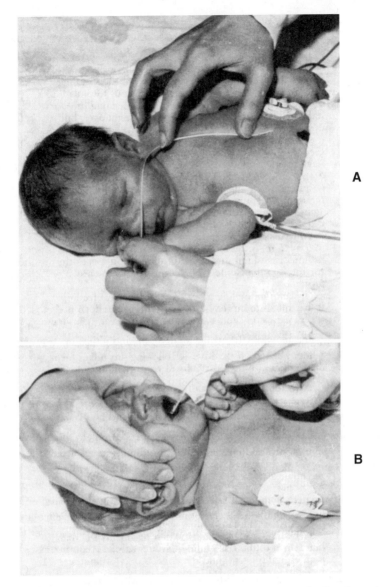

Figure 11-2 Gavage feeding. **A,** Measuring tube for nasogastric feeding from tip of nose to earlobe and to midpoint between end of xiphoid process and umbilicus. **B,** Inserting the tube. (From Wong DL, et al: *Whaley and Wong's Nursing care of infants and children,* ed 6, St. Louis, 1999, Mosby.)

4. Observe for signs of readiness for oral feeding
   a. Strong, coordinated suck and swallow
   b. Gag and rooting reflexes present and strong
   c. Spontaneous sucking on tube, hands, or pacifier
   d. Signs of hunger as feeding time approaches and signs of satiety after feeding are exhibited

5. Gradually advance newborn to oral feeding; progress from one method to the next until oral feedings are well-tolerated and can provide adequate nutrition and hydration

V. Hyperbilirubinemia

A. **Definition—increased level of unconjugated bilirubin from the inability of the newborn's liver to break down and excrete the bilirubin produced by RBC destruction** (see Chapter 10, p. 267)

B. **Types**
  1. Physiologic hyperbilirubinemia-jaundice appears after the first 24 hours of life, especially in
     a. LBW newborns
     b. Newborns of diabetic mothers
     c. Newborns who have difficulty with feeding immediately after birth
  2. Pathologic hyperbilirubinemia-jaundice appears during the first 24 hours of life, with levels increasing at a more rapid pace and to higher levels; it is associated with hemolytic disease
     a. Rh incompatibility: an Rh-positive newborn is exposed to antibodies formed by an Rh-negative mother and transmitted to the newborn transplacentally; the antibodies destroy the newborn's Rh-positive RBCs
     b. ABO blood type incompatibility: usually noted in mothers with blood type O who have newborns who are type A or B; experience less difficulty than the Rh-incompatible newborn

C. **Prevention**
  1. Initiate early and frequent feedings to stimulate the gastrocolic reflex and facilitate bowel elimination; bilirubin is excreted in stool rather than being reabsorbed into the circulation
  2. Administer RhoGAM to all unsensitized (negative indirect Coombs' test) Rh-negative mothers who give birth to Rh-positive newborns with a negative direct Coombs' test or who experience a pregnancy-related event that can lead to exposure of her blood to that of her fetus. Examples include abortion, amniocentesis, and chorionic villus sampling.

D. **Treatment: must be instituted promptly to reduce increasing bilirubin levels and facilitate its excretion before the levels become so high that bilirubin invades the brain and causes permanent damage (*kernicterus,* or bilirubin encephalopathy)**
  1. **Phototherapy:** light source of fluorescent bulbs is placed 18 to 20 inches above the newborn to facilitate bilirubin breakdown for excretion
     a. Place undressed newborn under the lights for full skin exposure; a small diaper or genital covering may be used to collect urine and stool

    b. Cover eyes completely
        (1) Close eye lids before patches are applied
        (2) Remove patches after taking the newborn out from the lights to
            (a) Check eyes for discharge, excess pressure, corneal irritation, and edema
            (b) Facilitate visual stimulation and eye contact with parents and family
    c. Do not apply lotions, creams, or oils to the skin
    d. Feed frequently at 2- to 3-hour intervals to:
        (1) Maintain hydration by replacing fluid lost from the skin and liquid stools
        (2) Enhance excretion of bilirubin by facilitating elimination
        (3) Provide water supplementation if needed
    e. Observe stools, which often are loose, green, and more frequent
    f. Assess temperature at least every 4 hours because the newborn is prone to cold stress and hyperthermia
        (1) Skin is exposed to air, increasing heat loss
        (2) Newborn is usually sleepy and lethargic, which decreases heat-producing muscular activity
        (3) Radiant warmer may be used
        (4) Lights along with a radiant warmer may increase body temperature
    g. Change position every 2 hours so that all skin surfaces are exposed
    h. Assess effectiveness of treatment
        (1) Monitor progress of jaundice
        (2) Collect blood to determine bilirubin levels noting increasing or decreasing levels
        (3) Discontinue treatment when downward trend in bilirubin occurs
    i. Fiber-optic panel or blanket that wraps around newborn is now available
        (1) Newborn can be held and cuddled
        (2) Patches are not required
        (3) Home treatment is possible because the unit is portable
    j. Teach parents about
        (1) Hyperbilirubinemia: why it occurs and the effects it can have on the newborn
        (2) Treatment: what is used, how it works, and why it is important
        (3) Instructions are required to reduce parental anxiety and prepare parents for early discharge because jaundice may appear at home: what to look for and what to do
    k. Document all care measures, time under phototherapy, and observations of status

2. Exchange transfusion: small amount (5 to 20 ml) of the newborn's blood is removed and replaced slowly with a comparable amount of compatible donor blood. This process is continued until 75% to 85% of infant's total blood volume is exchanged.
   a. Removes sensitized RBCs and bilirubin and corrects anemia that occurs from hemolysis
   b. Used to treat severe hyperbilirubinemia, especially when it is unresponsive to phototherapy

VI. Nursing interventions to facilitate the attachment process and reduce stress in families with a sick newborn

A. **Attachment process is often delayed or inhibited by separation from or limited contact with the newborn as a result of physical care requirements**
   1. Early attachment has long-term implications for the newborn's future growth and development and relationship with the family
   2. Newborn requires stimuli that promote development, including touch and auditory and visual stimuli
   3. Parents unprepared to cope with a high-risk newborn may experience
      a. Anxiety about the changing health status and uncertain future of their newborn
      b. Reluctance to establish a relationship with a newborn that might die; anticipatory grieving
      c. Role conflict as they attempt to meet the needs of their newborn, each other, children at home, their jobs, and themselves
      d. Guilt, blame, and anger: Why did this happen? What did we, or you, do wrong? What could we, or you, have done differently during pregnancy?
      e. Concern about finances
   4. Children at home experience
      a. Disappointment that the baby did not come home
      b. Worry about the baby's status influenced by parental anxiety
      c. Feeling of abandonment by their parents

B. **Nursing interventions**
   1. Provide time for parents to communicate, encouraging them to freely discuss their feelings and concerns without fear of judgment
   2. Introduce parents to their newborn
      a. Explain the purpose of all the equipment and procedures
      b. Keep parents informed of the newborn's status; repeat as needed because parents are anxious, which may interfere with understanding and learning
      c. Help parents focus on the newborn rather than all the equipment by pointing out the newborn's behaviors
      d. Encourage parents to touch and interact with their newborn
      e. Provide parents private time with their newborn

3. Establish flexible visiting hours; encourage parents to participate in the newborn's care
   a. Collect breast milk for gavage feedings
   b. Help with procedures
   c. Bring in clothes, toys from home, and photographs; helps establish the newborn's identity
   d. Reinforce the parents' care efforts
4. Involve the siblings
   a. Allow visitation
   b. Prepare children for the neonatal intensive care unit (NICU) environment
   c. Encourage touch and interaction
   d. Provide explanations
5. Initiate a discharge plan as soon as the newborn is admitted to the NICU; earlier discharge of newborns with special needs is a growing trend
   a. Teach parents what they need to know to care for their newborn in the home; provide time for practice
   b. Discuss home preparations that may have to be made
   c. Involve the social worker, community health nurses, and home care agencies as appropriate
   d. Make referrals to support groups of parents who have had similar experiences

WEB Resources

http://www.perinatal.com
　Phoenix Perinatal Associates provides information for heath care providers and clients related to high-risk pregnancy and birth.

http://www.nationalshareoffice.com
　Share—Pregnancy and Infant Loss Support, Inc., is a nonprofit group whose purpose is to benefit bereaved families.

http://www.bizjet.com/jnn
　Journal of Neonatal Nursing (JNN) is the official journal for the Neonatal Nurses Association. A table of contents for recent issues is included. Guests can access summaries of articles and download one selected full text article for each issue. Subscribers can access and download full text of all articles.

REVIEW QUESTIONS

1. Small for gestational age newborns experience difficulty adapting to extrauterine life as a result of which physiology?
   1. Anemia
   2. Hyperglycemia
   3. Limited subcutaneous fat
   4. Inadequate surfactant

2. Preterm newborns exhibit which characteristics?
   1. Assume a flexed posture when at rest
   2. Exhibit the scarf sign
   3. Provide resistance when the heel is brought to the ear
   4. Possess an abundance of brown fat

3. During care of a preterm newborn, nurses must be alert for which physiologic response?
   1. Hypercalcemia
   2. Premature closure of the ductus arteriosus and foramen ovale
   3. Meconium aspiration syndrome
   4. Hypoglycemia

4. To create a thermoneutral environment for a preterm newborn, the nurse should follow which guideline?
   1. Keep the newborn under a radiant warmer at all times
   2. Cover the newborn with a light blanket when under the warmer
   3. Warm all surfaces and objects that come in contact with the newborn
   4. Avoid bathing the newborn

5. The nurse can enhance the preterm newborn's tolerance for gavage feeding by which action?
   1. Instilling fluid at a rate of 4 ml/min
   2. Allowing the newborn to suck on a pacifier during the feeding
   3. Keeping the newborn under the radiant warmer during the feeding
   4. Weighing the newborn before and after the feeding

ANSWERS, RATIONALES, AND TEST-TAKING TIPS

Rationales	Test-Taking Tips

1. Correct answer: 3

Limited subcutaneous fat increases the newborn's risk for cold stress. SGA newborns have an excess of RBCs from exposure to hypoxia in utero. Hypoglycemia occurs from poor intrauterine nutrition and formation of nutrient stores. Inadequate surfactant production is associated with prematurity.

The clue in the question is "extrauterine life environment." Think of environmental factors rather than internal factors. If you put the options in either of these categories—internal or environmental—only option 3 is more aligned with environmental. The other three options are definitely internal factors. Select option 3.

2. Correct answer: 2

Preterm newborns have limited muscle tone that allows for the elbow to be brought past the midline of the chest (scarf sign) and the heel to the ear with no resistance. Preterm newborns tend to assume an extended posture when at rest. Brown fat is limited in preterm newborns. Therefore, they have an increased risk for hypothermia and cold stress.

The approach is to eliminate three options and to end up with the correct answer. The clue in option 1 is "flexed posture," which is found in a term newborn. The clue in option 3 is "resistance." With normal muscle tone, resistance is found when odd positions of the extremities are attempted. In option 4, avoid focusing on brown fat. Instead, focus on the clue "abundance of. . . fat." This would not be the case for a preterm newborn. Select the only option left, option 2, even though you have no idea of what it is. This is a situation in which you eliminate three options based on what you know.

3. Correct answer: 4

Nutritional deficits such as hypocalcemia and hypoglycemia are common because of the limited gestation time to form nutrient stores. Fetal circulatory shunts must close at birth. The hypoxia from the inadequate respiration interferes with closure of the shunts in the

Associate a preterm newborn as being born premature without adequate physiologic equipment. Thus, think in terms of preterm as a hyposituation. Remember to focus on what you know rather than selecting an option you know little about or one for which you cannot recall the details.

Rationales	Test-Taking Tips

preterm newborn. Respiratory distress syndrome with limited surfactant production is most likely to occur. Meconium aspiration is more likely to occur in postmature newborns.

4. Correct answer: 3

Once temperature is stabilized the newborn can be wrapped and taken out of the warmer to be fed, held, and cuddled. Only the head and sometimes the feet are covered when the newborn is under the warmer. Newborns can be bathed carefully to preserve skin integrity. Precautions must be taken to prevent heat loss by keeping the unbathed area covered and bathing the newborn under the warmer.

Eliminate option 1 with the clue at the end of the statement, "at all times." This action would be impossible to do. Option 2 sounds good. However, think about the activity of a newborn—the blanket would not likely be kicked off. Blankets are not used under a warmer since hypothermia is a risk and visibility of the newborn's condition would be obscured. Option 3 sounds most reasonable. Option 4 is impractical, as is option 1.

5. Correct answer: 2

Fluid should be instilled at 1 ml/min while holding and cuddling the newborn. Weighing the newborn gives an indication of the effectiveness of the fluid intake but does not enhance tolerance for the feeding.

Keep in mind the focus of the question as you read the options. The focus in this question is about the feeding or the GI system. Look for the option that has the GI intervention. The only one given is option 2.

12

Nursing Care of Children with Neurologic Disorders

FAST FACTS

1. Irritability and lethargy are early findings indicative of changes in the neurologic status of infants and young children.
2. The degree of neurologic involvement is directly related to the anatomic level of the defect.
3. The therapeutic level of phenobarbital is 10 to 40 μg/ml for seizure prevention maintenance.
4. The infant and young child demonstrates a different response to head injury as compared with an adult because of a larger head size, larger blood volume, and softer, thinner brain tissue.
5. Superficial reflexes and deep tendon reflexes (DTRs) normally are not tested in infants and young children.
6. Half of all cases of spina bifida cystica occur as a result of folic acid deficiency.

CONTENT REVIEW

I. Overview: neurologic system
   A. General concepts
      1. Structure and function
         a. Neurologic system includes:
            (1) Central nervous system (CNS), composed of cerebrum, cerebellum, brain stem, and spinal cord (Table 12-1, p. 332)
            (2) Peripheral nervous system, consisting of motor (efferent) and sensory (afferent) nerves

TABLE 12-1	Structure, Function, and Dysfunctions of the Brain	
Structure	**Function**	**Effects of Dysfunction**
Cerebrum	Consciousness, thought process, memory Sensory input Motor activity	Dependent on specific site involved
Frontal lobes	Motor activity Social interaction Abstract thinking Expressive language	Anterior damage—personality changes; posterior damage—impaired movement of body part Memory defects Language defects
Parietal lobes	Sensation Somatic interpretation	Language dysfunction Lower motor and sensory loss Aphasia
Cerebellum	Muscle movement: coordination and refinement	Ataxia Nystagmus Dystonia
Basal ganglia	Automatic control of lower motor centers	Athetosis Tremors at rest, nonintention
Diencephalon	Forms reticular activating system (RAS)	Stupor
Thalamus	Sensory impulse relay station to cerebral cortex	Altered consciousness
Hypothalamus	Control center for involuntary activities; Blood pressure Satiety Hunger Temperature regulation Sleep regulation	Coma Weight loss, anorexia Endocrine disorders
Brainstem Midbrain	Gives rise to cranial nerves Connection between hindbrain and forebrain Holds nuclei for cranial nerves III, IV, part of V	Stupor, coma Altered consciousness Decerebrate posturing Neurologic hyperventilation
Pons	Respiratory center (pneumotaxic center) Cranial nerves V-VIII	Deep, rapid, or periodic breathing Impaired muscle function supplied by the nerves (V through VIII)
Medulla	Respiratory center Cranial nerves IX, X, XI, XII	Biot's respiration Flaccid muscle tone Absence of deep tendon, gag and corneal reflexes

Modified from Wong, DL. et al: *Whaley and Wong's nursing care of infants and children,* ed 6, St Louis, 1999, Mosby.

(3) Autonomic nervous system, composed of sympathetic and parasympathetic systems
b. CNS controls and regulates body functions, which include the five senses
c. Peripheral nervous system is composed of:
  (1) 12 pairs of cranial nerves
  (2) 31 spinal nerves named for the portion of the spinal cord from which they emerge
    (a) Cervical
    (b) Thoracic
    (c) Lumbar
    (d) Coccygeal
d. Autonomic nervous system provides involuntary control of functions, including respiration and digestion
2. Development
a. Two thirds of brain cell growth occurs in fetal life; the nervous system continues to grow rapidly during infancy and early childhood and slows during late childhood and adolescence
b. The brain and spinal cord are among the first structures to be identified during intrauterine life
c. Myelinization—the development of a myelin sheath around a nerve fiber
  (1) Follows a cephalocaudal and proximodistal sequence
  (2) Occurs rapidly in infancy and continues throughout childhood
  (3) Reaches completion in late adolescence
3. Brain anatomy and physiology
a. Bones of the cranium encase the brain; three layers of **meninges,** the membranous covering of the brain and spinal cord
  (1) Dura mater (outer)
  (2) Arachnoid mater—delicate avascular layer
  (3) Pia mater (inner)—delicate layering that adheres to the outer surface of the brain. Note that the subarachnoid space, which is filled with cerebropinal fluid (CSF), lies between the pia mater and arachnoid membrane.
b. Brain, blood, and CSF maintain pressure equilibrium inside the skull
c. Blood supply to the brain is furnished by internal carotid arteries and vertebral arteries, which form the circle of Willis
d. The blood-brain barrier consists of walls of capillaries in the CNS and functions to slow or prevent the passage of various chemical compounds, radioactive ions, and disease-causing organisms from the blood into the CNS
e. CSF is manufactured in the choroid plexus of the ventricular network, which includes:
  (1) Lateral, third, and fourth ventricles
  (2) Foramina of Luschka and Magendie
  (3) Aqueduct of Sylvius

Box 12-1
Levels of Consciousness in Pediatrics

Full consciousness: awake and alert, orientated to time, place, and person; behavior is
  appropriate for age
Confusion: impaired decision-making skills
Disorientation: confusion regarding time and place and decreased LOC
Lethargy: limited spontaneous movement and sluggish speech
Obtundation: can be aroused with stimulation
Stupor: remains in a deep sleep, responsive only to vigorous and repeated stimulation
Coma: no motor or verbal response to noxious (painful) stimuli
Persistent vegetative state: permanent loss of function of the cerebral cortex; eyes
  follow objects only by reflex or when attracted to the direction of loud sounds; all
  four limbs are spastic but can withdraw from painful stimuli; hands show reflexive
  grasping and groping; the face can grimace, some food may be swallowed, and the
  child may groan or cry but utter no words.

Modified from Hazinski MF: *Care of the critically ill child,* ed 2, St. Louis, 1992, Mosby.

4. Spinal cord anatomy
   a. Vertebral column, consisting of 31 vertebrae, encases the spinal
      cord; vertebrae divided into segments
      (1) Cervical
      (2) Thoracic
      (3) Lumbar
      (4) Sacral and coccygeal
   b. Meninges cover the spinal cord
   c. Anterior, posterior, and radicular arteries supply blood to the
      spinal cord
5. Level of consciousness (LOC)
   a. Site of consciousness is located in the reticular activating
      system of the brainstem
   b. LOC assessment gives the earliest indication of improvement
      or deterioration in neurologic status (Box 12-1 and
      Figure 12-1)
6. Increased intracranial pressure (ICP)
   a. Description—condition that occurs when balance in the
      volumes of brain, tissues, CSF, and blood is disrupted
   b. Causes—tumors, bleeding, infection, and edema of cerebral
      tissue; accumulation of CSF in the ventricular system
   c. Manifestations—vary with age (Box 12-2, p. 336)
B. **Assessment of the neurologic system**
   1. Pediatric considerations
      a. Congenital defects of the CNS are mostly the result of failures
         that occur during the critical period of organ development in
         the first trimester of intrauterine life

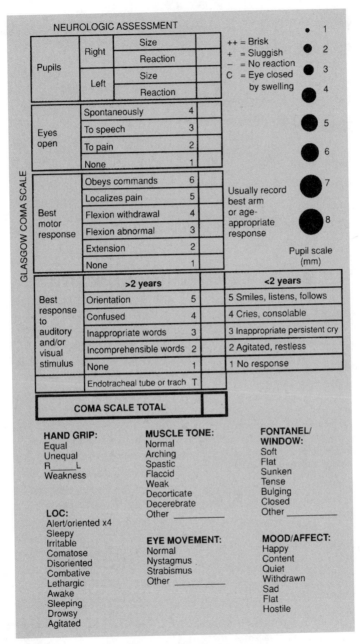

Figure 12-1   Pediatric Glasgow Coma Scale. (From Wong DL, et al: *Whaley and Wong's nursing care of infants and children,* ed 6, St. Louis, 1999, Mosby.)

Box 12-2

Clinical Manifestations of Increased Intracranial Pressure (ICP) in Infants and Children

Infants

Tense, bulging fontanel; lack of normal pulsations
Separated cranial sutures
Macewen's sign—percussion of head elicits a cracked-pot sound
Irritability
High-pitched cry
Increased occipitofrontal circumference
Distended scalp veins
Changes in feeding
Cries when held or rocked
"Setting sun" sign—eyes deviate with the iris downward to where a significant white part of the eye is found above the iris

Children

Headache
Nausea
Vomiting—often without nausea
Diplopia—double vision, blurred vision
Seizures

Personality and Behavior Signs

Irritability (toddlers), restlessness
Indifference, drowsiness, or lack of interest
Decline in school performance
Diminished physical activity and motor performance
Increased complaints of fatigue, tiredness; increased time devoted to sleep
Significant weight loss possible from anorexia and vomiting
Memory loss if pressure is greatly increased
Inability to follow simple commands
Progression to lethargy and drowsiness

Late Signs

Lowered level of consciousness
Decreased motor response to command
Decreased sensory response to painful stimuli
Alterations in pupil size and reactivity
Sometimes decerebrate or decorticate posturing
Cheyne-Stokes respirations
Papilledema

From Wong DL, et al: *Whaley and Wong's nursing care of infants and children*, ed 6, St. Louis, 1999, Mosby.

b. Because children less than 2 years of age are unable to follow directions, observations of the LOC and the reflex responses are used to gain information about neurologic status

2. Neurologic diagnostic procedures (Table 12-2, p. 338)
3. Health history
   a. Present health status
      (1) Assessment for these abnormal findings
         (a) Decreased LOC
         (b) Pain with activity; headache; pain in eyes or ears
         (c) Loss of balance, vertigo, dizziness, and unexplained falling
         (d) Weakness or numbness
         (e) School or learning difficulties
         (f) Seizure activity
      (2) Specific questions to ask
         (a) Has parent noticed any clumsiness, drowsiness, confusion, unsteady gait, or muscular weakness?
         (b) Has child experienced learning or school difficulty associated with attention to the task, interest, or ability to concentrate?
         (c) Has the child continued to grow and mature normally?
         (d) Does the child currently take any medications?
         (e) Are the child's immunizations up to date? Or which immunizations has the child had?
   b. Medical history (areas of concern)
      (1) Prenatal history
         (a) Exposure to teratogens
         (b) Medications taken
         (c) Drug or alcohol use
      (2) Birth history
         (a) Apgar score, fetal distress
         (b) Gestational age
         (c) Congenital anomalies
      (3) Postnatal development
         (a) Infections
         (b) Nutritional status
      (4) Developmental milestones
         (a) Age child attained each of the following: head control, grasping, sitting, crawling, walking, and toilet control
         (b) Speech or language: first words and progression to phrases and sentences versus age at the time
         (c) Performance of self-care activities
      (5) Trauma
         (a) Head, spinal cord injuries
         (b) Birth trauma
         (c) CNS insult

TABLE 12-2 **Major Neurologic Diagnostic Procedures in Pediatrics**

Procedure	Purpose	Indication	Developmental Considerations
Lumbar puncture	To obtain CSF for visualization, laboratory analysis, and pressure reading. To inject medication or spinal anesthesia. Contraindicated if findings of increased ICP are present	Meningitis, encephalitis, CNS hemorrhage	Child, toddler, or infant placed in side-lying position with knees and head flexed (fetal-like position)
Subdural tap	To remove accumulation of fluid from subdural hematomas and cerebral effusion. Relieves ICP	Subdural hematoma, cerebral effusion	Infant may be wrapped in mummy restraint. Infant must be placed in infant seat or semi-upright position following tap to decrease possibility of leakage. Older children may benefit from therapeutic play
Radiography	Reveals fractures, dislocations, spreading suture lines. Reveals degenerative changes	Trauma to skull, spinal column. Headaches. Congenital malformation	Noninvasive; machinery may be frightening and cold. Parent may need to accompany child
Computed Tomography (CT)	Horizontal and vertical cross section of brain may be visualized. Indicates tissue density	Neurologic trauma. Unconsciousness. Hydrocephalus. Lesions, tumors	Sedation usually necessary, since child needs to remain still. An infant may be fed 30 min before test to facilitate sleep. Child NPO before procedure
Electroencephalography (EEG)	Measures electrical activity of cerebral cortex	Determination of brain death. Diagnosis of seizures. Sleep abnormalities	Minimize external stimuli. Child must lie quietly during 45 minute procedure
Magnetic Resonance Imaging (MRI)	Evaluates soft tissue of brain and spinal column	Tumors, hemorrhages. Vascular disorders. Congenital malformations. Trauma, intracranial injury	Sedation may be required. Parent may remain with child to provide reassurance

Modified from Wong, DL, et al. *Whaley and Wong's nursing care of infants and children,* ed 6, St Louis, 1999, Mosby.

(6) Infection
    (a) Meningitis
    (b) Encephalitis
(7) Neurologic or psychiatric disorders
    (a) Hyperactivity
    (b) Autism
    (c) Seizure activity
(8) Specific questions to ask
    (a) In the past, has the child had a head injury or neurologic problems such as a seizure, tremor, or weakness?
    (b) Is there a history of prolonged labor or fetal distress?
c. Family history
  (1) Hereditary disorders
    (a) Muscular dystrophy
    (b) Huntington's chorea
    (c) Tay-Sachs disease
  (2) Neurologic disorders
    (a) Epilepsy
    (b) Seizure disorder
    (c) Mental retardation
4. Physical examination
  a. Mental status
    (1) Physical appearance and behavior
    (2) LOC
    (3) Attention span
    (4) Memory
    (5) Signs of anxiety or depression
    (6) Speech and language
  b. Cranial nerve testing
  c. Cerebellar function and proprioception
    (1) Evaluate coordination and fine motor skills
      (a) Spontaneous activity
      (b) Symmetry
      (c) Smoothness of movement
    (2) Evaluate balance using Romberg test for older children
    (3) Observe child's gait
  d. Sensory function: evaluation of sensory responses
    (1) Light touch—cotton ball stroked lightly across the cheek
    (2) Pain—skin lightly pricked with safety pin
  e. Muscular function: evaluation of muscle tone
    (1) Pull infant to sitting position using wrists
    (2) Use range of motion techniques
  f. Reflex testing
    (1) Superficial reflexes and deep tendon reflexes (DTRs) normally are not tested in infants and young children

        (2) Evaluation of common infant reflexes—rooting, sucking, extrusion, and Moro

    5. Relevant medications (Table 12-3)

II. Congenital disorders involving the CNS

  A. **Hydrocephalus**

    1. Definition—imbalance of CSF absorption or production caused by malformations, tumors, hemorrhage, infections, or trauma and resulting in head enlargement and increased ICP

    2. Two types of hydrocephalus

      a. Communicating

        (1) Occurs as result of impaired absorption within the subarachnoid space

        (2) Referred to as extraventricular—no interference of CSF within the ventricular system

      b. Noncommunicating

        (1) Obstruction of flow of CSF within the ventricular system—in the ventricles or from the ventricles into the subarachnoid space

        (2) Usually the result of developmental malformation—e.g., Arnold-Chiari malformations

    3. Etiology and incidence

      a. Most common cause of enlarged head circumference in children

      b. Associated with other congenital anomalies such as neural tube defects

    4. Pathophysiology

      a. CSF imbalance causes ventricular accumulation of CSF and pressure and results in dilation of ventricles and skull enlargement

      b. Complications

        (1) Increased ICP

        (2) Infection

        (3) Developmental delays

        (4) Obstruction of shunt

        (5) Skin breakdown

        (6) Sensory deficits

        (7) Mental retardation to various degrees

        (8) Seizure activity

    5. Assessment

      a. Questions to ask

        (1) Any changes in activity level or LOC?

        (2) Any difficulties encountered with feeding?

        (3) Any increases in head size or changes in fontanels noted?

      b. Age-specific assessment findings

        (1) Infant

          (a) Irritability and lethargy; feeds poorly

TABLE 12-3   Common Medications for CNS Disorders in Children

Medication and Indications	Route and Dosage	Side Effects	Nursing Implications
Antiepileptics Phenobarbital (Luminal) Tonic-clonic seizures	PO (seizures) 4-6 mg/kg/day	CNS: ataxia, drowsiness, irritability, headache GI: nausea, vomiting Liver: hepatitis, jaundice Genitourinary: renal damage Skin: rash, dermatitis Hematologic: bone marrow suppression Metabolic: hypocalcemia Respiratory: respiratory depression	Assess therapeutic plasma level: 10-40 µg/ml Assess LOC Assess respiratory status May be mixed with food Monitor vital signs, CBC, liver, and renal function studies when on long-term therapy Family education: Do not discontinue drug or increase dose Do not give with other drugs or ethyl alcohol May affect cognitive learning and motor speed May cause vitamin D and folic acid deficiency
Diazepam rectal gel (Diastat) Seizure activity in children over age 2 yr	Rectal: 2-5 yr, 0.5 mg/kg 6-11 yr, 0.3 mg/kg >12 yr, 0.2 mg/kg	CNS: depression, dizziness	For status epilepticus, IV Atevan, which has less respiratory depression in children over 2 years of age, and Valium are used. Rectal diazepam allows for easier administration to treat seizures in the home setting. For maintenance, oral antiepileptic therapy is used to suppress the seizure threshold.

Continued

TABLE 12-3 Common Medications for CNS Disorders in Children—cont'd

Medication and Indications	Route and Dosage	Side Effects	Nursing Implications
Antiepleptics—cont'd			
Phenytoin (Dilantin) Tonic-clonic seizures Complex partial seizures Simple partial seizures	PO 5-10 mg/kg/day	CNS: confusion, dizziness, drowsiness, insomnia Cardiovascular: cardiac arrest, bradycardia, hypotension Eyes, ears, nose, throat: gingival hypertrophy, slurred speech GI: nausea, vomiting, anorexia, diarrhea, weight loss Skin: hirsutism, rash, dermatitis Toxic effects: **Stevens-Johnson syndrome, thrombocytopenia**	Assess therapeutic plasma level (10-20 µg/ml) Family education: Stress compliance to prevent seizure activity Take with food to decrease GI upset Do not take with milk Stress importance of dental hygiene Monitor blood, liver, and renal studies in long-term therapy Advise family that child's urine may turn pink to brown in color
Osmotic Diuretic			
Mannitol (Osmitrol) Cerebral edema Increased intraocular pressure	IV: 0.5-1 g/kg (initial) 0.25-0.5 g/kg every 4-6 hr (maintenance)	CNS: headache, dizziness Cardiovascular: hypotension, tachycardia GI: nausea, vomiting Genitourinary: electrolyte imbalance Skin: rash, hives	Assess serum electrolytes and vital signs taking BP with child lying and standing Daily weights Assess for respiratory and neurologic status, changes in HR, rebound increased ICP Monitor for signs of hypovolemia

       (b) Progressive enlargement of head before fusion of cranial sutures

       (c) Bulging fontanels

       (d) Frontal bossing—prominent forehead

       (e) Dilation of superficial scalp veins

       (f) **Sunset eyes**—the infant's eyes appear to look only downward, with the sclera prominent over the iris

       (g) **Macewen sign**—percussion of the head elicits a cracked-pot sound

       (h) High, shrill cry and seizure activity are late signs

    (2) Older child

       (a) Headache

       (b) Nausea and vomiting

       (c) Spasticity of lower extremities

       (d) Altered school performance

  c. Diagnostic evaluation: diagnostic studies

    (1) Transillumination of the skull—in advanced cases, reveals light over the entire cranium

    (2) Skull radiograph—reveals widened fontanels and sutures

    (3) Magnetic resonance imaging (MRI)

    (4) Computed tomography (CT scan)—reveals fluid accumulation

6. Therapeutic management

  a. Medications

    (1) Diuretics—acetazolamide (Diamox) to decrease CSF production

    (2) Anticonvulsants—to limit seizure activity

    (3) Antibiotics—to treat infection, based on culture and sensitivity results

  b. Treatments: ventricular taps until surgery

  c. Surgery: depends on the type of hydrocephalus; may involve surgical removal of obstruction, resection of cyst, neoplasm or hematoma; mechanical shunt insertion into one of the lateral ventricles, usually the right ventricle; distal end placement into another body cavity to drain off excess CSF. Two types of shunts:

    (1) Ventriculoperitoneal (V-P)—CSF drains into the peritoneal cavity from the lateral ventricle; used most often in infants because excess tubing allows for growth (Figure 12-2, p. 344)

    (2) Ventriculoatrial (VA)—CSF drains into right atrium of the heart from the lateral ventricle, bypassing the obstruction; used in older children

  d. Shunt revisions: may be done electively during development or when shunt malfunctions

  e. Endoscopic ventriculostomy: used with a noncommunicating type; small opening is placed in third ventricle to drain excess CSF

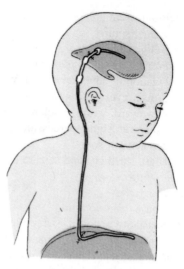

Figure 12-2   Ventriculoperitoneal shunt. (From Wong DL, et al: *Whaley and Wong's nursing care of infants and children,* ed 6, St. Louis, 1999, Mosby.)

    f. Complications in V-P shunting
        (1) Infection
           (a) Greatest risk occurs 1 to 2 months after placement
           (b) Signs include shunt malfunction, fever, and wound inflammation
        (2) Malfunction: kinking, plugging with exudate, or tube separation

 Warning!

Increased ICP and altered neurologic status present emergency situation in children with shunts.

        (3) Subdural hematoma occurs with a rapid increase in ICP
  7. Nursing management
    a. Acute care: presurgical
        (1) Nursing diagnoses
           (a) Risk for injury related to seizure
           (b) Potential altered cerebral tissue perfusion
        (2) Expected outcomes
           (a) Potential for injury will be reduced
           (b) Child will have no or minimal skin breakdown
           (c) Child will develop no further signs of increased ICP
           (d) Family will be able to discuss hydrocephalus, presurgical procedures, and shunting treatment
        (3) Interventions
           (a) Assess for signs of increased ICP: evaluate LOC using the Pediatric Glasgow Coma Scale (see Figure 12-1, p. 335)

(b) Monitor vital signs every 2 to 4 hours or more often if indicated

(c) Measure head circumference daily; assess fontanels every 4 hours for bulging

(d) Position head to prevent skin breakdown; carefully support head when feeding and turning; elevate head of the bed 30 degrees

(e) Observe seizure precautions; keep oxygen and suction equipment nearby

(f) Prepare family for the child's surgery

(g) Explain procedures and treatments

b. Acute care: postsurgical

    (1) Nursing diagnosis: risk for injury or infection related to the presence of a shunt

    (2) Expected outcome: incisional healing without signs of infection or injury

    (3) Interventions

        (a) Monitor vital signs and neurologic status, and assess for increased ICP

        (b) Monitor for signs of infection at incision site every 4 hours; report changes as noted

⚠ Warning!

Nurses must carefully monitor signs of CSF infection: increased temperature, poor feeding, vomiting, decreased responsiveness, seizure activity, and inflammation at the wound site.

        (c) Place on nonoperative side; position according to physician's orders

        (d) Keep child flat to avoid rapid reduction of intracranial fluid

        (e) If increased ICP is present, surgeon will order head of the bed to be elevated 15 to 30 degrees to enhance gravity flow through the shunt

        (f) Monitor input and output; maintain NPO as ordered

8. Evaluation

a. Questions to ask child's family

    (1) What are signs of shunt malfunction?

    (2) What are findings of increased ICP?

    (3) When would you call the physician or take the child to the emergency department?

b. Evaluation of expected outcomes

    (1) Child remains free of infection and signs of increased ICP

    (2) Parents verbalize understanding of discharge teaching: signs of infection and increased ICP, shunt procedure and

malfunctioning, and methods to promote growth and development

(3) Child maintains stable neurologic status

(4) Incisional site heals

(5) Family uses community agencies for information and support

B. Spina bifida—myelodysplasia

1. Definition: CNS defect that occurs as a result of the neural tube's failure to close during embryonic development

2. Common neural tube defects (NTDs) (Figure 12-3)

   a. Spina bifida occulta: posterior vertebral arches fail to close in lumbosacral area

      (1) Spinal cord remains intact

      (2) Usually not visible; nevi, dimple, or lipoma may be present

      (3) Meninges are not exposed on skin surface

      (4) Neurologic deficits usually are not present

   b. Spina bifida cystica: protrusion of spinal cord, its meninges, or both

      (1) Meningocele: protrusion involves meninges and a saclike cyst that contains CSF in the midline of the back, usually in the lumbosacral area

         (a) No involvement of spinal cord

         (b) Absence of neurologic deficits

      (2) Myelomeningocele: same as the meningocele plus a portion of the spinal cord

         (a) Involves the spinal cord

         (b) Sac is covered by a thin membrane that is prone to leakage or rupture

         (c) Neurologic deficits are evident

         (d) Mainly involves lumbar or lumbosacral area

3. Etiology and incidence

   a. Half of all cases occur as a result of folic acid deficiency in women

> **⚠ Warning!**
>
> The American Academy of Pediatrics recommends a folic acid intake of 0.4 mg/day for all women of childbearing age.

   b. Factors involved include heredity, environment, valproic acid (anticonvulsant) ingestion by the mother, and maternal heat exposure (hot tubs, saunas)

4. Pathophysiology

   a. Fusion failure of vertebral laminae of the spinal column or separation of already closed neural tube from increased CSF pressure

   b. Various degrees of neurologic dysfunction are present, depending on which portion of the spinal cord is involved. If it is below the second lumbar vertebrae, partial to total motor impairment results in flaccidity, partial paralysis of the lower extremities, and loss of elimination control.

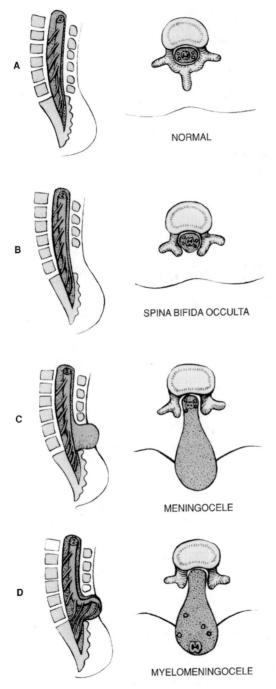

Figure 12-3 Spina bifida. Midline defects of osseous spine with varying degrees of neural herniations. **A,** Normal. **B,** Spina bifida occulta. **C,** Meningocele. **D,** Myelomeningo-cele. (From Wong DL, et al: *Whaley and Wong's nursing care of infants and children,* ed 6, St. Louis, 1999, Mosby.)

  c. Complications
   (1) Meningitis
   (2) Immobility
   (3) UTI
   (4) Mental retardation, cerebral palsy, and epilepsy
   (5) Latex allergy
  d. Associated defects
   (1) Hydrocephalus
   (2) Misshapen lower extremities and muscle atrophy
 5. Assessment
  a. Assessment findings depend on spinal cord involvement
   (1) Visible spinal defect
   (2) Flaccid paralysis of legs
   (3) Altered bladder function (neurogenic bladder)
   (4) Altered bowel function: lack of bowel control, rectal prolaspse

⚠ Warning!

Avoid the use of rectal route for temperature assessment. Obtain an axillary or tympanic temperature reading.

   (5) Joint deformities occur in utero: dislocated hip, scoliosis, kyphosis, and talipes valgus or varus—deformities that involve the foot and ankle (splay or club foot) (see Ch. 18, p. 525)
  b. Diagnostic procedures
   (1) Laboratory tests
    (a) In utero—increased alpha-fetoprotein (AFP) or maternal serum alpha-fetoprotein (MS-AFP) in the amniotic fluid may indicate NTD
    (b) Culture and sensitivity—urine and CSF to identify causative organism in complications of meningitis and UTI
   (2) Diagnostic studies
    (a) Ultrasonography—done at 16 to 18 weeks' gestation
    (b) Transillumination of sac—ability to transilluminate indicates meningocele; inability to transilluminate indicates myelomeningocele
    (c) CT scan and MRI—differentiate between various neural tube defects
 6. Therapeutic management
  a. Medications
   (1) Antibiotics used prophylactically or to treat existing infection
   (2) Urinary tract antiseptics: used to prevent UTIs
   (3) Antispasmodics and cholinergic blocking agents: oxybutynin chloride (Ditropan), propantheline bromide (Pro-Banthine) used to control bladder spasms

(4) Alpha-sympathetic agonists (imipramine hydrochloride [Trofranil]—a tricyclic antidepressant, or, pseudoephedrine [Sudafed]): used to enhance urinary sphincter competence

(5) Laxatives: bisacodyl (Dulcolax) and stool softeners, docusate calcium (Surfak), and enemas and fiber supplements: used to achieve degree of bowel continence

b. Treatments

(1) Correction of orthopedic deformities: casting, bracing, traction, surgery, and physical therapy

(2) Use of customized mobility devices

(3) Bladder and bowel: surgery and training programs such as clean intermittent catheterization (CIC)

c. Surgery: defect closure usually done within 24 to 72 hours

7. Nursing management

a. Acute care: presurgical

(1) Nursing diagnoses

(a) Impaired skin integrity, risk for infection related to presence of sac

(b) Risk for injury to the delicate spinal lesion

(c) Impaired physical mobility

(2) Expected outcomes

(a) Sac remains free of trauma and infection

(b) Family verbalizes knowledge about the defect, surgical procedure, and care required

8. Interventions

(a) Assess spinal column for presence of defect

(b) Monitor vital signs and neurologic status every 2 to 4 hours

(c) Protect sac: cleanse sac with the use of sterile technique and sterile saline; cover with sterile gauze moistened with solution as ordered (sterile saline, antibiotic, silver nitrate); handle gently during feedings and diaper changes; position to avoid pressure on the sac; apply protective devices if necessary to avoid stool contamination

⚠ Warning!

Sac rupture increases the risk of CNS infection.

(d) Maintain prone position using diaper rolls or small sandbags

(e) Observe for early signs of infection and increased ICP every 4 hours

(f) Prepare family for surgery and related procedures by the provision of information

9. Acute care: postsurgical
  (1) Nursing diagnoses
    (a) Alteration in urinary elimination: neurologic impairment
    (b) Risk for infection: incision site and UTI
    (c) Body image disturbance
    (d) Altered bowel elimination: constipation
  (2) Expected outcomes
    (a) Surgical wound remains intact and infection-free
    (b) Parents list methods to monitor child for UTI
    (c) Child and family member exhibits proficiency in (self-)catheterization
    (d) Child establishes pattern of bowel evacuation
  (3) Interventions
    (a) Assess vital signs and neurologic status every 2 to 4 hours
    (b) Monitor hydration: input and output, IV fluids as ordered
    (c) Monitor incision site for signs of infection every 4 hours
    (d) Monitor for urinary retention and stress incontinence
    (e) Assess child for signs of a UTI; hematuria
    (f) Perform intermittent catheterization every 3 to 4 hours
    (g) Administer antispasmodics, anticholinergics as ordered
    (h) Assist child to establish regular toileting habits to prevent constipation and impaction
a. Concerns about latex allergy—sneezing, wheezing, or the development of a rash when handling latex products
  (1) Nursing diagnosis: risk for injury
  (2) Expected outcomes:
    (a) Child will not experience adverse effects of latex allergy
    (b) Children with hypersensitivity to latex will be identified

> ⚠ **Warning!**
>
> Children with spina bifida are at high risk for latex allergy because of repeated exposure during surgery and bladder catheterizations.

  (3) Interventions
    (a) Identify latex-sensitive clients through careful assessment
    (b) Place high-risk and hypersensitive individuals in a latex-free environment
    (c) Use latex-free products in the client care setting

10. Evaluation
   a. Questions to ask to the child's family
      (1) Which findings should you report to a physician?
      (2) Which are the problems of care or growth and development that you expect or have encountered?
      (3) Do you see any barriers in your home that may hinder your child's mobility?
      (4) Does your child exhibit signs such as sneezing, rashes, or wheezing when handling latex products (gloves, bandages, catheters)?
   b. Behaviors to observe that indicate effective care
      (1) Child has decreased incontinence
      (2) Child adheres to individualized rehabilitation program
      (3) Child exhibits no signs of infection
   c. Evaluation of expected outcomes
      (1) Presurgical—sac integrity is maintained and sac remains free from infection
      (2) Postsurgical—surgical wound in the process of healing
         (a) Symptoms of increased ICP and hydrocephalus are detected early
         (b) Latex allergy is prevented or identified
      (3) Discharge—family members, child, or both
         (a) Comply with daily care and therapy regimen
         (b) Are receptive to assistance from community agencies as indicated
         (c) Integrate the child's care regimen into the family's routine
         (d) Verbalize normal growth and development behaviors
         (e) Identify rationale, steps to perform, and the schedule for the catheterization program

III. Acquired disorders involving the CNS
A. Meningitis
1. Description—inflammation of meninges from a bacterial or viral infection (aseptic)
2. Most common bacterial causes—*Hemophilus influenzae* (type B), *Streptococcus pneumoniae,* and *Neisseria meningitidis*
3. Etiology and incidence
   a. Peak incidence is between 6 and 12 months of age
   b. 90% of cases occur between 1 month and 5 years of age
4. Pathophysiology
   a. Organisms invade the CNS as a result of trauma or are carried to the CSF from other sites of infection such as the middle ear, nasopharynx, or sinuses
   b. Aseptic meningitis, caused by a virus, is associated with other diseases such as measles, mumps, and herpes

    c. Complications

       (1) Deafness and blindness

       (2) Developmental delays, learning disorders, and attention deficit–hyperactivity disorder

       (3) Weakness and paralysis of facial and other muscles, and seizures

       (4) Cerebral palsy and mental retardation

5. Assessment

    a. Questions to ask

       (1) Have there been recent episodes of a middle ear or sinus infection?

       (2) Has there been any recent exposure to communicable or viral disorders?

    b. Age-specific assessment findings

       (1) Infants and young children

         (a) Fever and chills

         (b) Irritability, shrill cry, and lethargy

         (c) Poor feeding and vomiting

         (d) Seizures

 Warning!

A child with a petechial or pruritic rash needs to be evaluated for meningococcal meningitis.

       (2) Older children

         (a) Irritability, headache, and photophobia

         (b) Fever

         (c) Nuchal rigidity; **Opisthotonos:** a prolonged spasm consisting of extreme hyperextension of the body during which the head and heels are bent backward and the body is bowed forward in infants

         (d) Drowsiness, stupor, and coma

         (e) Seizures

         (f) Positive **Brudzinski's** and **Kernig's** signs

    c. Diagnostic procedures

       (1) Laboratory tests

         (a) Lumbar puncture (LP)—Caution: done only if signs of increased ICP are absent, to prevent herniation of the brain stem

           (i) Bacterial: cloudy CSF; increased WBC—polymorphonuclear leukocytes, increased protein, decreased glucose, increased pressure reading

           (ii) Viral: slight increased WBC and protein; usually normal glucose and clear CSF

         (b) Cultures: CSF, blood, urine, and nasopharynx—identification of causative organism

(c) Serum glucose—drain shortly before the LP to compare it with the glucose level of the CSF

(d) CBC: markedly increased WBC in bacterial; mildly elevated WBC in viral

(2) Diagnostic studies—CT scan identifies abscess, effusion, and hydrocephalus

6. Therapeutic management
   a. Medications
      (1) Antibiotics—to treat causative organism or prevent opportunistic infection
      (2) Anticonvulsants—to prevent seizures (see Table 12-3, p. 342)
      (3) Corticosteroid—dexamethasone (Decadron, Dalalone) to decrease ICP
      (4) Antipyretic—usually acetaminophen (Tylenol) to decrease fever
   b. Treatments
      (1) Correction of fluid deficits
      (2) Electrolyte replacement

7. Nursing management
   a. Nursing diagnoses
      (1) Risk for injury related to seizure activity
      (2) Altered cerebral tissue perfusion
      (3) Hyperthermia related to infection
   b. Expected outcomes
      (1) Child exhibits a neurologic status that returns to baseline parameters for age
      (2) Child will remain free of injury secondary to cerebral edema and shock
      (3) Child's body temperature returns to baseline for age
   c. Interventions
      (1) Assess neurologic status: LOC, pupillary response, vital signs, for infants the head circumference every 2 to 4 hours; measure input and output every 8 hours
      (2) Monitor for seizure activity with implementation of seizure precautions (see Box 12-4, p. 362)
      (3) Isolate child to protect others from infection
      (4) Administer antibiotics and steroids promptly; administer antipyretic for a temperature above 102° F as ordered
      (5) Provide comfort measures: a quiet, calm environment, minimal handling, dim lighting, and restricted visitation
      (6) Provide tepid sponge baths, hypothermia blanket, or cool environmental temperature for fever
      (7) Restrict fluid intake by mouth for the first 48 hours to decrease ICP, if applicable
      (8) Maintain IV therapy as ordered
      (9) Provide frequent rest periods

(10) Elevate head of bed to 30 degrees; prevent neck flexion or head-neck out of alignment, which may hinder CSF drainage with resultant increased ICP

(11) Encourage fluid intake by mouth as condition permits

8. Evaluation

9. Questions to ask family

(1) Which precautions will you take to prevent recurrence of infection?

(2) Which findings should you report to your physician?

a. Evaluation of expected outcomes

(1) Parent administers antibiotic correctly

(2) Disease process is resolved without long-term complications

(3) Family maintains follow-up visits to physician or clinic

(4) Child demonstrates appropriate growth and developmental milestones for age

B. Head trauma

1. Description—An open or closed injury to the cranium and its contents; the types are concussions, contusions, skull fractures, cerebral edema, and vascular damage

2. Etiology and incidence

a. Injury frequently is due to mechanical force

b. Falls are the leading cause of head injury in toddlers, preschoolers, and school-aged children

c. Child abuse is the cause of severe head injury in children under 1 year of age

d. Adolescents most often receive head injuries in motor vehicle accidents

e. Infants and toddlers are particularly vulnerable to head trauma because of proportionately large head size

f. The injury may be classified as localized or generalized

3. Pathophysiology

a. Injury depends on force of impact

b. Specific types of head injuries

(1) Concussion—a temporary and reversible neuronal dysfunction characterized by post-traumatic amnesia

(2) Contusion and laceration—involve superficial tears and bruising of cerebral tissue, especially in occipital, temporal, and frontal lobes

(3) Fractures—linear, depressed, compound, basilar, and diastatic types

c. Complications

(1) **Epidural hemorrhage**—arterial bleeding with findings evident within 24 to 48 hours

(2) **Subdural hemorrhage**—venous bleeding; common in infancy from falls or violent shaking; findings may not be evident for weeks or months

Box 12-3
Clinical Manifestations of Acute Head Injury

Minor Injury

May or may not lose consciousness
Transient period of confusion
Somnolence
Listlessness
Irritability
Pallor
Vomiting (one or more episodes)

Signs of Progression

Altered mental status (e.g., difficulty rousing child)
Mounting agitation
Development of focal lateral neurologic signs
Marked changes in vital signs

Severe Injury

Signs of increased ICP
  Increased head size (infant)
  Bulging fontanel (infant)
Retinal hemorrhage
Extraocular palsies (especially cranial nerve VI)
Hemiparesis
Quadriplegia
Elevated temperature (sometimes)
Unsteady gait (older child)
Papilledema (older child)

Associated Signs

Skin injury (to area of head sustaining injury)
Other injuries (e.g., to extremities)

From Wong DL, et al: *Whaley and Wong's nursing care of infants and children*, ed 6, St Louis, 1999, Mosby.

        (3) Cerebral edema
        (4) Postconcussion syndrome—symptoms vary with age and are mainly behavioral changes and seizures
    4. Assessment
        a. Initial questions to ask
            (1) What was the sequence of events for the trauma?
            (2) Did the child lose consciousness? Loss of consciousness suggests a risk for arterial bleeding.
            (3) How did the child respond?
            (4) Is there a history of a previous head injury?
        b. Assessment findings depend on severity (Box 12-3)

c. Diagnostic procedures (see Table 12-2, p. 338)
   (1) Electroencephalogram (EEG)—reveals seizure activity secondary to trauma
   (2) Opthalmoscopic examination—detects retinal hemorrhage

 Warning!

Children with retinal hemorrhage and subdural hematoma require further evaluation for child abuse, particularly in infants for "shaken baby syndrome."

5. Therapeutic management
   a. Medications (see Table 12-3, p. 342, for osmotic diuretics and antiepileptics)
      (1) Sedatives: chloral hydrate (Aquachloral) to manage restlessness
      (2) Analgesics: acetaminophen (Tylenol) for headache
6. Treatments
   a. Oxygen therapy
   b. Surgery—in the event of hemorrhage or skull fracture
7. Nursing management
   a. Nursing diagnosis: altered tissue perfusion or impaired gas exchange related to inadequate respiratory effort
   b. Expected outcomes
      (1) Maintain adequate perfusion and gas exchange
      (2) Minimize cerebral oxygen requirements
   c. Interventions
      (1) Assess neurologic status every 1 to 2 hours: LOC using the Glasgow Coma Scale (see Figure 12-1, p. 335)
      (2) Monitor the vital signs hourly; check neurovascular status, and central venous pressure, if applicable
      (3) Assess for abnormal posturing and unusual behaviors
      (4) Monitor for signs of increased ICP
      (5) Monitor oxygen and carbon dioxide levels by way of arterial blood gases or pulse oximetry for oxygen saturation
      (6) Maintain IV fluids, and monitor input and output as ordered
      (7) Maintain child on bed rest, with head of bed elevated to 30 degrees; if an infant, place in an infant or a car seat that is secured firmly
      (8) Administer sedatives or osmotic diuretics as ordered
   d. Nursing diagnosis: pain related to head injury
   e. Expected outcome: promote comfort and relieve anxiety
   f. Interventions
      (1) Assess pain level using appropriate pain rating scale for age
      (2) Administer analgesics and sedatives as ordered
      (3) Decrease environmental stimuli

8. Evaluation
   a. Questions to ask the child's family
      (1) What are your concerns about long-term care?
      (2) What has the physician discussed about rehabilitation?
   b. Behaviors to observe
      (1) Parents appropriately monitor and support the child during the acute phase
      (2) Family members ask questions about condition, treatment, outcome, and home care
   c. Evaluation of expected outcomes
      (1) Maintenance of respiratory function with an improved neurologic status attained
      (2) Family members verbalize specific plans for rehabilitation or have contact with a support group for persons with head injury

IV. Seizure disorders

A. Description—seizures are sudden, transient alterations in brain function resulting from excessive levels of electrical activity in the brain; may also be a symptom of other pathologic conditions, without cause identification. Epilepsy is a chronic seizure disorder produced by excessive neuronal discharges

B. Classified as either partial or generalized, depending on the area of brain involvement (Table 12-4, p. 358)

C. Etiology and incidence
   1. Most seizures are idiopathic in origin
   2. Seizures can be congenital or acquired from brain injury before or after birth
   3. High incidence occurs in the first two years of life

D. Pathophysiology
   1. Seizure activity caused by a group of hyperexcitable cells that produce spontaneous discharge
   2. Physiologic stimuli such as an abnormal glucose level or electrolyte imbalance play a contributing role

E. Assessment
   1. Questions to ask
      a. Have any unusual behaviors been noted: irritability, poor feeding, tugging at ear, or inattention to events or activities? How long ago? Is there a pattern of occurrence?
      b. Is there a family history of seizure activity?
      c. Does the child experience an **aura** before any seizure activity?
   2. Assessment findings (see Table 12-4, p. 358)
      a. Ictal: sudden acute onset such as a convulsion
      b. Postictal: drowsiness, confusion, aphasia, sensory and motor impairment

TABLE 12-4 Comparison of Simple Partial, Complex Partial, and Absence Seizures

Clinical Manifestations	Simple Partial	Complex Partial	Absence
Age of onset	Any age	Uncommon before age 3 yrs	Uncommon before age 3 yrs
Frequency (per day)	Variable	Rarely over 1-2 times	Multiple
Duration	Usually less than 30 sec	Usually >60 sec, rarely <10 sec	Usually <15 sec, rarely >30 sec
Aura	May be sole manifestation of seizure	Frequently	Never
Impaired consciousness	Never	Always	Always, brief loss of consciousness
Automatisms	No	Frequently	Frequently
Clonic movements	Frequently	Occasionally	Occasionally
Postictal impairment	Rare	Frequently	Never
Mental disorientation	Rare	Common	Unusual

From Wong DL, et al: *Whaley and Wong's nursing care of infants and children,* ed 6, St. Louis, 1999, Mosby.

c. Status epilepticus: child does not regain consciousness between tonic-clonic seizures; potential for these complications:
 (1) Acid-base imbalances: severe metabolic and respiratory acidosis
 (2) Respiratory depression and tissue hypoxia
 (3) Hypotension
3. Diagnostic procedures
 a. Laboratory tests
 (1) Lumbar puncture (LP)—CSF abnormality caused by trauma or infection. Note that LP is not performed if increased ICP is suspected—a sudden decrease in pressure of CSF may result in herniation of the brain through the foramen magnum at the base of the skull.
 (2) CBC—increased WBC if infection is present
 (3) Lead level—reveals increased levels, which may be the cause of the seizures
 (4) Urine—reveals the cocaine metabolite benzoylecgonine
 b. Diagnostic studies
 (1) EEG—detects abnormal electrical activity and patterns specific to the seizure type
 (2) CT scan—may reveal brain tumors, trauma, or infection as the cause of the seizure

F. Therapeutic management
1. Medications: antiepileptics
 a. Raise seizure threshold
 b. During active seizures, lorazepam (Ativan) or diazepam (Valium) are given; for maintenance therapy, phenytoin (Dilantin) or phenobarbital are commonly given by mouth (see Table 12-3, p. 342)
2. Treatments
 a. Surgery—removal of hematoma or tumor if known to cause seizures; removal of the eliptogenic area for repetitive, incapacitating seizure activity
 b. Follow-up serum drug levels—done particularly for evaluation of therapeutic levels of antiepileptics every month or as directed
 c. Vagal nerve stimulation—for children over 12 years of age who have partial seizures and are not able to achieve effective drug therapy control

G. Nursing management
1. Nursing diagnoses
 a. Risk for injury related to seizure activity
 b. Risk for aspiration related to altered LOC
2. Expected outcomes
 a. Child has a reduced risk for injury
 b. Child maintains respiratory function

3. Interventions
   a. Assess frequency, duration, and type of seizure activity

 Warning!

Status epilepticus is an emergency situation that requires immediate interventions to prevent brain injury or death.

   b. Observe for these items:
     (1) Change in LOC
     (2) Activity preceding seizure
     (3) Presence of aura
     (4) Pupillary reaction postseizure
     (5) Incontinence of bowel, bladder, or both during or after seizure activity
     (6) LOC before and after a seizure
   c. Assess respiratory effort, RR, signs of respiratory distress, and skin color
   d. Place child in side-lying position in bed. Make sure the bed is in a low position, the side rails are up and padded, and all sharp and small objects have been removed from reach.
   e. If not in bed during a seizure, assist to the floor and remove harmful objects

 Warning!

Do not attempt to place objects such as an airway into the mouth or to restrain the client during seizure activity. Loosen clothing and protect the client from injury.

   f. Stay with client
   g. Administer antiepileptics as ordered
H. Evaluation
  1. Questions to ask
   a. What are your concerns about long-term care?
   b. What are your questions about the medication schedule, effects, or follow-up with the physician?
  2. Behaviors to observe
   a. Keeps scheduled appointments with physician or at clinic
   b. Statements about the description of seizure and behaviors afterward
   c. Reports signs of medication side effects
  3. Evaluation of expected outcomes
   a. Injury is prevented
   b. Respiratory function is maintained
   c. Family states correct information about the disorder, treatments, and medication regimen
   d. Therapeutic serum levels of the antiepileptic is maintained

V. Home care: family education topics and referrals
A. Hydrocephalus
1. Shunt maintenance: signs of shunt malfunction, infection, increased ICP, and when to notify physician or take the child to the emergency room; importance of follow-up visits to physician; need for shunt modification as child grows
2. Incision site: signs of local inflammation, irritation, or pressure
3. Medications: administration of seizure medications as ordered
4. Activity: avoid participation in contact sports
5. Referrals: National Hydrocephalus Foundation, childhood development programs

B. Spina bifida
1. Elimination: bladder and bowel training including clean intermittent catheterization technique; signs of UTI
2. Skin care: positioning and range-of-motion exercises
3. Mobility: use assisted living devices; lower extremity flexibility: muscle stretching, positioning to provide hip support, and range-of-motion exercises
4. Growth and development: inform parents that overprotective behavior may hinder milestone attainment
5. Safety: importance of having latex-sensitive child wear medical-alert identification
6. Referrals: Spina Bifida Association, occupational and physical therapy

C. Meningitis
1. Disease process: pathology, need for follow-up
2. Medications: administration of antibiotics: explain dosages, times, and side effects
3. Activity: need for adequate rest periods, rationale for isolation to prevent spread of disease, suggest age-appropriate activities to promote stimulation and continued development

D. Head trauma

> ⚠ **Warning!**
>
> If child is to be managed at home, parents must be instructed to check the child every 1 hour for changes in level of responsiveness; if asleep, child needs to be awakened for the assessments.

1. Observations: Instruct parents when to seek further medical attention (see Seizure Disorder below)
2. Medications: avoid the use of sedatives or analgesics
3. Referrals: National Head Injury Foundation, Brain Injury Association, and home health and social services with specialization in rehabilitation and long-term care

E. Seizure disorder
1. Safety: teach seizure precautions (Box 12-4, p. 262)
2. Medication: medication schedule, side effects, importance of compliance with maintaining therapeutic serum levels for

Box 12-4
Seizure Precautions

The extent of precautions depends on the type, severity, and frequency of the seizures. Precautions may include:
  Side rails raised when child is sleeping or resting
  Side rails and other hard objects padded
  Waterproof mattress or pad on bed or crib
Appropriate precautions during potentially hazardous activities:
  Swimming with a companion
  Use of protective helmet and padding during bicycle riding, skateboarding, and
    inline skating
  Supervision during use of hazardous machinery or equipment (older children)
Have the child carry or wear medical identification.
Alert other caregivers to the need for any special precautions.

From Wong DL, Hockenberry-Eaton M, Wilson D: *Whaley and Wong's nursing care of infants and children,* ed 6, St. Louis, 1999, Mosby.

antiepileptics; importance of dental care during phenytoin (Dilantin) therapy, vitamin D and folic acid during phenobarbital and phenytoin (Dilantin) therapy

3. Follow-up: laboratory testing for therapeutic serum drug levels
4. Referrals: Epilepsy Foundation of America

WEB Resources

www.efa.org
  Epilepsy Foundation of America. This website includes the mission statement of the Epilepsy Foundation, its history, local affiliates, and event calendar. It provides information for families about programs, services, and research. Site features a Kid's Club. Educational topics include first aid for seizures, tips for safe living, seizure medications, and surgery.

www.cdc.gov/ncip/duip
  Division of Unintentional Injury of the National Centers for Injury Prevention and Control. Informational site for injury-related topics: motor vehicle accidents and head injury. Includes recommendations for prevention, use of a bike helmet, injury statistics, and references.

REVIEW QUESTIONS

1. An infant is scheduled for surgery to repair myelomeningocele. Preoperatively, which of these nursing diagnoses should receive priority in the infant's care?
    1. Altered family processes
    2. Risk for infection
    3. Knowledge deficit
    4. Altered growth and development

2. A child exhibits seizure activity. Which of these actions should the nurse take?
    1. Attempt to restrain the child with pillows around the arms
    2. Insert a padded tongue blade into the mouth between seizures
    3. Use pillows to prevent the child from hitting hard or sharp objects
    4. Suction the mouth with intermittent suction as needed to maintain the airway

3. An infant's diagnosis is myelomeningocele. To protect the sac from infection, which of these actions is appropriate?
    1. Change diapers as soon as they are soiled
    2. Apply sterile, dry dressings to sac
    3. Elevate the head of the crib to a high Fowler's position
    4. Place the infant in a supine position at all times

4. Immediately after the insertion of a ventriculoperitoneal (V-P) shunt, the nurse should expect to position the infant in which manner?
    1. On the operative side, with the head of crib elevated
    2. On the nonoperative side, with the crib flat
    3. Supine, with the head of the crib elevated
    4. Supine, with the crib flat

5. A child diagnosed with meningitis is restless and irritable when first hospitalized. To promote the child's comfort, which of these actions should the nurse take?
    1. Encourage the parent to stay with the child only at night
    2. Keep environmental noise to a minimum
    3. Tell the parents that the child will be in a supine position for the next 12 hours
    4. Postpone all scheduled testing until further notice

6. A child is admitted to the pediatric unit for seizure activity. The physician orders phenobarbital (Luminal). The nurse provided the parents with instructions about correct administration of this medication. The nurse would evaluate the teaching as effective when the parents identify the need to have which of these actions?
1. Skip a dose if the child vomits
2. Discontinue the medication when seizure activity stops
3. Double the next dose if the child misses a dose
4. Notify the physician if severe headaches or skin rashes occur

7. Before discharge, the parents have been given instructions about the signs of a blocked shunt in an infant. Which of these statements by the parents indicates a correct understanding of home care parameters?
1. "We will notify the physician if we observe irritability and a bulging soft spot."
2. "We will notify the physician if the baby's temperature is 99 degrees."
3. "Urine retention and cool skin are signs of a blocked shunt."
4. "Vomiting and diarrhea are signs of a blocked shunt."

8. An infant is diagnosed with pneumococcal meningitis. The parents question the mode of transmission for this infectious agent. The nurse reviews the child's history. Which of these causes should be considered?
1. Chicken pox
2. Middle ear infection
3. Lyme disease
4. Urinary tract infection (UTI)

9. During an infant's postoperative assessment after the surgical correction of a myelomeningocele, the nurse observes a bulging anterior fontanel and measurements were recorded of an increased head size. Based on these findings the nurse knows the infant is at imminent risk for the development of which condition?
1. Encephalitis
2. Hydrocephalus
3. Meningitis
4. Fluid overload

10. With the consideration of the client's diagnosis of myelomeningocele, an infant is most likely to have which of these findings?
1. Dyspnea and cardiac abnormalities
2. Fecal continence and microcephalus
3. Genitourinary and orthopedic abnormalities
4. Meningeal sac everted and located in the thoracic region

ANSWERS, RATIONALES, AND TEST-TAKING TIPS

Rationale	Test-Taking Tips

1. Correct answer: 2

Many myelomeningocele sacs are at risk for rupture during delivery or transport. Any opening increases the risk for infection. Although it is important for parents to understand the nature of a spinal defect and its impact on the child's growth, development, and family life, the immediate preoperative priority is the prevention of infection.

The use of Maslow's hierarchy of needs can be applied here—the physiologic needs are the first priority before the psychosocial needs. Option 2 is a physiologic need, whereas option 4 is both physical and psychological. Option 2 is the best answer in this given situation. A clue in the stem is the timeframe of "preoperatively." Note that all of the options are correct answers. Put in an order of priority, the sequence would be option 2, 3, 4, and then 1.

2. Correct answer: 3

The child, as with any client during seizure activity, must be protected from injury. The convulsing client should not be moved or restrained during a seizure. Force should not be exerted in an attempt to place solid objects between the teeth or to suction for airway maintenance during or immediately after a seizure. These actions may stimulate another seizure.

Avoid misreading the options. Note that the options have two parts so you may have placed more emphasis on the second part than on the first part. If you did, you probably missed selection of the correct answer. Another approach is to simply look at the verbs in a group: restrain, insert, prevent, and suction. It is obvious that the action is prevention. Associate that seizures need safety as a priority to minimize or avoid injury to the client.

3. Correct answer: 1

The myelomeningocele sac must remain free of urine or stool contamination. Therefore, frequent diaper changes are essential. Dressings applied to the sac are to be moistened, usually with sterile normal saline, to prevent drying of the sac. Ideally, the infant in a

Look for clues in the options. Eliminate option 2, which has the word "dry," making it incorrect. Eliminate option 3, which has "high Fowler's" for crib position. Use common sense—if this elevation were done the infant would slide down to the flat part of the crib. Eliminate option 4, because it has

Rationale	Test-Taking Tips

prone or partially prone-to-side-lying position is placed in a low Trendelenburg position to reduce spinal fluid pressure in the sac. The hips are flexed to avoid pressure on the defect. Range of motion exercises may need to be done to prevent hip flexion contractures.

the absolute "at all times," which means no other position can be used.

4. Correct answer: 2

After this type of surgery, the infant is positioned on the nonoperative side to prevent pressure on the shunt valve and the pressure areas of the operative site. The crib is kept flat to prevent complications from a rapid reduction of intracranial fluid. Placed on the operative side, there is risk of increased pressure on the shunt valve. An elevated head of the bed can cause a rapid decrease in ICP. The items in options 3 and 4 are incorrect answers.

Remember the basic principles of postoperative care for clients with cranial and eye surgery. Position the client on the nonoperative side for the prevention of increased pressure in the surgical area. The timeframe is also important to note: immediate postprocedure care.

5. Correct answer: 2

The room should be kept as quiet as possible and the environmental stimuli kept to a minimum. Most children are sensitive to noise, bright lights, and other environmental stimuli such as odors. The parents should be encouraged to stay with the child as much as possible and not just at night. The parents should be involved in the child's care as much as possible to decrease separation anxiety. Usually the child

Eliminate options 1 and 4 with the use of common sense—test postponement is usually an incorrect action, as is just having the parents stay at night. Option 3 is incorrect—the child will not be able to assume a comfortable supine position, and special positioning for 12 hours has nothing to do with this type of problem.

assumes a side-lying position because of nuchal rigidity and the tendency to hyperextend the neck with an opisthotic position. Acute meningitis is a medical emergency and tests should not be postponed. Early recognition of the causative organisms through testing is essential. Expedient therapy with medication prevents death and disability.

6. Correct answer: 4

Parents need to know the adverse reactions to the seizure medication phenobarbital (Luminal). Severe headache and skin rash are side effects that need to be reported. The other options reflect a need for more education. The family should be taught the need to continue the medication regularly without interruption, not to double the dose if one is missed, and to notify the health professional when the child has an illness such as vomiting.

If you have no idea of the correct answer, cluster the options under the theme of inappropriate medication guidelines. Key words about the medication dose in options 1, 2, and 3 are: "skip," "discontinue," and "double."

7. Correct answer: 1

Parents need to recognize signs that indicate shunt malfunction. These include irritability and a bulging anterior fontanel, both of which are signs of increased ICP. A temperature of 99° F is not significant to warrant notification of the physician. A temperature of 102° F or higher, especially in children, requires physician notification. The grouped findings in options 3 and 4 are not specific to a blocked shunt. However,

Associate "blocked shunt" with the result of increased pressure. Select option 1, which has the key terms "irritability" and "bulging soft spot." Did you read option 1, select it then go on to the next question? You were lucky in this case. Avoid missing questions from this type of poor reading pattern. When you are tempted to skip reading some options, immediately force yourself to go option 4 to read the options in the reverse order: options 4, 3, 2, and 1. This simple action will keep

Rationale	Test-Taking Tips

vomiting and especially projectile vomiting would indicate increased ICP and should be reported.

your mind more alert and allow you to select the best answer.

8. Correct answer: 2

Meningitis and other intracranial complications can be extensions of an infection from the middle ear or mastoid. Middle ear infections are frequently bacterial infections. Varicella virus causes chicken pox. Lyme disease is caused by a spirochete, which enters the skin through a tick bite. *Escheria coli* and other gram-negative organisms common to the anal, perineal and perianal regions cause most UTIs.

If you have no idea of the correct option, try the common sense approach by using anatomic locations. Select the given area that is closest to the brain—option 2, the middle ear.

9. Correct answer: 2

The anomaly most frequently associated with myelomeningocele is hydrocephalus. A bulging fontanel and increased head size are consistent with increased ICP caused by blockage of CSF. In options 1, 3, and 4, the findings are not consistent with post-op complications after the correction of a myelomeningocele. Bacterial meningitis is a complication of otitis media.

Note that options 1 and 3 contain the suffix "itis," suggesting inflammation; this is not a typically a postoperative problem. Select option 2 rather than option 4, because fluid overload is more often indicated by abnormal pulmonary or cardiac findings.

10. Correct answer: 3

Myelomeningocele, a neural tube defect (NTD), is one of the most common causes of a neurogenic bladder. Orthopedic anomalies of the hip, knee, and

Note that if option 2 was read quickly, you may have misread "continence" as "incontinence" and selected it even though microcephalus is not found with this condition.

foot are possible depending on
the location of the spinal
lesion. The findings in option 1
are not consistent with an
NTD. Fecal incontinence, not
fecal incontinence, and
hydrocephalus are most often
evident in clients with
myelomeningocele. The largest
number of these defects are
located in the lumbar or
lumbosacral region.

13

Nursing Care of Children with Cardiovascular Disorders

FAST FACTS

1. Clinical consequences of congenital defects include congestive heart failure (CHF) and hypoxemia.
2. Early signs of CHF are tachycardia, tachypnea, fatigue, a change in play behavior, irritability, sudden weight gain, respiratory distress, and sweating of the scalp in infants during feedings.
3. Before administering digoxin, assess the apical pulse rate for a full minute. Hold the medication and notify the physician when the pulse rate is below the normal range for age: 90 to 110 beats per minute for an infant, and 70 to 85 beats per minute for older children.
4. The therapeutic serum level for digoxin is 0.8 to 2.0 µg/L.
5. Hypokalemia increases the risk of digoxin toxicity.
6. First signs of digoxin toxicity in older children are bradycardia and upset stomach; in young children it is tachycardia; and in infants it is poor feeding. Other signs of digoxin toxicity are anorexia, nausea, vomiting, diarrhea, ECG changes of extra beats, and heart block.
7. Selection of the correct size of blood pressure cuff is essential. The cuff width should cover about two thirds of the upper arm.

CONTENT REVIEW

I. Cardiovascular (CV) system overview

A. **General concepts**
1. The heart lies in the thoracic cavity; in infants and children the heart lies more horizontally in the chest
2. The apex of the heart extends into the fourth left intercostal space (ICS) until 7 years of age
3. Fetal oxygenation of blood occurs in the placenta

B. **Review of heart structure and function**
1. Structure
   a. **Pericardium**—tough, double-walled sac that protects the heart
   b. Three layers of heart wall
      (1) **Epicardium**—thin outermost layer covering the surface of the heart
      (2) **Myocardium**—middle layer of heart wall responsible for the pumping action of the ventricles; consists of striated muscle fibers
      (3) **Endocardium**—innermost layer; lines the inner chambers of the heart and covers the heart valves
   c. Four chambers
      (1) Right and left atria—act as reservoirs for blood returning from the veins
      (2) Right and left ventricles—pump blood to the lungs (right) and throughout the body (left)
   d. Left and right sides of the heart are divided by the cardiac septum
      (1) The left heart consists of the left atrium, mitral valve, left ventricle, and aorta
      (2) The right heart consists of the right atrium, tricuspid valve, right ventricle, and pulmonary artery
   e. Two sets of valves
      (1) Atrioventricular—tricuspid and mitral
      (2) Semilunar—pulmonic and aortic
   f. Pressure differences between the right and left sides of the heart regulate blood flow through the heart and into the systemic circulation. If there are defects in this system, the blood flows from an area of great pressure to an area of least pressure.
   g. Great vessels: arteries and veins located in a cluster at the base of the heart
      (1) The aorta carries oxygenated blood out from the left ventricle to the body
      (2) The superior and inferior vena cavae carry unoxygenated blood from the upper and lower body, respectively, to the right atrium
      (3) The pulmonary artery leaves the right ventricle, branches, and carries unoxygenated blood to pulmonary vasculature in the lungs

(4) The pulmonary vein returns oxygenated blood from the pulmonary vasculature to the left atrium

2. Function and fetal development
   a. The primary purposes of the CV system are to pump oxygen and nutrients throughout the body and to remove the end-products of metabolism
   b. The heart develops between 4 and 8 weeks' gestation
   c. Fetal vascular resistance is high
   d. Fetal structures provide for a pattern of intrauterine circulation
      (1) Foramen ovale—pumps blood from the right to the left atrium
      (2) Ductus arteriosus—shunts blood from the pulmonary artery to the descending aorta
      (3) Ductus venosus—shunts most of the blood supply around the fetal liver
   e. Circulatory changes that result in postnatal circulation (Figure 13-1, p. 374)
      (1) Dilation of the pulmonary vessels and decreased pulmonary vascular resistance occur as the lungs expand at birth
      (2) An increase in systemic vascular resistance occurs, causing an increased pressure in the left side of the heart when the umbilical cord is clamped
      (3) Closure of the foramen ovale usually occurs shortly after birth
      (4) Closure of the ductus arteriosus usually occurs by the fourth day of life

3. Basic concepts of cardiac physiology
   a. To provide effective oxygen transport to the tissues of the body, the heart must maintain adequate cardiac output (CO) pumped per unit of time:
      Cardiac Output equals Stroke Volume times Heart Rate
   b. Stroke volume is the amount of blood ejected by the heart during any one contraction; it is influenced by
      (1) **Preload**—the volume or fiber length of the ventricles at rest before contraction
      (2) **Afterload**—resistance the ventricles encounter during contraction
      (3) **Contractility**—ability of the heart muscle to act as an efficient pump through myocardial fiber shortening

II. Assessment
A. Health history
1. Questions to ask parents
   (1) Does the infant tire easily during feeding or play?
   (2) Does the child perspire during activity or for no reason?
   (3) Does the child have frequent infections?
   (4) Does the child nap longer than expected?
   (5) Does the child squat rather than sit when at play?
   (6) Does the child turn blue during crying episodes?

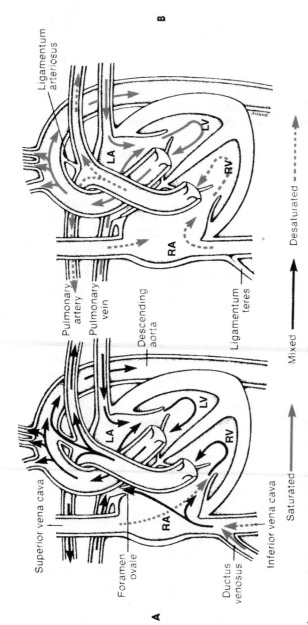

Figure 13-1 Changes at birth. **A,** Prenatal circulation. **B,** Postnatal circulation. RA, right atrium; LA, left atrium; RV, right ventricle; LV, left ventricle. Although four pulmonary veins enter the LA, for simplicity, this diagram shows only two. (From Wong DL, et al: *Whaley and Wong's nursing care of infants and children,* ed 6, St. Louis, 1999, Mosby.)

         (7) Does the child experience leg pains while running?

         (8) Is the child's weight gain as expected?

  2. Present problem(s)

    a. Fatigue, leg pain, or cramps

    b. Frequent respiratory infections

  3. History

    a. Congenital cardiac defect

    b. Cardiac surgery or evaluation

    c. Rheumatic fever

    d. Mother's health during pregnancy: rubella or other infections in the first trimester; drug or alcohol use

    e. Apgar score, gestational age, and complications at birth

    f. Down syndrome

  4. Family history

    a. Heart disease or hypertension

    b. Hyperlipidemia

    c. Congenital heart defects

B. Physical examination

  1. Sequence

    a. Observation of the child's general appearance

      (1) Positioning

      (2) RR and respiratory effort

      (3) Nail configuration for clubbing; skin and nail color

    b. Inspection of the anterior chest precordium

      (1) Note obvious bulging, especially on the left side, which could indicate cardiac enlargement; assess for symmetry of both sides of the rib cage

      (2) Apical impulse or point of maximum intensity may normally be seen in thin children at the fourth intercostal space (ICS), left midclavicular line (MCL)

    c. Palpation of the precordium

      (1) The apical impulse is normally felt in the lateral position at the left MCL and the fourth ICS in children under 7 years of age, and at the left MCL and the fifth ICS in children over 7 years of age

      (2) Thrills are produced by blood flowing through a narrowed or an abnormal opening (as with septal defects)

    d. Palpation of the nail bed base until blanching and check for capillary refill time, which is normally 1 to 3 seconds

    e. Auscultation of the following sites for rate, rhythm, pitch, location, and intensity of S_1 and S_2 heart sounds in this sequence

      (1) Aortic area—the second right ICS near the sternum; S_2 is louder than S_1

      (2) Pulmonic area—the second left ICS near the sternum

      (3) Erb's point—the second and third left ICS near the sternum

      (4) Tricuspid area—the fifth right and the left ICS close to the sternum; S_1 is louder than the preceding S_2

(5) Mitral or apical area—will be located at the fourth ICS until 7 years of age, and the fifth ICS after age 7 years; S_1 is the loudest

   f. Auscultation of murmurs, pericardial rubs, extra heart sounds—S_3, which may be normal in children, and S4

2. Pediatric considerations

   a. A venous hum heard at the medial end of the clavicle and the interior border of the sternocleidomastoid muscle usually is insignificant

   b. Rheumatic fever accounts for most of the acquired murmurs in childhood

   c. Sinus dysrhythmias in which the HR increases with inspiration and decreases with expiration are considered normal in children

   d. Priority findings during the examination of a child with known heart disease are:

     (1) Weight gain—to include over which period of time

     (2) Edema—periorbital, peripheral

     (3) Respiratory status—tachypnea

     (4) Cyanosis—central, peripheral

     (5) Enlarged or distended neck veins in older children

     (6) Clubbing of fingers and toes

     (7) Murmurs, bruits, and thrills

     (8) Developmental delays

   e. Selection of the correct size of blood pressure cuff is essential: the cuff width should cover about two thirds of the upper arm

C. Diagnostic and laboratory tests

1. Cardiac catheterization—reveals abnormal communication between the heart chambers, as well as pressure differences and abnormal blood gas sampling in the chambers; helps in the location of a septal defect

2. Electrocardiography (ECG)—reveals atrial and ventricular hypertrophy, as well as dysrhythmias

3. Echocardiography—reveals any changes in valve function, great vessel location, and size and any presence of shunting within the heart

4. CBC

   a. Increased hematocrit and hemoglobin called *polycythemia,* and RBCs possibly from chronic hypoxia

   b. Decreased platelets or thrombocytopenia

5. Arterial blood gas levels—aid in evaluating acid-base balance, oxygen saturation, oxygen level, and carbon dioxide level

6. Prothrombin time (PT), activated partial thromboplastin time (aPTT)—indicates altered clotting mechanism if increased

D. Medications: priority drug classifications (Table 13-1)

TABLE 13-1 Commonly Used Cardiovascular Medications for Children

Medication and Indications	Route and Dosage	Side Effects	Nursing Implications
Cardiac glycoside, antidysrhythmic Digoxin (Lanoxin) CHF Atrial fibrillation	Oral digitizing dose: Infant, 30 μg/kg Age <2 yr, 40-50 μg/kg Age >2 yr, 30 μg/kg Maintenance dose (in 2 divided doses): Infant, 8-10 μg/kg Age <2 yr, 10-12 μg/kg Age >2 yrs, 8-10 μg/kg	CNS: fatigue, weakness, headache CV: tachycardia, bradycardia, dysrhythmias GI: anorexia, nausea, vomiting Sensory: blurred vision, halos	Monitor vital signs, ECG Assess serum glycoside level (0.8-2.0 μg /L) Monitor serum potassium level if also on diuretic Assess hepatic and renal function Administer medications same time daily Take apical pulse for 1 full minute before giving dose Withhold dose if pulse is below or above parameters for age group Monitor for signs of digoxin toxicity: in young children, tachycardia; in older children, bradycardia, upset stomach, vomiting, in infants poor feeding *Parent teaching:* Take pulse for 1 full min and record before giving medication; hold if HR <110/min or >140/min, unless other parameters have been set by physician Correct measurement and dose administration Keep medicine container in locked cabinet Know signs of CHF

Continued

TABLE 13-1 Commonly Used Cardiovascular Medications for Children—cont'd

Medication and Indications	Route and Dosage	Side Effects	Nursing Implications
Antihypertensive, B-adrenergic blocker			
Propranolol (Inderal) Hypertension Supraventricular dysrhythmias	Oral: 0.5-1 mg/kg/day in 2 doses; increase as necessary to 1-5 mg/kg/day in 2-4 doses	CNS: insomnia, dizziness, memory changes CV: bradycardia, hypotension GI: nausea, vomiting, diarrhea Respiratory: bronchospasm Skin: rash, alopecia	Take apical and radial pulses before administering; notify physician of sustained HR changes Monitor central venous pressure, ECG, and BP during IV infusion Weigh child daily and notify physician if increased Administer before meals or 2 hr after meals to increase absorption *Parent teaching:* Teach how to take pulse before administration and to administer with meals
Antihypertensive: ACE inhibitor			
Captopril (Capoten) Hypertension Heart failure	Oral: 300 µg/kg titrated initial dose; increase by 300 µg/kg in 8- to 24-hr intervals as needed (children on diuretics or with renal dysfunction should initially receive 150 µg /kg titrated initial dose)	CNS: dizziness, headache CV: hypotension, tachycardia, chest pain, palpitations GI: nausea, vomiting, constipation Genitourinary: proteinuria, renal dysfunction Skin: rash, urticaria Hematologic: neutropenia, agranulocytosis	Assess baseline vital signs Take BP before administration Administer 1 hr before meals Take daily weight, monitor input and output Monitor urine for protein Monitor serum potassium levels *Parent teaching:* Report weight gain of >2 lb/wk and edema, especially periorbital Avoid rapid position changes Administer medication 1 hr before meals Report any sign of infection

Diuretic, loop

Furosemide (Lasix)
 	
Severe CHF
 	
Chlorothiazide (Diuril)
 	
CHF
Hypertension
	Oral:
	2 mg/Kg as single dose, may increase by 1-2 mg/kg at 6-8 her; 1-2 mg/kg initially (up to 5-6 mg/kg per day)
		CNS: headache, dizziness, weakness
		CV: orthostatic hypotension, weak pulse
		GI: nausea, vomiting, anorexia, dry mouth
		Metabolic: hypokalemia, acid-base imbalance
		Hematology: thrombocytopenia
		Skin: photosensitivity, rash
			Assess baseline vital signs, especially BP, lying and standing
			Monitor serum electrolytes, blood glucose, uric acid
			Assess hydration status, daily weights
			Monitor for signs of hypokalemia (confusion, weakness, muscle cramps, anorexia)
			Parent teaching:
			Administer early in day to prevent nocturia
			Administer same time daily
			Encourage potassium-rich foods
			Report weight changes to physician:
			  Infant: >50 g/day
			  Child: >200 g/day
			  Adolescent: >500 g/day
			Child should change from lying to standing positions slowly

Diuretic, potassium-sparing

Spironolactone (Aldactone) CHF Hypertension	Oral: 1.5-3.3 mg/kg/day in 1-4 doses	CNS: headache, lethargy, confusion GI: nausea, vomiting, diarrhea Metabolic: hyperkalemia, hyponatremia Skin: rashes	Monitor input and output, daily weights Monitor serum potassium and sodium levels Monitor BP throughout treatment *Parent teaching:* Avoid excess potassium in child's diet Know signs of hyperkalemia Report sore throat, fever, bleeding, or bruising to physician

III. Congenital heart disease
A. **Cardiac defects**
1. Two classification methods (Figure 13-2)
   a. Acyanotic-cyanotic
      (1) Acyanotic: congenital abnormalities of the heart in which mainly oxygenated blood enters the systemic circulation
      (2) Cyanotic: abnormalities in which unoxygenated blood mixes with oxygenated blood and enters the systemic circulation. Cyanotic events occur as a result of a right-to-left shunt.
   b. Hemodynamics (Box 13-1)
B. **Etiology and incidence**
1. Mostly unknown; prenatal factors include:
   a. Teratogenic exposure during first trimester of pregnancy: rubella, drugs, and alcohol
   b. Maternal type I diabetes
   c. Maternal age of over 40 years
2. Genetic factors are also implicated; certain chromosome aberrations are associated with increased risk of cardiac defects: Down and Holt-Oram syndromes
3. Most common acynotic defect: ventricular septal defect (VSD) accounts for 32% of all defects
4. Most common cyanotic defect: tetralogy of Fallot accounts for 4% of all defects
C. **Pathophysiology** (see Box 13-1)
D. **Assessment** (see Box 13-1)

Text continued on p. 383

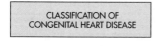

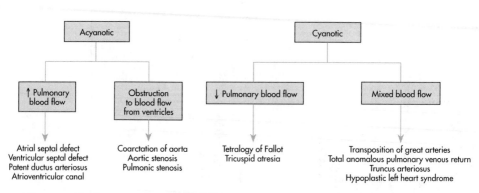

Figure 13-2 Comparison of acyanotic-cyanotic and hemodynamic classification systems of congenital heart disease. (From Wong DL, et al: *Whaley and Wong's nursing care of infants and children,* ed 6, St. Louis, 1999, Mosby.)

Box 13-1
Review of Cardiac Defects

Defects with Increased Pulmonary Blood Flow

Ventricular septal defect (VSD)

Altered hemodynamics and pathophysiology: opening between ventricles; oxygenated blood shunted from the left to the right ventricle

Assessment findings: CHF; failure to thrive; frequent respiratory infections; holosystolic murmur at the left lower sternal border

Therapeutic management: surgical repair of a large VSD using a Dacron patch; small defects may be closed with purse string sutures

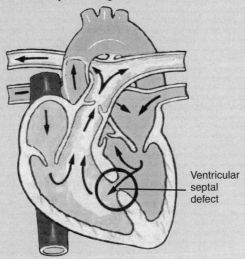

Ventricular
septal
defect

Atrial septal defect (ASD)

Altered hemodynamics and pathophysiology: an opening between the atria allows oxygenated blood to be shunted from the left to the right atrium

Assessment findings: mostly asymptomatic; crescendo-decrescendo, systolic ejection murmur

Therapeutic management: direct surgical closure with a Dacron patch

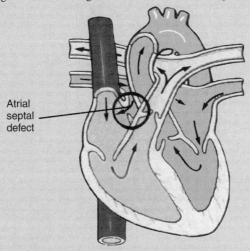

Atrial
septal
defect

Modified from Wong DL, et al: *Whaley and Wong's nursing care of infants and children,* ed 6, St. Louis, 1999, Mosby.

Continued

Box 13-1
Review of Cardiac Defects—cont'd

Defects with Increased Pulmonary Blood Flow—cont'd

Patent ductus arteriosus (PDA)

Altered hemodynamics and pathophysiology: oxygenated blood shunted from the aorta into the pulmonary artery

Assessment findings: characteristic machinery-like murmur at the mid to left upper sternal border; widened pulse pressure

Therapeutic management: surgical division or ligation of patent vessel (thoroscopic procedure allows clipping of ductus without thoracotomy); nonsurgical placement of coils to occlude PDA (done in the cardiac catheterization laboratory); indomethacin is administered to preterm infants and some newborns to constrict the ductus to promote closure

Defects Obstructing Blood Flow from Ventricles

Coarctation of aorta (COA)

Altered hemodynamics and pathophysiology: collateral circulation bypasses the coarcted area to supply blood to the lower extremities; left ventricular pressure and workload are increased

Assessment findings: failure to thrive; weak or absent femoral pulses; systolic murmur; hypertension in the upper extremities and lowered BP in the lower extremities; fatigue, headaches, and leg cramps

Therapeutic management: resection of the coarcted portion with end-to-end anastomosis of the aorta or enlargement of the constricted section using a graft

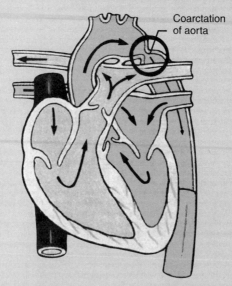

Coarctation of aorta

Modified from Wong DL, et al: *Whaley and Wong's nursing care of infants and children,* ed 6, St. Louis, 1999, Mosby.

Box 13-1
Review of Cardiac Defects—cont'd

Defects Obstructing Blood Flow from Ventricles—cont'd

Aortic stenosis (AS)
Altered hemodynamics and pathophysiology: stricture in aortic outflow causes
resistance to ejection of blood from the left ventricle; elevated left ventricular
systolic pressure; left ventricular hypertrophy
Assessment findings: systolic murmur; fatigue and syncope; decreased pulse pressure
Therapeutic management: aortic valvotomy surgical repair

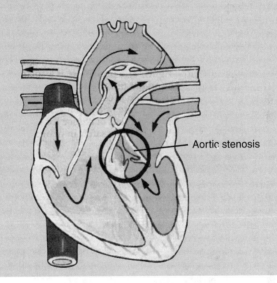

Aortic stenosis

Continued

E. **Therapeutic management**
   1. Medications (see Table 13-1, p. 378)
      a. Diuretics—chlorothiazide (Diuril), spironolactone (Aldactone),
         and furosemide (Lasix)
      b. Cardiac glycosides—digoxin (Lanoxin)
      c. Electrolyte replacement—potassium (Klorvess)
      d. Bronchodilators—beta-adrenergic stimulant dilates the
         bronchioles: isoproterenol (Isuprel) increases CO
      e. Prostaglandins—keep the ductus arteriosus open in premature
         infants until surgical intervention is possible
   2. Treatment: conservative until surgery
   3. Surgery: refer to Box 13-1 (pp. 381-385) for surgical procedures
      performed for various defects

Box 13-1
Review of Cardiac Defects—cont'd

Defects with Decreased Pulmonary Blood Flow

Tetralogy of Fallot (TOF)—Defect consists of four anomalies:
Altered hemodynamics and pathophysiology: unsaturated (unoxygenated) blood is shunted through the VSD directly into the aorta; increased right ventricular pressure
Assessment findings: hypoxemia; cyanosis that increases with activity; hypercyanotic **"tet" spells;** systolic murmur and thrill in the upper left sternal border; digital clubbing; growth retardation
Therapeutic management: palliative care for those who are unable to have complete repair involves increasing pulmonary blood flow (Blalock-Taussig shunting procedure); surgical repair involves complete VSD closure, resection of stenosis, and enlargement of the right ventricular output tract.

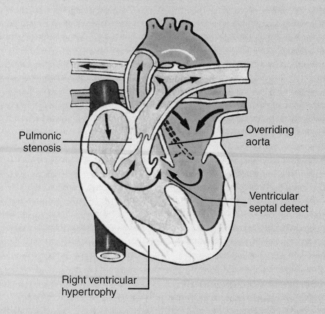

Pulmonic stenosis

Overriding aorta

Ventricular septal detect

Right ventricular hypertrophy

Tricuspid atresia
Altered hemodynamics and pathophysiology: failure of the tricuspid valve to develop; decreased pulmonary blood flow and increased left-to-right shunting; no communication between the right atria and right ventricle
Assessment findings: cyanosis present at birth; tachycardia, dyspnea, digital clubbing; chronic hypoxemia; and continuous murmur in the aortic area

Modified from Wong DL, et al: *Whaley and Wong's nursing care of infants and children,* ed 6, St. Louis, 1999, Mosby.

Box 13-1
Review of Cardiac Defects—cont'd

Defects with Decreased Pulmonary Blood Flow—cont'd

Therapeutic management: neonates may receive prostaglandin E infusion for maintaining PDA; palliative surgery involves shunt placement to increase blood flow to the lungs

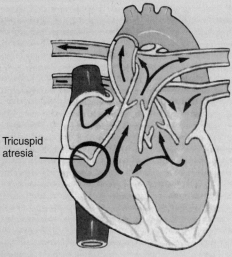

Tricuspid atresia

Mixed Blood Flow

Transposition of the great arteries

Altered hemodynamics and pathophysiology: the pulmonary artery leaves the left ventricle and aorta and exits from the right; the defect results in two separate circulations; only mixing of saturated and unsaturated blood occurs by way of defects that may exist: VSD, ASD, and PDA

Assessment findings: depend on defect—cyanosis occurs early; cardiomegaly; CHF; murmur if VSD is present

Therapeutic management: complete surgical repair includes arterial switch, Mustard, or Rastelli procedure; palliative care: Rashkind balloon atrial septostomy during catheterization to provide mixing of blood; Prostaglandin E temporarily increases blood mixing

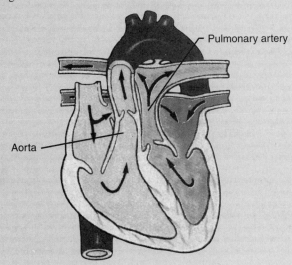

Pulmonary artery

Aorta

F. Nursing management: child with congenital cardiac defect
1. Nursing diagnoses
   a. Decreased CO
   b. Activity intolerance
2. Expected outcomes
   a. Child returns to or maintains stable vital signs
   b. Child maintains adequate tissue perfusion as evidenced by pink color, warm extremities, and strong pulses
   c. Child maintains an optimal activity level within limitations imposed by the disease process
   d. Parents promote growth and development for the child's age and condition
3. Interventions
   a. Assess HR for a full minute (both apical and peripheral pulses). Note rate, quality, rhythm, and pulse deficit. Assess vital signs and skin color changes during activity, and compare these assessments with the resting state.
   b. Assess BP while child is at rest; use properly sized cuff
   c. Assess level of fatigue and contributing factors
   d. Administer cardiac glycosides as ordered. Monitor the child for signs of digoxin toxicity. Withhold medication if pulse falls below or exceeds set limits for the child's age, or if vomiting occurs.
   e. Maintain cardiac monitoring as needed
   f. For hypercyanotic spell, position the child into a knee-chest or squatting position to reduce venous return to the right side of the heart; administer morphine subcutaneously or through existing IV line; administer oxygen as ordered
   g. Allow rest periods between activities; provide a calm and quiet environment
   h. Provide age-appropriate toys and activities that do not require high-energy expenditure
4. Cardiac surgery
   a. Presurgical care
      (1) Nursing diagnoses
         (a) Knowledge deficit
         (b) Parental anxiety
      (2) Expected outcomes
         (a) The child and family verbalize knowledge of the basic structure and function of the heart with description of the defect
         (b) The child and family members state the rationales and their roles related to various equipment and procedures associated with cardiac surgeries
      (3) Interventions
         (a) Assess the child and the family's readiness to learn

      (b) Assess the child and the family's previous experience and present knowledge base

      (c) Provide preoperative education based on knowledge from the initial assessment findings; include visits to the areas where the child and family will be before, during, and after surgery

      (d) Use age-appropriate explanations for various procedures and equipment

      (e) Encourage the child and family to express feelings and concerns about surgery

      (f) Reinforce information provided by the cardiac surgeon or anesthesiologist

  b. Postsurgical care

    (1) Nursing diagnoses

      (a) Risk for decreased CO

      (b) Risk for ineffective airway clearance

      (c) Risk for infection

    (2) Expected outcomes: child demonstrates improved cardiovascular and respiratory function

      (a) Adequate tissue perfusion: capillary refill time of 3 to 5 seconds

      (b) Stabilization of vital signs

      (c) Clear lungs on auscultation

      (d) Adequate urine output

      (e) Arterial blood gases within normal range

5. Interventions

  a. Assessment of the cardiac function includes:

    (1) Vital signs and LOC

    (2) Central venous and pulmonary artery pressures: left atrial pressure is 0 to 8 mm Hg; normal central venous pressure is 0 to 5 mm Hg

    (3) Heart sounds

    (4) Peripheral pulses

    (5) Renal function (input and output, specific gravity of urine, creatinine, and BUN)

  b. Monitor effort, rate, and depth of respirations; assess for the presence of dyspnea or wheezing

  c. Assess child for temperature elevation, and an increase in WBC count, HR, or RR

  d. Monitor the ventilator settings to deliver the appropriate tidal volume and oxygen percentage

  e. Monitor the arterial blood gas results

  f. Assess the amount of pulmonary secretions

  g. Monitor chest tube drainage and patency

  h. Turn the child and perform suction as necessary

  i. Provide chest physiotherapy as ordered

      j. Have the extubated child cough and breath deeply every hour

      k. Monitor the condition of the incision and IV sites for signs of infection

      l. Have the child avoid contact with visitors and staff who have infections

      m. Administer antibiotics as ordered

      n. Use proper hand-washing technique

G. Evaluation

  1. Questions to ask parents

      a. Tell me about your plans for the child's care at home: Medications? Activity? School?

      b. How do you deal with your anxiety and fears?

  2. Family behaviors to observe:

      a. Measures taken to ensure prevention of infection

      b. Statements indicating effective coping techniques are being used

      c. Statements indicating a positive outlook concerning the child's condition

  3. Evaluation of expected outcomes

      a. The child exhibits improved cardiac status, including HR and BP within 10% of baseline

      b. The child exhibits improved respiratory status, including clear lung sounds and arterial blood gases within normal limits for age

IV. Congestive heart failure (CHF)

A. Description—in this cardiac disorder the heart is unable to deliver adequate blood to the systemic circulation to meet the body's demands

B. Commonly, 90% of infants with congenital cardiac defects develop CHF within the first year of life

C. Etiology and incidence: CHF is the result of congenital heart disease; other causes for CHF include:

  1. Pulmonary embolism or chronic lung disease

  2. Hemorrhage or anemia

  3. Cardiomyopathies

  4. Severe emotional or physical stress

D. Pathophysiology

  1. Basic defect is the decrease in the intrinsic contractility of the myocardium; caused by prolonged increased pressure (afterload) or volume overload

  2. Causes are classified according to these changes:

      a. Volume overload: left-to-right shunts cause right ventricular hypertrophy

      b. Pressure overload: occurs from obstructive lesions, for example, coarctation of aorta and aortic valvular stenosis

      c. Decreased contractility: involves disorders that directly affect the contractility of myocardium, for example, cardiomyopathy and severe anemia

        d. High cardiac demands: the body's need for oxygenated blood exceeds CO, for example, in sepsis and hyperthyroidism

   3. CHF in children most commonly manifests with bilateral failure; unilateral failure is not typical

   4. Compensatory mechanisms are activated as the heart attempts to meet the body's demands

        a. Cardiac: hypertrophy and dilation of the cardiac muscle

        b. Noncardiac: sympathetic nervous system stimulation:

           (1) Catecholamine release—increased force and rate of myocardial contraction

           (2) Decreased renal perfusion—activates the renin-angiotensin-aldosterone system to cause water and sodium retention

   5. As compensatory mechanisms fail, CHF findings occur from decreased myocardial contraction and CO and increased preload and afterload

E. Assessment

   1. Assessment findings of CHF can be divided into three groups:

        a. Impaired myocardial function

        b. Pulmonary congestion

        c. Systemic venous congestion (Box 13-2, p. 390)

⚠ Warning!

The earliest signs of CHF are tachycardia (during rest or slight activity), tachypnea, fatigue with less play activity, irritability, or scalp sweating in infants.

   2. Diagnostic procedures

        a. Laboratory results

           (1) Arterial blood gas values—low partial pressure of oxygen (PO_2) and pH, high partial pressure of carbon dioxide (PCO_2)

           (2) Serum electrolytes changes—hyponatremia, hypochloremia, and hyperkalemia

           (3) Digoxin level—monitor for toxicity and regulate dosage; therapeutic level is 0.8 to 2.0 µg/L

⚠ Warning!

Initial signs of digoxin toxicity in older children are bradycardia and upset stomach; in young children, sign is tachycardia; and in infants, sign is poor feeding.

        b. Diagnostic studies

           (1) Chest x-ray film—reveals pulmonary congestion and cardiomegaly

           (2) ECG—reveals ventricular hypertrophy

F. Therapeutic management

   1. Medications (see Table 13-1, p. 377)

        a. Cardiac glycosides—increase the force and decrease the rate of cardiac contractions to improve cardiac pumping performance

Box 13-2
Clinical Manifestations of Congestive Heart Failure

Impaired Myocardial Function

Restlessness

Weakness

Tachycardia

Sweating (inappropriate)

Decreased urine output

Fatigue

Anorexia, poor feeding in infants

Pale, cool extremities

Weak peripheral pulses

Decreased BP

Gallop rhythm

Cardiomegaly

Pulmonary Congestion

Tachypnea

Dyspnea

Exercise intolerance

Orthopnea

Cough, hoarseness

Cyanosis

Wheezing

Infants

    Nasal flaring

    Grunting

    Sternal/intercostal retractions

    Plus any of the findings listed

Systemic Venous Congestion

Weight gain

Hepatomegaly

Peripheral edema, especially periorbital

Ascites

Neck vein distention (older children)

Modified from Wong, DL, Hockenberry-Eaton M, Wilson D: *Whaley and Wong's nursing care of infants and children,* ed 6, St Louis, 1999, Mosby.

    b. Diuretics: furosemide (Lasix)—control excessive fluid retention and decrease preload

    c. Angiotensin-converting enzyme (ACE) inhibitors—inhibit the function of the kidney's renin-angiotensin system

    d. Electrolytes: with loop or thiazide diuretic therapy—give potassium chloride for replacement

    e. Sedative-analgesic: morphine—give to decrease energy expenditure and dilate bronchi in the event of acute pulmonary edema

  2. Treatments: supplemental cool humidified oxygen for shortness of breath (SOB), fluid restriction, and diet control

  3. Surgery: unnecessary unless underlying cause needs to be corrected

G. Nursing management

  1. Nursing diagnoses

    a. Decreased CO

    b. Ineffective breathing pattern

    c. Activity intolerance

    d. Fluid volume excess

    e. Altered nutrition: less than body requirements

2. Expected outcomes

    a. Heartbeat is strong, regular, and within limits for age; respirations remain in normal limits

    b. Adequate CO, a decrease in the prolonged P-R interval, and a decrease in ventricular rate will be obtained

Age	HR Range
1 wk–3 mo	100-220
3 mo–2 yr	80-150
2-10 yr	70-110
10 yr–adolescence	55-90

    c. Therapeutic digoxin level will be maintained: 0.8 to 2.0 µg/L

    d. Adequate caloric and protein intake will be provided to support growth

    e. Anxiety is reduced; rest is promoted

    f. Child will exhibit evidence of fluid loss—frequent urination, weight loss to within normal limits

3. Interventions

    a. Assess apical HR for a full minute every 2 hours

    b. Monitor digoxin level with an observation for findings of digoxin toxicity

    c. Record strict input and output to maintain fluid restriction, as ordered; assess for edema

    d. Assess heart sounds for abnormal or new sounds and peripheral pulses for changes to weakness every 2 hours

    e. Monitor for potassium levels below 3.5 mol/L

    f. Administer diuretics and digoxin as ordered: withhold digoxin dose if:

        (1) HR is less than 100 beats per minute (bpm) or greater than 160 bpm for infants

        (2) HR is less than 70 bpm or greater than 140 bpm for children up to 10 years of age

        (3) HR is less than 60 bpm or greater than 120 bpm for children older than 10 years of age

    g. Weigh child daily at the same time, in the same clothing or without clothing, and before eating

    h. Feed infant 2 ounces every 2 to 3 hours as ordered; use gavage feeding if needed

    i. Allow rest periods after activity; avoid disturbance of the child during rest periods

    j. Maintain infants in a neutral thermal environment, with frequent position changes

    k. Add prescribed formula additives such as Polycose, medium-chain triglyceride (MCT) oil

H. **Evaluation**
   1. Questions to ask parents
      a. Are the child's pulses, extremity color, and skin temperature adequate?
      b. Has the child's breathing improved?
      c. Have the family's anxiety and fears decreased?
      d. Is the child's energy level increased?
   2. Behaviors to observe
      a. Parents understand to report SOB and sweating, especially during rest
      b. Parents monitor the child for anxiety associated with SOB and activity intolerance

V. Acquired heart disease: rheumatic fever

A. **Description—an inflammatory disease after an infection caused by Group A beta-hemolytic streptococci**
B. **Commonly affects many body systems**
   1. Musculoskeletal: joints—knees, elbows, ankles, and wrists
   2. Cardiac muscle and valves
   3. CNS—chorea
   4. Integument—macular rash on the trunk and extremities
C. **Etiology and incidence**
   1. In most cases, an antecedent upper respiratory infection is present 3 weeks before the onset of symptoms
   2. May occur at any age; primarily occurs in mid to late childhood
   3. Increased frequency among males; seasonal outbreaks are observed in late winter and early spring
D. **Pathophysiology**
   1. Streptococci, present in the upper respiratory system, release toxins and enzymes that cause an inflammatory reaction in the connective tissue of the heart, joints, and skin
   2. Edema and cellular infiltration of the lymphocytes occur
   3. *Aschoff's bodies,* rounded nodules containing multinucleated cells and fibroblasts, are localized in the mitral valve area of the myocardium
E. **Assessment**
   1. Assessment findings
      a. Cardiac: chest pain, tachycardia, systolic murmur, carditis, CHF, and cardiomegaly
      b. *Polyarthritis*—multijoint inflammation; *arthralgia*—joint pain
      c. *Chorea*—involuntary, purposeless, rapid motions such as raising and lowering the shoulders, grimacing
      d. Macular rash on the trunk and extremities
      e. Subcutaneous nodules over the bony prominences such as the joints, scalp, and spine
      f. General—low-grade fever, with an oral temperature of 99° F to 100° F; epistaxis; weakness; and fatigue

2. Diagnostic procedures
   a. Laboratory results
     (1) Antistreptolysin O titer—elevated titers over 333 Todd units
     (2) Erythrocyte sedimentation rate—elevated
     (3) C-reactive protein—elevated for Group A beta-hemolytic streptococci
     (4) Throat culture—positive
   b. Diagnostic studies
     (1) Diagnosis—made using Jones criteria (Box 13-3)
     (2) ECG—prolonged PR interval and tachycardia

F. Therapeutic management
1. Medications
   a. Antibiotics—penicillin, erythromycin, penicillin G benzathine, or sulfadiazine as prophylactic therapy against recurrence
   b. Salicylates—decrease inflammation; usually a 2-week course; are gradually withdrawn; specifically used in rheumatic fever; not usually prescribed in the pediatric age group, especially with or after viral diseases because of the risk of Reye syndrome
   c. Prednisone—for children with carditis and valvulitis

Box 13-3
Guidelines for Diagnosing an Initial Attack of Rheumatic Fever (Jones Criteria, 1992 Update)*

Major Manifestations
Carditis
Polyarthritis
Chorea
Erythema marginatum
Subcutaneous nodules

Minor Manifestations
Clinical findings:
  Arthralgia
  Fever
Laboratory findings:
  Elevated acute-phase reactions
  Erythrocyte sedimentation rate
  C-reactive protein

Supporting Evidence of Antecedent Group A Streptococcal Infection
Positive throat culture or rapid streptococcal antigen test
Elevated or increasing streptococcal antibody titer

*If supported by evidence of a preceding Group A streptococcal infection, the presence of two major manifestations or of one major and two minor manifestations indicates a high probability of acute rheumatic fever.
From Jones Criteria Update: *JAMA* 1992, 268(15):2070.

2. Treatments
   a. Bed rest during the acute febrile phase
   b. Limited physical exercise in children with carditis

G. Nursing management
   1. Nursing diagnoses
      a. Pain
      b. Risk for injury
   2. Expected outcomes
      a. Child has joint pain relieved or controlled for minimal discomfort in the acute phase
      b. Child limits movement that causes discomfort
      c. Child recovers without cardiovascular or mobility complications
   3. Interventions (for carditis, see nursing care of the child with CHF, p. 390)
      a. Assess severity of pain in the joints involved with the use of a pediatric pain rating scale
      b. Assess nonverbal signs of pain: crying, irritability, and refusal to move
      c. Administer analgesics or anti-inflammatory agents as ordered
      d. Maintain bed rest during the acute phase when the temperature is increased
      e. Reposition the child every 2 hours to maintain body alignment; move the child gently while supporting the joints
      f. Use bed cradle over affected extremities to decrease skin and joint irritation
      g. Provide age-appropriate quiet activities for diversion

H. Evaluation
   1. Questions to ask parents
      a. What will you do before the application of braces on the child's teeth?
      b. What is your plan for giving the medication in school and at home?
   2. Behaviors to observe
      a. Compliance with the antibiotic regimen
      b. Compliance with the methods to protect joints from pain
   3. Evaluation of expected outcomes
      a. Child verbalizes that joint pain is controlled or relieved
      b. Family demonstrates preventive measures to avoid recurrence of disease

VI. Home care: family education topics and referrals
A. Congenital cardiac defects
   1. Disease process: treatments, long-term care; cardiac complications such as right and left heart failure; inform parents when to call the physician: unexplained fever, change in child's behavior
   2. Cyanotic episodes: explain the rationale for knee-chest or squatting position; administration of oxygen

3. Medications: administration of prescribed medications, including digoxin:
   a. Measure the exact dose
   b. Administer slowly and toward the back of the mouth
   c. Administer at regular intervals: every 12 hours, 1 hour before or 2 hours after feedings
   d. Explain when to withhold dose and what to do if a dose is missed, or if the child vomits
   e. Describe the early signs of drug toxicity
   f. Advise when to notify the physician
   g. Advise that if an overdose is given, call the physician immediately
4. Activity: physical activity and limitations; selection of age-appropriate activities suited to condition; allow adequate time for task completion to promote self-esteem and independence
5. Growth and development: review age-related developmental tasks and provide parental guidance information: appropriate limit setting, provision for discipline, meeting the child's emotional needs

B. CHF
1. Condition and treatments: signs and symptoms of CHF and when to notify the physician; feeding techniques and nutritional requirements; positioning
2. Medications: see cardiac defects
3. Activity: importance of energy conservation, need for adequate rest and sleep; examples of quiet age-appropriate activities
4. Referrals: for congenital heart disease, American Red Cross; for cardiopulmonary resuscitation training, the local chapter of Pediatric Advanced Life Support (PALS)

C. Rheumatic fever
1. Medication: administration of antibiotics; compliance with prescribed antibiotic regimen
2. Long-term care: need for prophylactic antibiotic (daily oral, monthly IM) therapy before dental, upper respiratory, and urologic procedures; importance of follow-up care because the child is susceptible to recurrence

WEB Resources

www.tchin.org
  Children's Health Information Network provides information and resources to families of children with congenital and acquired heart disease. Features include support groups and national event information; also provides a Resource Room that categorizes educational materials.

www.ohsu.edu
  This site is sponsored by the Congenital Heart Research Center at Oregon Health Sciences University in Portland. It is dedicated to understanding the role of fetal heart development in congenital heart defects. Cliniweb International provides links to citations for articles on various congenital heart defects.

REVIEW QUESTIONS

1. A mother has been given instructions about the administration of pediatric digoxin (Lanoxin). The physician has ordered the medication to be administered bid. Which of these statements by the parent indicates an understanding of these instructions?
   1. "I'll give the medication with feedings around breakfast and lunch times."
   2. "I'll mix the medication with formula."
   3. "I'll give another dose if the baby vomits."
   4. "I'll give the medication before feedings, 12 hours apart."

2. A presurgical plan of care has been established for a child before corrective surgery for tetralogy of Fallot. Which of these nursing diagnoses should receive priority in the child's care during the immediate postsurgical period?
   1. Alteration in elimination
   2. Impaired gas exchange
   3. Knowledge deficit
   4. Altered family processes

3. An infant recently admitted to the pediatric unit has been diagnosed with a ventricular-septal defect (VSD). During the shift physical assessment of this infant, the nurse should expect which of these findings?
   1. Cyanosis and increased anterior-posterior diameter of the chest
   2. Extreme difficulty feeding and irritability
   3. Machine-like murmur and shortness of breath (SOB)
   4. Systolic murmur and no other significant signs

4. A child diagnosed with rheumatic fever is prescribed aspirin. What is the purpose of this medication in this situation?
   1. To decrease fever
   2. To prevent headache
   3. To prevent clot formation
   4. To reduce inflammation

5. A 3-month-old infant is brought to the emergency department. His mother states that he has trouble eating, is coughing, and breathing irregularly. The nurse assesses a RR of 60, with sternal retractions and an apical rate of 168. An x-ray film reveals enlargement of the heart. Which of these nursing diagnoses should receive priority in this infant's plan of care?
   1. Impaired gas exchange
   2. Altered fluid balance
   3. Decreased cardiac output (CO)
   4. Altered nutrition

6. A toddler has been diagnosed with coarctation of the aorta. With consideration of the child's diagnosis, the nurse should expect which of these findings?

1. Bounding bilateral femoral pulses
2. BP is higher in the upper extremities
3. Machine-like murmur
4. Weak, thready unilateral radial pulse

ANSWERS, RATIONALES, AND TEST-TAKING TIPS

Rationales	Test-Taking Tips

1. Correct answer: 4

Digoxin administration guidelines include giving the medication at regular intervals, usually 12 hours apart, and 1 hour before or 2 hours after feedings. Digoxin is given on an empty stomach for best absorption, 1 hour before or 2 hours after feedings. Medication is not to be mixed with the formula, because refusal to take the entire amount results in an inaccurate intake of the dose. If the child vomits, digoxin guidelines indicate a second dose should not be given. The physician should be notified.

If you have no idea of the correct option, select the most complete one, option 4. Other clues in terms of main themes can alert you to incorrect answers. In option 1, the time interval is the clue. In option 2, the clue is "mix" the drug with food without specific amounts being stated. Only in rare circumstances are medications mixed with specific small amounts of foods or fluids. If the client has a gastric tube, then it is appropriate to mix drugs with liquids because the total amount is easily given. The clue in option 3 is the abnormal event, vomiting. Medications usually are not repeated after emesis.

2. Correct answer: 2

Use Maslow's hierarchy of needs to prioritize that physiologic needs should be addressed before psychosocial needs. The need for adequate gas exchange is the priority physiologic need in the immediate postsurgical period, rather than an elimination concern. Psychosocial needs are not a priority at this time.

Cluster options 3 and 4 under psychological needs. Between the remaining options, options 1 and 2, physiologic needs, a cardiopulmonary need is more important in the immediate postoperative period than a gastrointestinal need. The timeframe is important to note in this question. It is the clue to the correct answer. Option 1 would be more important for home care.

3. Correct answer: 4

One of the characteristic signs of VSD is a loud, harsh, pansystolic murmur heard best at the lower left sternal border. The findings in option 1 are consistent with cystic fibrosis (CF); those in option 2 are

First note that the problem is with the heart. Thus, eliminate options 1 and 2, which are not directly related to the heart. Then think about anatomy. Maybe even draw a picture of a normal heart, then a VSD. In a VSD, mixing of

consistent with CHF, abnormal GI conditions, or both; those in option 3 are consistent with patent ductus arteriosus (PDA)—the turbulent flow of blood from the aorta through the PDA to the pulmonary artery. The classic characteristics of PDA are a machinery-like murmur and SOB.

oxygenated and unoxygenated blood occurs. Most likely more blood will be shunted from the high-pressure system—the left ventricle—to the low-pressure system—the right ventricle. Thus, most of the arterial blood from the left ventricle will carry oxygen to the body and minimal systemic effects will occur.

4. Correct answer: 4

Salicylates are used to control or minimize inflammation, especially in joints. Although salicylates are effective in decreasing a fever associated with this disease process, the primary purpose is to decrease inflammation that can cause pathologic connective tissue changes. Headache is not a major finding in rheumatic fever. Aspirin is not given as an antiplatelet or anticoagulant in this disease.

Recall that a major problem in rheumatic fever is joint inflammation. Associate this effect with rheumatoid arthritis in which high doses of aspirin are used effectively to control or minimize joint inflammation. Pain relief is a secondary gain from the anti-inflammatory effect. Avoid an emotional reaction from your knowledge that aspirin is not given to children to prevent Reye syndrome. Remember the most important criteria: "aspirin is not given to a child *during or after a viral infection.*"

5. Correct answer: 3

The goals in infants with CHF are to improve cardiac function, remove accumulated fluid and sodium, and decrease the cardiac workload. The result is improved CO. Because of poor weight gain and activity intolerance, infants with CHF may demonstrate developmental delays. However, developmental delays are not a priority in emergency situations. Also, no information is given in the stem to support the selection of any of the other nursing diagnoses.

The key words in the stem that indicate an immediate physiologic need are "sternal retractions," "respirations of 60," "HR of 168," and "enlarged heart." All these findings point to an immediate cardiopulmonary physiologic need. The clue in the stem is the result of the x-ray for an enlarged heart, which suggests heart failure. No other findings are given to support the selection of options 1, 2, or 4.

Rationales	Test-Taking Tips

6. Correct answer: 2

Coarctation of the aorta (COA), a narrowing of the aorta, usually is first identified at a routine physical examination by upper extremity hypertension. In those body areas that receive blood from vessels proximal to the defect, the BP is elevated. In COA, the pulses are bounding in body areas that receive blood from vessels proximal to the narrowed aorta. The site of the narrowing is usually the thoracic or descending aorta. Femoral pulses are usually weak or absent in COA. The finding in option 2 is characteristic of PDA.

Eliminate option 3 because the problem is in the aorta and a murmur is not likely to be found there. Eliminate option 1 by using an educated guess that problems in the aorta will more likely result in weak femoral pulses, not bounding pulses. Eliminate option 4 because it has a narrow focus—unilateral and only the radial pulse. Select option 2.

14

Nursing Care of Children with Hemotologic and Immunologic Disorders

FAST FACTS

1. Children with iron deficiency anemia exhibit pallor, fatigue, dyspnea, and tachycardia.
2. In sickle cell anemia, conditions of decreased oxygen tension and increased blood viscosity cause the hemoglobin to form sickle-shaped cells.
3. Hemophilia is transmitted as an X-linked disorder.
4. When administering oral ferrous sulfate, an iron supplement, use a straw or a dropper to avoid staining the teeth.
5. The Z-track technique is recommended for administration of IM iron preparations.

CONTENT REVIEW

I. Overview of the hematologic system
A. Review of anatomy and physiology
1. The hematologic system includes blood and blood-forming tissue
   a. Two components of blood
      (1) Plasma—the fluid portion, including the solutes:
         (a) Albumin
         (b) Electrolytes

(c) Proteins—clotting factors, globulins, antibodies, and fibrinogen
            (2) Formed elements—cellular portion
                (a) RBCs
                (b) WBCs
                (c) Platelets (thrombocytes)
    b. Blood-forming organs
        (1) Red bone marrow or myeloid tissue
        (2) Lymphatic system
            (a) Lymph
            (b) Lymphatic vessels
            (c) Lymphatic structures—thymus, tonsils, spleen, and lymph nodes
    c. All of the formed elements of blood are formed in the myeloid tissue in postnatal life
    d. In infants and children, bones contain red marrow. After adolescence, only the ribs, sternum, vertebrae, and pelvis produce cells; the remainder of bone marrow becomes yellow from fat deposits
2. Function of the hematologic system and its formed elements
    a. This complex system is responsible for cell oxygenation, removal of the end-products of metabolism, immune protection, clotting, and heat regulation
    b. Functions of RBCs
        (1) Transport hemoglobin, which provides oxygen to the cells
        (2) Hemoglobin portion acts as an acid-base buffer
        (3) Carbonic anhydrase allows carbon dioxide to react with blood to be transported to the lungs
    c. Functions of WBCs
        (1) Neutrophils and monocytes—are phagocytes involved in inflammatory reactions
        (2) Eosinophils—are involved in allergic or hypersensitivity reactions
        (3) Basophils—are responsible for histamine release that increases blood vessel permeability to WBCs at the site of an injury
    d. Functions of platelets
        (1) Form clots
        (2) Release serotonin, a vasoconstrictor, at the site of injury to decrease blood flow out from the injured site
B. **Assessment**
    1. Summary of major laboratory and diagnostic studies
        a. Components of a complete blood count (CBC)
            (1) RBCs, hematocrit and hemoglobin (H&H): measure the oxygen-carrying capacity of the blood

       (2) WBCs: used to diagnose infection; will be elevated in infections and are especially significant in bacterial infections

       (3) Differential WBCs: used to diagnose bacterial, fungal, and viral infections

       (4) Mean corpuscular volume and mean corpuscular hemoglobin: used to diagnose iron deficiency anemia

       (5) Platelet count: determines bleeding potential severity

  b. Diagnostic tests

       (1) Bone marrow aspiration—used to diagnose leukemia, aplastic anemia, and thrombocytopenia

       (2) Bone marrow biopsy—used to obtain a more accurate diagnosis of similar items as in bone marrow aspiration

2. Health history

  a. General considerations

       (1) Activity: lack of energy, tires easily, and SOB

       (2) Diet and other factors

          (a) Lack of iron in the diet

          (b) Poor growth, appetite, or both

          (c) Tendency to bruise and bleed easily

          (d) Recurrent infections

          (e) Illness in siblings

       (3) Immunization is up to date. If not up to date, collect further information.

  b. Family considerations for a history of:

       (1) Bleeding tendencies

       (2) Recent infections and anemia

       (3) Malignancy

       (4) Maternal HIV

3. Physical examination—findings provide indication of hematologic dysfunction

  a. Lymph: inspect and palpate the lymph nodes for tenderness and enlargement

  b. Skin: pallor, petechiae, cyanosis, ecchymoses, purpura, and clubbing of nails

  c. Neurologic: lethargy and irritability

  d. GI: hepatosplenomegaly

  e. Oral cavity: pallor and bleeding

  f. Musculoskeletal: bone pain, joint swelling, and pain

II. Mechanisms of immunity

A. Functions of the immune system

1. Responds to foreign substances or antigens with:

  a. Nonspecific immune defenses—generalized response to any antigen

  b. Specific immune defenses—responds selectively to an antigen

2. Skin is the first line of defense for protection of the body

B. **Components of the immune system**
   1. Primary lymphoid organs: thymus and bone marrow
   2. Secondary lymphoid organs: lymph nodes and spleen
C. **Mechanisms of immunity**
   1. Humoral immunity—specific mechanism involves antibody production and the B-lymphocyte; immune process occurs outside of cells
   2. Cell-mediated immunity—specific mechanism involves immune processes within the cell mediated by T-lymphocytes; T-lymphocyte functions
      a. Viral, fungal, protozoan, and some bacterial protection
      b. Graft rejection
      c. Skin hypersensitivity
      d. Malignant cell surveillance

III. Anemias

A. **Sickle cell anemia (SCA)**
   1. Description: severe, chronic anemic disorder
      a. Homozygous form of a group of inherited diseases in which the normal adult hemoglobin (hemoglobin A) is replaced by a variant form (hemoglobin S)
      b. Abnormal hemoglobin results in abnormally shaped and increased fragility of RBCs
   2. Incidence and etiology
      a. 8% of Black Americans are carriers of the sickle cell trait
      b. SCA may be present in persons of Hispanic and Mediterranean descent
      c. Sickling is not found until late infancy from the presence of fetal hemoglobin
   3. Mode of transmission: *autosomal recessive disorder—both parents must be carriers of the sickle cell trait;* each pregnancy has a one in four chance or producing a child with SCA
   4. Pathophysiology
      a. In hemoglobin S, the defect is a substitution of valine for glutamine on the beta polypeptide chain of the globin portion
      b. Erythrocytes containing hemoglobin S become sickle-shaped in situations of decreased oxygen tension, decreased hydration, and temperature elevation
      c. Sickled RBCs are crescent-shaped, have reduced oxygen-carrying capacity, and decreased life span
      d. Sickled RBCs are rigid; they cause trapping and increased blood viscosity, capillary stasis, and thrombosis; eventually, tissue ischemia and necrosis result

e. Sickle cell crises are periods of exacerbation in which disease symptoms are most acute
  (1) Three major types of sickle cell crises
    (a) Vaso-occlusive—painful episodes marked by vessel occlusion, ischemia, and necrosis caused by pooling of blood and clumping of cells
    (b) Splenic sequestration—large quantities of blood are pooled in the liver and spleen
    (c) Aplastic—decreased RBC production, usually results from a virus (human parvovirus)
  (2) Other complications
    (a) Megaloblastic anemia—from an excessive need for folic acid and B_{12}
    (b) Hyperhemolytic crisis—increased rate of RBC destruction
    (c) Stroke—occurs when sickled cells block the major blood vessels of the brain
    (d) Chest syndrome—sickling occurs in small vessels in the lungs, causing severe chest pain, fever, and anemia
    (e) Septicemia—streptococcal pneumonia and *Haemophilus influenzae,* type B cause an overwhelming infection

5. Assessment
  a. Assessment findings: tissue ischemia and necrosis that result from an increased blood viscosity and RBC destruction; Figure 14-1, p. 406, provides the major sites affected
  b. Diagnostic procedures: laboratory tests
    (1) Hemoglobin electrophoresis (fingerprinting)—detects homozygous and heterozygous forms of the disease and percentages of various hemoglobin forms
    (2) Sickle-turbidity test (Sickledex)—screening test for hemoglobin S
    (3) Blood smear—may reveal the sickled shape of RBCs, rather than normal, the biconcave disk
    (4) Antenatal screening—possible through amniocentesis
  c. Pediatric complications
    (1) Delayed growth, development, and onset of puberty
    (2) Impaired fertility
    (3) *Priapism*
      (a) Definition: prolonged or constant penile erection that is often painful and seldom associated with sexual arousal, which may result from urinary calculi
      (b) Cause: microcirculating obstruction and engorgement of the penis
      (c) Treatment: bed rest, sedation and analgesics

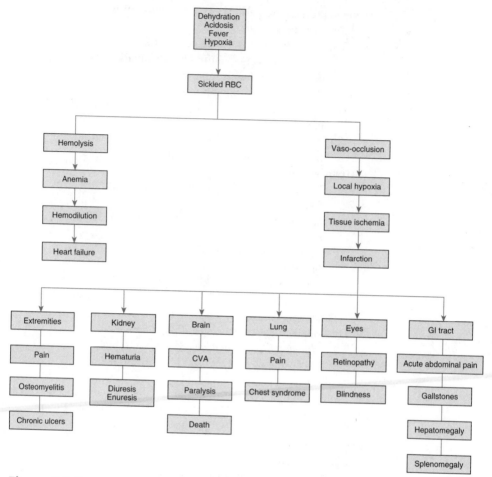

Figure 14-1 Tissue effects of sickle cell anemia. (From Wong DL, et al: *Whaley and Wong's nursing care of infants and children,* ed 6, St. Louis, 1999, Mosby.)

> ⚠️ **Warning!**
>
> Avoid administration of meperidine hydrochloride (Demerol, Pethidine) because of seizure risk.

       (4) Enuresis—incontinence of urine, especially at night
6. Therapeutic management
   a. Medications
      (1) Analgesics to control the severe pain during a crisis: opioids such as morphine and oxycodone (Percocet, Tylox)—orally, parenterally or via PCA pump
      (2) Antibiotics to treat the existing infection

     b. Treatments
        (1) Rest
        (2) Oxygen administration
        (3) Fluid and electrolyte replacement, usually aggressive
        (4) Blood replacement
        (5) Bone marrow transplantation—in research stages

7. Nursing management
     a. Nursing diagnoses
        (1) Altered tissue perfusion—renal, cerebral, and peripheral
        (2) Risk for fluid volume deficit
        (3) Risk for injury and infection
     b. Expected outcome
        (1) Optimal circulatory blood flow with delivery of oxygen and nutrients to all organs
        (2) Child maintains adequate hydration
        (3) Child remains infection-free
     c. Interventions
        (1) Assess for signs of hypoxia: irritability, restlessness, agitation, and hyperventilation, along with increased apical pulse and RR, confusion, and cyanosis
        (2) Monitor input and output, and daily weights
        (3) Assess for signs of infection and dehydration (dry mucous membranes and skin, poor skin turgor, decreased urine output)
        (4) Encourage the child to drink fluids every 2 hours. Use 5 oz/kg of body weight as a minimum fluid requirement and increase by 50% during periods of stress or exercise.
        (5) Provide rest periods to decrease oxygen expenditure
        (6) Administer blood products as ordered; assess for a transfusion reaction
        (7) Perform passive range-of-motion exercises every 4 to 6 hours
        (8) Isolate child from sources of infection; administer antibiotics, as ordered
     d. Nursing diagnosis: pain
     e. Expected outcome: child verbalizes absence of or minimal pain
     f. Interventions
        (1) Devise pain prevention schedule including the use of opioids
        (2) Assess for location, severity, duration, and quality of pain
        (3) Assess intensity of pain with the use of an age-appropriate pain rating scale
        (4) Administer analgesics as ordered—oral; if in crisis use an IV or a client-controlled analgesia pump; avoid administration of meperidine (Demerol, Penthidine)
        (5) Apply warmth to the affected area

> ## ⚠ Warning!
> Avoid the use of ice or cold compresses, which may cause vasoconstriction and further sickling.

    (6) Encourage relaxation techniques, deep breathing exercises, and guided imagery

    (7) Gently handle painful joints and extremities; provide support with pillows and maintain in alignment with the rest of the body

  8. Evaluation

    a. Questions to ask parents

      (1) How does this hospitalization differ from others?

      (2) Which resources do you need at home?

    b. Behaviors to observe

      (1) Parent's participation in pain evaluation, hydration, and pain-relief measures

      (2) No evidence of further sickling during assessments

      (3) Child verbalizes relief of pain

    c. Evaluation of expected outcomes

      (1) Family verbalizes knowledge of disease, cause, and methods to prevent crises

      (2) Family seeks genetic counseling and support from appropriate agencies

B. Aplastic anemia

  1. Description: disorder characterized by bone marrow failure and the depletion of all formed elements of the blood

  2. Etiology: causes of acquired aplastic anemia

    a. Drugs, including antibiotics and antineoplastic agents

    b. Infection, including hepatitis and human parvovirus

    c. Chemicals: benzenes and petroleum products

    d. Radiation

  3. Incidence

    a. May be acquired or inherited; Fanconi's syndrome is associated with a congenital variety of aplastic anemia

    b. In children, occurs between 3 and 5 years of age

  4. Pathophysiology

    a. Decreased production of blood cells

    b. Replacement of cellular elements of bone marrow with fat

    c. Results in pancytopenia: severe anemia (decreased H&H), leukopenia (decreased WBC), and thrombocytopenia (decreased platelets)

  5. Assessment

    a. Assessment findings—related to the degree of bone marrow failure

      (1) Petechiae from decreased platelets

      (2) Ecchymosis and pallor

      (3) Fatigue

(4) Recurrent infections

(5) Bleeding: epistaxis is more common

   b. Diagnostic procedures

      (1) Laboratory studies

         (a) CBC—reveals macrocytic anemia

         (b) Platelets—decreased count

      (2) Diagnostic studies: bone marrow aspiration and biopsy; reveal replacement of red bone marrow by fatty, yellow marrow

  6. Therapeutic management

    a. Medications

      (1) Globulins: antilymphocyte globulin (ALG) and antithymocyte gloulin (ATG)

      (2) Androgen therapy: to stimulate erythropoiesis

      (3) Immunosuppressive agents: cyclophosphamide (Cytoxan)

      (4) Cyclosporine: for those who do not respond to ATG

    b. Treatments

      (1) Total body irradiation or thoracoabdominal irradiation

      (2) Transfusion of blood products

      (3) Bone marrow transplantation

  7. Nursing management and evaluation: refer to nursing care of the child with leukemia, p. 414

IV. Hemophilia

A. Description: a group of blood coagulation disorders that are related to a clotting factor deficiency

  1. Two common forms of hemophilia

    a. Hemophilia A (classic)—deficiency of factor VIII

    b. Hemophilia B (Christmas disease)—deficiency of factor IX

  2. Classified into three groups, according to the severity of factor deficiency: severe, moderate, and mild

  3. Hemophilia A accounts for 75% of all cases

B. Mode of transmission

  1. Transmitted as an X-linked recessive disorder

  2. Frequent pattern of transmission is between an unaffected male and a female who carries the trait for hemophilia

C. Incidence: occurs almost always in males: incidence is 1 in 10,000 male births

D. Pathophysiology

  1. Factors VIII and IX are the plasma proteins necessary for the formation of fibrin clots at the site of vascular injury

  2. Prolonged bleeding into any body tissue marks the disease

E. Assessment

  1. Assessment findings

    a. In infancy

      (1) Prolonged bleeding after circumcision

      (2) Ecchymoses over bony prominences

   a. Throughout life
    (1) Subcutaneous hemorrhages
    (2) Hemarthrosis—bleeding into a joint
    (3) Frequent bruising and bleeding
    (4) Joint pain and stiffness
    (5) Epistaxis
    (6) Bleeding from oral mucosa
   b. Complications
    (1) Airway obstruction from bleeding into the oral cavity or the thorax
    (2) Hepatitis from factor replacement
    (3) AIDS
    (4) Muscle atrophy from hemarthrosis
  2. Diagnostic procedures: laboratory studies
   a. Factor assay—reveals deficiency in clotting factors VIII and IX to confirm the diagnosis
   b. Coagulation tests: increased activated partial thromboplastin time (aPTT), increased thrombin-clotting time
   c. Coagulation screening: decreased platelet count, increased bleeding time
   d. Thromboplastin generation test: reveals the ability to generate thromboplastin
   e. Prenatal diagnosis possible through amniocentesis; carrier detection possible with the use of DNA testing

F. Therapeutic management
  1. Medications
   a. Analgesics and antipyretics: to control pain and lower temperature
   b. Nonsteroidal anti-inflammatory drugs (NSAIDs): to decrease inflammation of hemarthrosis
   c. Corticosteroids: to control hematuria, hemarthrosis, and chronic synovitis
   d. Epsilon-aminocaproic acid: to prevent clot destruction; for use in trauma or oral surgery
  2. Treatment: factor replacement—administer plasma products such as factor VIII concentrate, DDAVP (1-deamino-8-D-arginine vasopressin), and fresh frozen plasma

G. Nursing management
  1. Nursing diagnoses: risk for injury related to hemorrhage
  2. Expected outcomes
   a. Prevention of bleeding by avoidance of trauma
   b. Child receives prompt, appropriate care should bleeding occur
  3. Interventions
   a. Administer factor replacement or other products such as (DDAVP) as ordered

   b. Inform parents of the need for selected medical and age-appropriate exercise regimens to strengthen muscles and joints
   c. Apply pressure to the site of injury for at least 15 minutes
   d. Elevate the bleeding site above the level of the heart for 12 to 24 hours; immobilize the affected limb
   e. Place cold compresses to promote vasoconstriction
   f. Monitor the child's factor VIII and PTT levels at least once daily
   g. Encourage selection of iron-rich foods: provide sample menus, a food list, and dietary consultation
4. Nursing diagnoses
   a. Pain related to bleeding into tissues
   b. Risk for impaired physical mobility related to joint hemorrhage
5. Expected outcomes
   a. Child verbalizes absence or control of pain
   b. Child maintains optimal mobility within limitations of the disease, with an absence of immobility complications
6. Interventions
   a. Assess for joint pain, swelling, and decreased range of motion
   b. Assess mobility status: joint mobility, pain, stiffness, swelling, muscle tone, and assisted daily living
   c. Assess for complications of immobility
   d. Administer nonaspirin analgesics, such as acetaminophen as ordered
   e. Immobilize the affected extremity; apply ice to the painful area
   f. Use a bed cradle over the affected extremity
   g. Provide opportunities for age-appropriate activities, within activity restrictions
   h. Provide active and range-of-motion exercises every 2 to 4 hours, as needed
   i. Exercise unaffected joints to maintain mobility

⚠ **Warning!**

Passive range-of-motion exercises are never performed after the acute phase of a bleeding episode to avoid any stretching of the joint capsule. Active range-of-motion exercises allow the client to control pain tolerance.

H. Evaluation
1. Questions to ask parents
   a. In preparation for home care, what other information or resources do you need?
   b. Which findings do you need to monitor and which need to be reported to the physician?

2. Behaviors to observe
   a. Child verbalizes reduction or absence of pain
   b. Child participates in assisted daily living with an absence of immobility complications
3. Evaluation of expected outcomes
   a. Parents report signs of bleeding to the physician or clinic
   b. Parents state measures to prevent trauma and bleeding episodes
   c. Parents properly adhere to the protocol for administration of concentrates or plasma protein

V. Leukemia

A. **Description: term given to a group of malignant diseases of the blood-forming tissue and lymphatics; characterized by** *proliferation of immature WBCs* **in the bone marrow**
B. **Classification**
   1. Classification is determined by the prevalent cell type and level of maturity using these terms:
      a. Lympho—refers to lymphoid or the lymphatic system
      b. Myelo—refers to involvement of the bone marrow
      c. Blastic and acute—involves immature cells
      d. Cystic and chronic—involves mature cells
   2. Two common childhood forms
      a. Acute lymphocytic leukemia (ALL): divided into 3 subtypes
      b. Acute nonlymphocytic leukemia (ANLL) or acute myelocytic leukemia (AML): divided into 7 subtypes
C. **Etiology and incidence**
   1. The peak onset is between 2 and 6 years of age
   2. The most common form of childhood cancer, ALL accounts for one third of cancers in white children
D. **Pathophysiology** (Figure 14-2)
   1. Immature WBCs proliferate and invade various organs of the body, particularly the vascular organs, liver, and spleen
   2. Immature cells (or "blasts") compete with normal cells for nutrients and depress bone marrow function to cause:
      a. Anemia—from decreased RBCs
      b. Infection—from neutropenia
      c. Bleeding tendencies—from decreased platelets
E. **Assessment**
   1. Assessment findings
      a. From the invasion of bone marrow
         (1) Infection
         (2) Blood in urine and emesis
         (3) Bone pain; bones weaken with results of fractures
         (4) Fever
         (5) Poor wound healing
         (6) Pallor

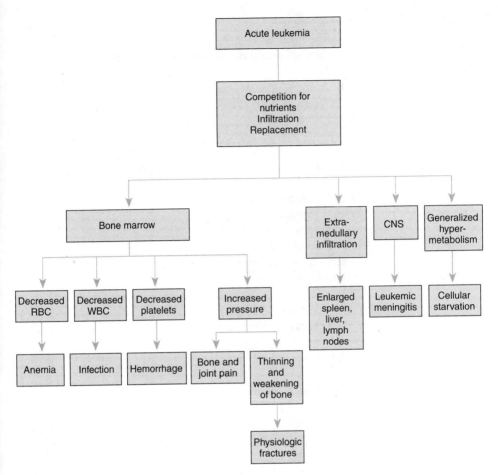

Figure 14-2   Principal sites of tissue involvement in leukemia. (From Wong DL, et al: *Whaley and Wong's nursing care of infants and children,* ed 6, St. Louis, 1999, Mosby.)

      (7) Fatigue
      (8) Epistaxis
      (9) Abdominal pain
    (10) Petechiae
  b. From the infiltration of organs
      (1) Hepatosplenomegaly
      (2) CNS: headache, vomiting, increased ICP, lower extremity weakness
2. Diagnostic procedures
  a. Laboratory tests
      (1) Peripheral blood smear—contains immature WBCs
      (2) CBC—reveals anemia, neutropenia, and thrombocytopenia; done weekly or monthly during maintenance therapy

    b. Diagnostic studies
      (1) Lumbar puncture—assesses CNS involvement
      (2) Bone marrow aspiration—reveals the presence of blast cells
      (3) Bone scan—assesses the degree of bone involvement
      (4) CT scan—reveals the degree of organ involvement

F. Therapeutic management
1. Medications: chemotherapeutic agents, with or without cranial radiation (Table 14-1). The four phases are:
    a. For induction: to decrease the leukemic cells and to achieve remission
      (1) IV vincristine and L-asparaginase
      (2) Oral prednisone
    b. For intensification or consolidation: to treat the leukemic cells that have invaded the child's body
      (1) High dose methotrexate, L-aspariginase, cytarabine, and intermediate-dose methotrexate
      (2) IV agents given during first 6 months of treatment
    c. Prophylactic for CNS of high-risk children
      (1) Intrathecal hydrocortisone
      (2) Intrathecal methotrexate
      (3) Intrathecal cytarabine
    d. For maintenance to preserve remission
      (1) Oral 6-mercaptopurine daily
      (2) Weekly IM methotrexate
2. Additional medications: anti-gout agents—allopurinol (Zyloprim): to control the severity of hyperuricemia during chemotherapy at any level of therapy
3. Treatments: radiation in combination with chemotherapy, as outlined above; bone marrow transplantation

G. Nursing management
1. Nursing diagnoses
    a. Alteration in nutrition (less than body requirements) related to nausea, vomiting and decreased appetite associated with chemotherapy
    b. Altered oral mucous membranes, impaired skin integrity
    c. Risk for infection
2. Expected outcomes
    a. Child has minimal or absent side effects from chemotherapy, commonly nausea and vomiting
    b. Child is protected from exposure to pathogenic organisms
    c. Child's oral mucous membranes remain intact
3. Interventions
    a. Use good hand-washing technique before and after contact with the child
    b. Assess the child for the side effects of chemotherapy

Text continued on p. 417

TABLE 14-1 Commonly Used Chemotherapeutic Agents in Pediatrics

Medication and Route	Indications	Side Effects	Nursing Implications
Actinomycin-D Route: IV	Wilms tumor Ewing's sarcoma	Nausea, vomiting, diarrhea Stomatitis Alopecia Thrombocytopenia	Monitor IV infusion to avoid extravasation Monitor vital signs and assess for signs of infection Assess oral mucosa and hemetest stools
Cytosine arabinoside (Cytarabine) Route: IV, IM, intrathecal	ALL ANLL Prophylaxis CNS therapy	Nausea, vomiting, anorexia Stomatitis Rash, alopecia Hyperuricemia Hepatitis	Monitor for drug toxicity and infection Monitor liver and kidney function test results: ALT, SGOT, creatinine Observe for fluid and electrolyte imbalances
Dacarbazine (DTIC) Route: IV	Neuroblastoma Ewing's sarcoma	Nausea, vomiting Myelosuppression Fatigue, malaise	Monitor infusion to avoid extravasation Administer IV fluids to avoid imbalances Monitor vital signs and observe for infection
L-asparaginase (Elspar) Route: IM, IV	ALL induction	Nausea, vomiting Headache, fever Anaphylaxis Liver function impairment Toxicity: liver dysfunction, hyperglycemia, renal failure, pancreatitis	Observe for 30-60 min on initiating medication for signs of anaphylaxis Monitor liver function test results Check daily weight
Mercaptopurine (6-MP) Route: PO, IV	ALL maintenance therapy	Nausea, vomiting Leukopenia GI ulceration, anorexia Rash, pigmentation	Assess baseline liver function test results Observe for signs of infection Recommend good oral hygiene Observe for signs of bleeding

Continued

TABLE 14-1	Commonly Used Chemotherapeutic Agents in Pediatrics—cont'd		
Medication and Route	**Indications**	**Side Effects**	**Nursing Implications**
Methotrexate Route: PO, IV, IM, intrathecal	ALL	Nausea, vomiting Photosensitivity Myelosuppression Hepatotoxicity (on high-dose therapy)	Assess baseline hepatic function test results Avoid vitamins, tetracycline, phenytoin (Dilantin), chloramphenicol Avoid exposure to ultraviolet light
Prednisone Route: PO	ALL maintenance therapy	Weight gain Cushing's states Hypertension Impaired wound healing Increased appetite	Obtain baseline height and weight Report any sudden weight gain Teach not to stop drug abruptly Encourage diet low in sodium
Vincristine Route: IV	ALL maintenance therapy Neuroblastoma	Neurotoxicity Constipation Leukopenia Alopecia Paralytic ileus Fever	Assess baseline CBC and bilirubin Monitor input and output, weight Assess neurologic status Assess vital signs Assess bowel elimination
Cyclophosphamide (Cytoxan, CTX) Route: PO, IV, IM	ALL, Wilm's tumor, Ewing's sarcoma	Nausea, vomiting Gross hematuria Immunosuppression	Force fluids Encourage frequent voiding Teach to report symptoms of burning on urination, hematuria

c. Administer an antiemetic 30 minutes before chemotherapy is given; an antiemetic is commonly continued for up to 1 day after the chemotherapy has been completed

d. Assess the oral mucosa for pain, ulcers, lesions, stomatitis, and any effects on changes in eating patterns

e. Assess for bleeding from any orifice; check urine and stool for blood; monitor platelet, WBC, H&H, and neutrophil counts

f. Assess for signs of infection

g. Provide mouth rinses and a soft toothbrush; apply topical xylocaine, as ordered, before eating

h. Provide a nutritionally complete diet for age and a diet based on the child's preferences

i. Isolate the child from persons with upper respiratory or other infections

4. Nursing diagnosis: body-image disturbance related to hair loss and other physical changes

5. Expected outcomes

a. Child adapts to limitations of a chronic illness

b. Parents seek out social services and psychological counseling as necessary

6. Interventions

a. Assess the family for feelings about a chronic illness with encouragement to express concerns about lifestyle changes

b. Provide privacy

c. Observe the child for signs of withdrawal, regression, and other behavioral changes

d. Prepare the family and child for body appearance changes

e. Encourage the family to allow the child to participate in safe peer activities

H. Evaluation

1. Questions to ask parents

a. Which changes will be made in your lifestyle?

b. How have you prepared for long-term care?

2. Behaviors to observe

a. Child participates in appropriate school and peer activities

b. Parents seek out social services or other resources

c. Parents and child exhibit behaviors to prevent breakdown of the oral mucosa

3. Evaluation of expected outcomes

a. Family verbalizes feelings about a chronic disorder, with discussion of long-term implications in positive terms

b. Child's oral mucosa remains intact

VI. Acquired immune deficiency syndrome (AIDS)

A. Description: disorder caused by HIV type 1 and characterized by a generalized dysfunction of the immune system

B. **Etiology: the causative agent, HIV, is present in blood and body fluids: semen, saliva, tears, vaginal secretions, and breast milk**
C. **Incidence**
   1. AIDS is the ninth leading cause of death in children between 1 and 4 years of age, and the seventh leading cause of death in adolescents and young adults between 15 and 24 years of age
   2. The current risk groups in pediatrics include recipients of multiple transfusions (hemophiliacs) and newborns of affected mothers
D. **Pathophysiology**
   1. HIV infects the CD_4 T-lymphocytes, which are responsible for cellular immunity, and may lie dormant or may proliferate; HIV then inactivates the immunity of that cell
   2. In pediatric AIDS, abnormal B-cell function is present early in the course of the disease. Thus, both cellular and humoral immunity are compromised.
   3. HIV attacks the macrophage and uses the cell to cross the blood-brain barrier
   4. Horizontal transmission of HIV is through contact with blood or body fluids and intimate sexual contact; vertical transmission occurs when HIV-infected woman passes infection to her infant
E. **Assessment**
   1. Assessment findings (Box 14-1)
      a. Infants: perinatally affected
         (1) T-lymphocytes infected by HIV
         (2) Hepatosplenomegaly
         (3) Opportunistic infections
         (4) Progressive encephalopathy
         (5) Microcephaly

Box 14-1
Common AIDS-Defining Conditions in Children

Pneumocystis carinii pneumonia
Lymphoid interstitial pneumonitis
Recurrent bacterial infections
Wasting syndrome
Candida esophagitis
HIV encephalopathy
Cytomegalovirus
Mycobacterium avium-intracellulare complex infection
Pulmonary candidiasis
Herpes simplex disease
Cryptosporidiosis

From Wong DL, et al: *Whaley and Wong's Nursing care of infants and children,* ed 6, St. Louis, 1999, Mosby.

    b. Infants: infected during the neonatal period
      (1) Failure to thrive
      (2) Developmental delays
      (3) Oral candidiasis
      (4) Diarrhea
      (5) Hepatosplenomegaly
      (6) Chronic interstitial pneumonia and cough
      (7) Chronic otitis media
    c. Children and adolescents
      (1) Malaise
      (2) Fatigue
      (3) Night sweats
      (4) Weight loss
      (5) Diarrhea
      (6) Fever
      (7) Regression of developmental milestones
      (8) Generalized lymphadenopathy
      (9) Nephropathy
      (10) Interstitial pneumonitis and *Pneumocystis carinii* pneumonia
      (11) Encephalopathy
  2. Diagnostic procedures: laboratory studies
    a. Enzyme-Linked Immunosorbent Assay (ELISA)—determines the response of antibodies to the HIV virus
    b. Western blot immunoassay—confirms the presence of HIV antibodies
    c. CBC—reveals an increased WBC with infection; decreased helper T cells
    d. Virus culture and polymerase chain reaction (PCR)—detects proviral DNA

F. Therapeutic management: medications
  1. Antiretrovirals—nucleoside reverse transcriptase inhibitors, nonnucleoside reverse transcriptase inhibitors and protease inhibitors
  2. Antibiotics—trimethoprim (TMP)/sulfamethoxazole (SMZ) (Bactrim Co-Trimoxzole, or Septra) to treat opportunistic infections (see Table 17-2, p. 507)
  3. Gamma globulin—to compensate for B-lymphocyte deficiency
  4. Immunizations: inactivated poliovirus (IPV) is given in the regular immunization schedule; varicella vaccination not given

G. Nursing management
  1. Nursing diagnosis: risk for infection
  2. Expected outcomes
    a. Child's risk of future infections is reduced
    b. Family verbalizes risk factors regarding disease acquisition and transmission

3. Interventions
   a. Provide a private room, avoiding exposure of the child to other illnesses
   b. Wash hands before entering and after leaving the room
   c. Assess for fever, malaise, fatigue, weight loss, vomiting and diarrhea, altered activity level, oral lesions, rash, and purulent drainage
   d. Wear gloves for care, especially when in contact with body fluids and when changing diapers
   e. Label contaminated articles and dispose of them according to hospital policy and Centers for Disease Control guidelines
   f. Administer immunizations, as ordered
   g. Administer antibiotics, as ordered
4. Nursing diagnosis: altered nutrition—less than body requirements
5. Expected outcome: child regains optimal nutritional status
6. Interventions
   a. Document child's weight with comparison to previous weight
   b. Assess oral cavity for the presence of *Candida albicans*
   c. Assess dietary and fluid intake and output
   d. Monitor serum and urine electrolytes, albumin, and glucose
   e. Provide a high-calorie, high-protein diet
   f. Administer dietary supplements or TPN as ordered
   g. Administer medications to treat *Candida albicans* infection

H. **Evaluation**
1. Questions to ask parents
   a. What are your plans for school and for social and home activities?
   b. What are your concerns about long-term needs and medications?
2. Behaviors to observe
   a. Child participates in family and peer activities
   b. Child attends school within limitations of the disease and treatment
3. Evaluation of expected outcomes
   a. Child remains free of opportunistic infections
   b. Family and child exhibit a reduction in anxiety and feelings of isolation
   c. Family seeks assistance from support group

VII. Home care: family education topics and referrals
A. **Sickle cell anemia (SCA)**
1. Disease process: causes of SCA; anatomy and physiology of RBCs; methods to prevent crises: avoid exposure to low oxygen tension and cold temperatures; and prognosis
2. Fluids: specific quantities of fluids needed to maintain hydration

3. Medication: proper method of antibiotic administration; the importance of routine immunizations, including pneumococcal and meningococcal vaccines

4. Safety: teach parents to protect child from known sources of infection and to report signs of infection to the physician without delay; stress measures to avoid sickling, and review signs of an impending crisis: fever, pallor, severe chest pain, respiratory distress, and seizure activity

5. Referrals: genetic counseling services; screening of family members; comprehensive sickle cell treatment clinic, Sickle Cell Disease Association

B. Hemophilia

1. Diet: encourage selection of iron-rich foods: provide sample menus, food list, importance of staying within the recommended weight guidelines

2. Blood factor replacement therapy: venipuncture technique; proper time and method of antihemolytic factor (AHF) administration

3. Safety: teach parents to recognize the symptoms of bleeding: pain, swelling, limited joint motion; inform parents of safety precautions for child: wearing medical identification, avoiding contact sports and aspirin-containing products, and wearing protective equipment; supportive measures when bleeding episode occurs; complications associated with hemarthrosis

4. Hygiene: use of soft toothbrush soaked in warm water before use; electric razor for shaving

5. Mobility: an exercise program; encourage participation in noncontact sports

6. Referrals: National Hemophilia Foundation; dietary consultation; genetic counseling; physical therapist; public health nurse

C. Leukemia

1. Safety: teach preventive measures such as hand washing, avoiding exposure to crowds and known sources of chicken pox; report signs of infection, mucosal irritation, hemorrhagic cystitis, and severe vomiting; avoid live virus vaccines

2. Activity: encourage participation in safe peer activities

3. Psychosocial: prepare the family and child for body appearance changes; observe the child for signs of withdrawal, regression, or other behavioral changes, encourage family and child to express concerns about lifestyle changes; maintain peer contacts to ease school re-entry

4. Referrals: social services and psychological counseling as necessary

D. HIV and AIDS

1. Disease process: protective measures to prevent infection: hand washing, avoidance of handling bodily fluids, use of gloves during diaper changes, use of bleach solution as a disinfectant—a 1:10 ratio of bleach to water

2. Safety: avoid exposure to known sources of infection; contact health professional immediately if exposed to childhood illness; provide peers and school personnel with information about the mode of transmission and safe activities
3. Activity: Encourage participation in family and school activities as much as possible
4. Diet: high in calories and protein
5. Referrals: home health care nursing service, local AIDS support groups, social service agencies

WEB Resources

www.pedhivaids.org
National Pediatric and Family Resource Center sponsored by the University of Medicine and Dentistry of New Jersey. Provides updates on medications and scientific information; serves professionals who care for children, and adolescents and families with HIV and AIDS. Includes recent publications, videos, and educational materials.

www.bmtinfo.org/html.htm
Provides information from experts in stem cell transmission.

www.oncolink.upenn.edu/disease/index_ped.html
Sponsored by University of Pennsylvania cancer specialists; includes information on Wilms tumor and neuroblastoma.

www.cdc.gov/nip/recs/child-schedule.pdf
This site provides the latest immunization schedule for infants and children. It also provides access to specific information on immunizations.

REVIEW QUESTIONS

1. A child with leukemia complains of fatigue. The nurse assesses the skin color as pallor. Considering the child's diagnosis, which of these laboratory results explains these assessment findings?
   1. Cerebrospinal fluid with elevated WBCs
   2. Hemoglobin of 8 g/dl
   3. Platelet count of 150,000/mm^3
   4. Serum sodium level of 130

2. A 9-year-old with sickle cell anemia has been hospitalized in vaso-occlusive crisis. Because the child complains of painful joints, which of these actions should the nurse take to promote the child's comfort?
   1. Apply ice compresses and elevate the affected extremities
   2. Apply heat packs and administer an ordered analgesic
   3. Provide cold compresses and administer aspirin
   4. Provide heat packs and passive range-of-motion exercises

3. To promote optimal functioning of a 14-year-old with hemophilia who has hemoarthrosis, the nurse's best action would be which of these?
   1. Elevate and immobilize the affected joint
   2. Institute active range-of-motion exercises to the affected joint during the acute phase
   3. Apply pressure to the area as needed
   4. Apply warm compresses to the affected joint

4. Which of these nursing diagnoses should receive priority during a vaso-occlusive crisis in a 15-year-old with sickle cell anemia?
   1. Decreased cardiac output (CO)
   2. Ineffective individual coping
   3. Alteration in comfort
   4. Ineffective airway clearance

5. Which of these instructions should the parents of a child who has recovered from a sickle cell crisis receive?
   1. Avoid contact with all children
   2. Isolate the child from known sources of infection
   3. Restrict the child's intake during the night
   4. Reinforce the basics of trait transmission

ANSWERS, RATIONALES, AND TEST-TAKING TIPS

Rationales	Test-Taking Tips

1. Correct answer: 2

In leukemia, bone marrow is infiltrated with proliferative immature cells. Decreased RBC production results in decreased hemoglobin and a diagnosis of anemia. The finding in option 1 is consistent with meningitis. This platelet count is within normal range, with a minimum of 150,000/mm³. A decreased platelet count, *thrombocytopenia,* has findings of bleeding or hemorrhage. A high count, *thrombocytosis,* has findings of clot formation such as thrombophlebitis of the legs or cerebral infarcts. A decrease in the serum sodium does not result in pallor or fatigue. Clinical findings of low serum sodium include confusion, hostility, and agitation.

Classic clinical findings of skin pallor, fatigue, and SOB are consistent with a diagnosis of anemia. Associate Leukemia with Little number values of substances produced in the bone marrow. In leukemia the bone marrow is busy producing massive volumes of immature WBCs. Thus, it has exhausted it ability to produce normal levels of RBCs, platelets, and mature WBCs. The results are decreased H&H and platelet counts and decreased mature WBCs, but an increase in immature white cells that results in a high white blood count.

2. Correct answer: 2

Pain management during a crisis includes analgesics, initial acetaminophen, and application of heat. Cold or ice compresses are not applied to the area because cold enhances the sickling of RBCs and local vasoconstriction, which promotes local hypoxia. Passive range-of-motion exercises promote circulation. However, the child's activity tolerance will dictate whether passive exercises are possible. Because the information given in the stem indicates the child is in pain, exercises are contraindicated.

Did you note that these are two-part options? Did you avoid selection of a wrong answer by reading the second part of the option first and the first part second? On reading the first part of each option, you see that you must decide between heat and cold. Then, read the second part of the options for clues. You must decide among these actions—to elevate, medicate, or move the extremity. Your common sense tells you not to move something that is hurting, so eliminate option 4. The information in the stem doesn't identify specific joints. Thus, option 1 is not a good choice. The

remaining two options indicate
medication for pain, which is a
correct action. Eliminate option 3
with aspirin because the client is a
child with an unknown cause of the
crisis, which could be a virus.

3. Correct answer: 1

During bleeding episodes, the joint
is elevated and immobilized to
prevent the crippling effects of
joint degeneration, which is a
specific problem with
hemarthrosis. Active
range-of-motion exercises are
begun *after* the acute phase.
Option 3 is too general to be
correct. Pressure to the area
must be applied for at least 10
minutes to allow for clot
formation. Cold instead of warm
packs or compresses are used to
promote vasoconstriction to stop
or minimize the bleeding.

Apply the basic principles for the care
of an injured or damaged extremity,
no matter what the cause—elevate
and immobilize. A clue in the stem
is "to promote optimal functioning."

4. Correct answer: 3

Vaso-occlusive crises are the result
of sickled cells that obstruct
blood vessels, and cause
occlusion of them, especially in
the joints. The results are
ischemia and necrosis. The
affected extremities are most
painful during the acute sickle
cell crisis. Comfort is a priority.
The nursing diagnoses in options
1 and 4 are inappropriate during
vaso-occlusive crisis. There is
insufficient data in option 2 to
support it as a nursing diagnosis.

Key words in the stem are
"vaso-occlusive crisis." Associate
this crisis with other conditions in
which there is occlusion of a vessel,
such as angina. This leads to the
selection of option 3, which is also
a priority for the client with angina.

5. Correct answer: 2

Infection is the major predisposing
factor in the development of a
sickle cell crisis. During the
infection and stress of the crisis,

Eliminate option 1, because it contains
the absolute term "all." This action
would be impossible to achieve.
Eliminate option 3, because there

Rationales	Test-Taking Tips
the body's immune system is compromised. The parents should understand the need to isolate the child from known sources of infection for at least a few weeks after hospitalization, until the immune system has recovered. Parents also must balance the developmental needs of the child and model living a normal life. Hydration is necessary for hemodilution, which prevents sickling. Fluids are not restricted. The action in option 4 is an appropriate intervention after the initial diagnosis when the child is old enough to understand the sickle cell disease process.	are only a few clinical events in which fluids are restricted—increased ICP, renal failure, and wetting the bed at night. Options 2 and 4 sound like good choices. One way to select the correct answer is to reread the stem. Note that an age is not given. Therefore, option 4 is probably incorrect. An age of the child would give you the clue for the ability of the child to understand. A second step is to select option 2 because it is a physiologic need, which has priority over the psychosocial need of option 4.

15

Nursing Care of Children with Respiratory Disorders

FAST FACTS

1. Postural drainage is performed before meals and at bedtime.
2. A positive sweat test is diagnostic for cystic fibrosis.
3. The therapeutic theophylline level is 10 to 20 μg/ml.
4. The most common upper respiratory tract infections are characterized as croup syndromes: acute laryngotracheobronchitis, acute spasmodic laryngitis, and acute epiglottitis.
5. Common infections of the lower airway include bacterial tracheitis, asthmatic bronchitis, bronchitis, bronchiolitis, and pneumonia.
6. Aspiration is more common into the right main stem bronchus and into the right middle lobe.
7. The consistency of sputum, that is, thick or sticky, is more important than its color.
8. The eustachian tube lies more horizontally and is shorter, wider, and straighter in infants, increasing the risk for infection that peaks between 6 months and 2 years of age.

CONTENT REVIEW

I. Respiratory system overview
A. Structure
1. The respiratory system is composed of these parts
   a. Upper respiratory tract (URT)
      (1) Nose—serves to filter and moisten air
      (2) Pharynx—contains tonsils; responsible for phonation

b. Considered either upper or lower respiratory tract:
   (1) Larynx—cartilaginous framework that contains the glottis and epiglottis
   (2) Trachea—smooth muscle structure supported by rings of cartilage. It divides into two primary bronchi, the left and right. The right is more vertical, with more frequent occurrences of aspiration than the left, which is more horizontal in position.
c. Lower respiratory tract, which is the reactive portion
   (1) Bronchial tree—divides into secondary bronchi as they enter the lung, which further divide into bronchioles
   (2) Lungs—mainly consists of alveoli
   (3) Lobes—the right lung has three lobes, and the left has two
2. Alveoli, the sites of gas exchange, are located within the lobules of the lungs. The space up to the alveoli is called *dead space*— meaning no gas exchange takes place.
3. Pulmonary capillaries surround the alveoli
4. The medulla oblongata maintains neurocontrol of breathing
5. The pulmonary and bronchial arteries supply blood to the lungs
6. The phrenic nerve innervates the diaphragm, the major muscle of respiration

B. Functions
1. The two primary functions of the respiratory structures are to supply oxygen to the cells and remove carbon dioxide, the end product of metabolism
2. The URT allows air into the lower respiratory tract; the URT purifies and humidifies the air
3. The mechanism of gas exchange occurs across the alveolar membrane to the pulmonary capillaries
4. The lungs serve as a buffering mechanism for alteration of carbon dioxide to maintain acid-base balance and provide a quick process to adapt to changes within minutes
5. Gas exchange occurs as result of three processes
   a. Ventilation—inspiration and expiration
   b. Diffusion—movement of gases across alveolar membrane that is dependent on the pressure gradient from areas of high to low concentration
   c. Perfusion—oxygenated blood is transported from the lungs to the body tissues at the capillary level

C. Pediatric considerations
1. Major anatomic differences that affect the ways infants and children respond to respiratory pathology
   a. Peripheral airways narrowly branch and cause easier airway obstruction
   b. Less alveolar area is available for gas exchange

    c. The eustachian tube lies more horizontally and is shorter, wider, and straighter in infants, increasing the risk of infection that peaks between 6 months and 2 years of age

    d. Right bronchi is straighter

D. Assessment

  1. Health history

    a. Focus of general questions

      (1) Home environment, including possible allergens; exposure to environmental hazards, chemicals, dust, animals, and cigarette smoke

      (2) Activity: exposure to respiratory infections; travel to a foreign country

      (3) Medications: current medications for breathing difficulties, allergy problems, ear infections, and sore throats

    b. Present health questions about the presence of these findings

      (1) Coughing

      (2) SOB

      (3) Tightness in the chest

      (4) Nasal congestion with a runny nose, and noisy respirations

      (5) Difficulty breathing

      (6) Apnea

      (7) Sudden onset of difficulty breathing, grunting with respirations, nasal flaring, and sternal or intercostals retractions indicate acute respiratory distress: call an ambulance or get the child to the nearest emergency room

    c. Medical history

      (1) Low birth weight (LBW); prematurity; use of ventilation-assistance devices

      (2) Thoracic surgery

      (3) Previous hospitalizations for pulmonary disease

      (4) Hyperactive airway disease

      (5) Chronic pulmonary disorders: cystic fibrosis (CF) and TB

      (6) Daily exposure to second-hand cigarette smoke

    d. Family history of TB, CF, allergy, atopic dermatitis, or smoking

  2. Physical examination

    a. Examination of the anterior and posterior chest

      (1) Breathing pattern and effort

      (2) RR and respiratory depth

      (3) Chest movement with breathing—use of accessory muscles, retractions

      (4) Skin color and chest wall configuration

    b. Palpate the chest for thoracic expansion, tactile fremitus, crepitus (grating sensation), and soreness

    c. Auscultate the chest for quality of and abnormal breath sounds, and vocal resonance in older children

    d. Nasal passage
      (1) Drainage
        (a) Consistency: if thick and sticky, it is more characteristic of infection
        (b) Color: clear is normal; white may indicate allergies; and yellow or greenish may indicate bacterial infection
      (2) Nasal flaring
  3. Diagnostic procedures
    a. Laboratory studies—CBC; arterial blood gases; sputum culture and sensitivity, sputum for acid-fast bacilli, which is specific for active TB; and throat culture and sensitivity (C&S)
    b. Diagnostic studies—pulmonary function study, chest x-ray film, oximetry, and bronchoscopy
 E. **Medications** (Table 15-1)

II. Infections and croup syndromes of the URT
 A. **Otitis media**
  1. Description: middle ear infection caused by bacteria or a virus; a very common disorder of early childhood
  2. Classified as acute otitis media (AOM) or otitis media with effusion (OME)
  3. Etiology and incidence
    a. Half of all children experience otitis media by 1 year of age
    b. Causative organisms of AOM: *Streptococcus pneumoniae* and *Haemophilus influenzae*
    c. The peak incidence is between 6 months and 2 years of age; occurs in winter months
  4. Pathophysiology
    a. Malfunction or obstruction of the eustachian tube causes fluid collection in the middle ear, negative middle ear pressure, and resulting effusion
    b. Factors that predispose young children to develop otitis media
      (1) The anatomic position of the eustachian tube: shorter, wider, and straighter
      (2) Undeveloped cartilage lining
      (3) Immature humoral defense system
      (4) Feeding position encourages the pooling of fluids and formula in the pharyngeal cavity
      (5) Environmental factors: passive smoking, daycare attendance
    c. Complications of otitis media: chronic otitis media, hearing loss, meningitis, eardrum perforation and scarring, *cholesteatoma* (cystic mass in the middle ear)
  5. Assessment
    a. Assessment findings
      (1) AOM
        (a) Fever, with temperature usually around 104° F (rectal), or 106° F (axillary)

TABLE 15-1 Commonly Used Pulmonary Medications for Children

Medication Route and Dosage	Indications	Side Effects	Nursing Implications
Bronchodilator			
Theophylline	Bronchial asthma	CNS: insomnia, agitation, tremors*	Administer with food to decrease GI upset
	Chronic bronchitis	GI: anorexia, nausea*, vomiting	Assess respiratory status
Route: oral	Emphysema	Hepatic: jaundice, hepatitis	Monitor daily serum drug levels
Liquid, sustained release tablets, capsules		Genitourinary: urinary retention	(10-20 μg/ml); toxicity: >20 μg/ml) or if symptoms persist
		Integumentary: rash, erythema	Parent teaching:
Dosage (maintenance):		CV: prolonged PR intervals, postural hypotension, tachycardia, hypertension	Administer at same time daily to maintain levels
Age 1-9 yr: up to 20 mg/kg/day			Report any CNS, CV, or GI side effects to physician
Age 9-16 yr: up to 16 mg/kg/day			
Salmeterol (Serevent)	Long-term prevention of asthma symptoms in children >12 yr	CNS: nervousness, restlessness, tremor	Not to be used for exacerbations
		CV: rapid HR, increased systolic BP	
Route:	Exercise-induced bronchospasm	Respiratory: pharyngitis, cough	
Inhalation			
Dosage:			
MDI: 2 puffs q 12			
Dry powder inhaler: 1 blister q 12			

*Common toxic effects

Continued

TABLE 15-1 Commonly Used Pulmonary Medications for Children—cont'd

Medication Route and Dosage	Indications	Side Effects	Nursing Implications
Beta-Adrenergic, Selective Beta₂-Agonist Metaproterenol (Alupent, Metaprel) Route: oral; syrup, tablets, MDI Dosage: Aged <6 yr: 1.3-2.6 mg/kg/day (syrup) Aged 6-9 yr: 10 mg qid (tablets) >9 yrs: 20 mg tid or qid >12 yr: MDI 2-3 inhalations q 3-4 hr; maximum 12 inhalations/day Nebulizer solution (5%) 0.3 ml in 2.5 ml NS q 4-6 hr	Bronchial asthma Bronchospasm	CNS: tremors, insomnia CV: tachycardia, dysrhythmia GI: nausea, vomiting	Assess respiratory status Do not crush tablet Shake canister well; wait 2 minutes before second inhalation Parent teaching: Proper usage and care of inhaler or spacer Have child demonstrate use of inhaler on return visit Inhaler should not be used more frequently than prescribed

Beta₂ Agonists

Drug	Uses	Side Effects	Nursing Considerations
Terbutaline (Brethine, Brethaire) Route: oral; tablets, MDI Dosage: >12 yrs: 2.5-5 mg tid (tablets) MDI: 2 inhalations (400 µg) q 4-6 hr Nebulizer or SC solution: 0.25 mg q 15-30 min	Asthma Emphysema	CNS: nervousness, lethargy, headache CV: palpitations, tachycardia, dysrhythmias GI: nausea, vomiting Sensory: dry nose and mouth, tinnitus	Assess respiratory status and baseline HR Do not crush time-released tablets Mix regular tablets with small amounts of food or fluid Parent teaching: Correct inhalation or injection technique Do not exceed dosage Do not use with other inhalants

Mast Cell Stabilizer

Drug	Uses	Side Effects	Nursing Considerations
Cromolyn sodium (Intal) Route: Inhalation Dosage: MDI: 2 puffs qid Spinhaler: 20 mg Intal capsules qid Nebulizer solution (20 mg/2 ml ampule): 1 ampule qid	Long-term control of asthma Prevents acute asthma attacks. It is a prophylactic asthmatic agent.	CNS: nervousness, restlessness, tremors CV: rapid pulse, pounding heart, increased systolic BP	Parent teaching: Monitor child's respiratory patterns, integrity of nasal and oral passages, throat irritation Irritation, mouth dryness, and cough may be reduced by gargling and rinsing mouth after each dose Drug has no effect once asthma attack begins. It is NOT to be used to TREAT an asthma attack.

Expectorants

Drug	Uses	Side Effects	Nursing Considerations
Guaifenesin (Robitussin-DM) Route: oral Dosage: 2-5 yr: 50-100 mg/hr (not to exceed 600 mg/day) 6-11 yr: 100-200 mg/hr (not to exceed 1.2 g/day)	Productive cough associated with upper respiratory tract infections	CNS: drowsiness GI: nausea, vomiting, diarrhea	Assess respiratory status, cough frequency and productivity Increase fluid intake; maintain hydration Instruct child in how to cough effectively Provide cool mist vaporizer

(b) Bulging and bright-red tympanic membrane

(c) Severe pain; very young children pull at the affected ear

   (2) OME

      (a) Fullness in the ear

      (b) Dull and retracted tympanic membrane

      (c) Serous fluid in the middle ear

 b. Diagnostic procedures

   (1) Laboratory studies—culture and sensitivity (C&S) of the purulent discharge for identification of the causative organism

   (2) Diagnostic studies

      (a) Tympanogram—measures the stiffness and compliance of the tympanic membrane

      (b) Audiometry—assesses the severity of a hearing loss

6. Therapeutic management

 a. AOM

   (1) Medications

      (a) Antibiotics—a 10- to 14-day regimen to eradicate the causative organism: sulfonamides and cephalosporins; 3rd generatioon cephalosporins given as single parenteral dose

      (b) Analgesics and antipyretics—to decrease fever and pain

   (2) Treatment: screening for hearing loss; after effective therapy decrease factors for increased risk of infection

   (3) Surgery: myringotomy—to relieve symptoms of severe pain and conductive hearing loss; adenoidectomy is performed if eustachian tube blockage is secondary to adenoid hypertrophy

 b. OME

   (1) Medications: antihistamines—decrease drainage and inflammation in the middle ear; clear the eustachian tube; additional course of antibiotics may be needed

   (2) Surgery

      (a) Myringotomy for persistent bilateral effusion

      (b) Insertion of tympanoplasty tubes to facilitate drainage and help ventilate the middle ear

7. Nursing management

 a. Nursing diagnosis: pain

 b. Expected outcomes

   (1) Absent or decreased pain after therapy

   (2) Child's rest needs are met

 c. Interventions

   (1) Assess verbal and nonverbal signs of pain: irritability, tugging at ear, and bulging tympanic membrane

   (2) Administer analgesics, antipyretics, and antibiotics as ordered

      (3) Position the child for comfort and drainage: lying on the affected side

      (4) Apply heat over the ear, with the child lying on the affected side

      (5) Cleanse the external canal with a sterile swab soaked in hydrogen peroxide

      (6) Have child avoid chewing during the acute period by offering a soft diet because chewing increases pain

      (7) Apply an ice bag over the affected ear to decrease swelling and pressure

8. Evaluation
  a. Questions to ask parents
    (1) Which water activities are allowed?
    (2) What are your concerns about the medications needed?
  b. Behaviors to observe
    (1) Child resumes normal activity level with the protection of the ears during water sports or swimming
    (2) Parents ask appropriate questions for follow-up care
  c. Evaluation of expected outcomes
    (1) Re-infection of middle ear is prevented
    (2) Child recovers from surgery or infection without complications

B. Epiglottitis
1. Description: acute inflammation of the epiglottis that involves supraglottic obstruction

⚠ Warning!
Because epiglottitis results in acute respiratory distress, it is an emergency situation.

2. Etiology and incidence
  a. Caused by a bacterial organism, usually *H. influenzae;* rarely, *Streptococcus*
  b. Most commonly affects children between 2 and 5 years of age
  c. Occurs most often in the winter season
3. Pathophysiology
  a. Bacteria invades the epiglottis and surrounding laryngeal area; inflammation and edema rapidly cause airway obstruction
  b. Sudden onset, within 4 to 12 hours

⚠ Warning!
Medical measures must be instituted rapidly or death may occur

4. Assessment
  a. Assessment findings
    (1) Early signs
      (a) Sore throat, difficulty or inability to swallow
      (b) Fever

(c) Toxic appearance: sudden onset of a temperature over 102.2° F; respiratory distress; tachypnea; inspiratory stridor; anxiety demonstrated by the child; dysphonia (muffled, hoarse voice), along with drooling and a posture of "chin thrust" outward to help keep the airway open

(2) Other signs indicative of epiglottitis: absence of a spontaneous cough, agitation, red and inflamed oral cavity, and drooling

b. Diagnostic procedures

(1) Laboratory studies

(a) Arterial blood gases—respiratory acidosis—decreased pH and PaO_2, increased $PaCO_2$

(b) Throat C&S—identifies causative organism

(2) Diagnostic studies

(a) Lateral neck x-ray film—to confirm diagnosis

(b) Direct laryngoscopy—performed in surgical suite

> ⚠️ **Warning!**
>
> Inspection of the throat should only be attempted when immediate intubation can be done because touching the throat with a tongue depressor can result in a laryngeal spasm with closure of the airway.

5. Therapeutic management

a. Medications

(1) Analgesics and antipyretics—to reduce fever and throat pain

(2) IV antibiotics—to treat infection

(3) Corticosteroids—to decrease inflammation

(4) Immunization: *Haemophilus* type B—to prevent occurrence

b. Treatments and surgery

(1) Oxygen therapy—via mask, cannula, or endotracheal tube to treat hypoxia; use high humidification to cool airway and decrease swelling

(2) Endotracheal intubation or tracheostomy, if the child is in severe respiratory distress

(3) Room humidifier with cool air in the early stage to help minimize airway swelling

6. Nursing management

a. Nursing diagnoses

(1) Ineffective airway clearance

(2) Ineffective breathing pattern

(3) Risk for fluid volume deficit

b. Expected outcomes

(1) Child will maintain patent airway

(2) Child will exhibit an absence of upper airway infectious process

        (3) Child's respiratory status will return to within normal parameters

        (4) Child will maintain fluid balance

  c. Interventions

        (1) Continuously assess respiratory status: vital signs and the presence of or changes in nasal flaring, stridor; dyspnea or drooling; use of accessory muscles, with seesaw breathing in infants

        (2) Assess breath sounds, skin color changes, and attempts to cough

        (3) Assess adequacy of child's respirations and any changes in energy with increase in fatigue

        (4) Avoid visualization of the epiglottis or taking a throat culture with tongue blade to prevent spasm of the epiglottis or larynx with the result of airway occlusion

        (5) Keep emergency intubation equipment at the child's bedside

        (6) Provide humidified supplemental oxygen

        (7) Maintain the child in an upright position

        (8) Assist with emergency procedures as needed

        (9) Provide tracheostomy care as indicated

       (10) Assess hydration status; record intake and output; check for dry mucous membranes and sunken eyes; administer and monitor IV fluids

  d. Nursing diagnosis: anxiety—parents and child

  e. Expected outcomes

        (1) Child and parental anxiety is decreased or minimized

        (2) Child's respiratory state returns to or toward the baseline

  f. Interventions

        (1) Assess the fear and anxiety levels of the child and parents

        (2) Provide a calm environment

        (3) Remain with child in the acute phase

        (4) Allow the parents to remain with the child

        (5) Inform the parents of the child's status and explain all procedures

        (6) Encourage the parents to express their fears

7. Evaluation

  a. Questions to ask parents

        (1) Which questions do you have about acute care?

        (2) What will you plan to do for a recurrence?

  b. Behaviors to observe

        (1) Parents' presence calms and supports child

        (2) Parents' and child's anxious behaviors decrease as respiratory distress is relieved

  c. Evaluation of expected outcomes

        (1) Child and family express decreased anxiety as the acute stage of the disease ends

        (2) Parents remain with the child to provide support

        (3) Child maintains calmer behavior, as air hunger is relieved

C. Laryngotracheobronchitis (LTB)

1. Description: most common form of croup; involves viral infection of the larynx, trachea, and bronchi (Table 15-2)
2. Etiology and incidence
   a. Caused by viruses associated with upper respiratory infection—parainfluenza virus: types 1, 2, and 3; respiratory syncytial virus; influenza virus: types A1, A2, and B; adenovirus; and rhinovirus
   b. Mainly affects boys; peak age of incidence is 9 to 18 months
   c. Occurs most often in winter months and begins at night
3. Pathophysiology
   a. Viral infection causes mucosal inflammation of the larynx and trachea, resulting in a narrowed airway
   b. As the child struggles to move air past the obstruction, negative pressure in the thoracic cavity increases and pulmonary vascular fluid leaks into the interstitial spaces, causing hypoxia
   c. Respiratory acidosis and respiratory failure eventually occur if treatment is delayed
4. Assessment
   a. Assessment findings: four stages of progression in LTB (Box 15-1, p. 440)
   b. Diagnostic procedures
      (1) Laboratory studies
          (a) Arterial blood gases—respiratory acidosis—decreased pH and PaO_2, increased $PaCO_2$
          (b) Throat culture reveals causative agent
          (c) CBC reveals leukocytosis; if WBC is over 10,000/mm^3, a bacterial infection is present
      (2) Diagnostic studies: chest and neck X-ray films to rule out epiglottitis
5. Therapeutic management
   a. Medications
      (1) Bronchodilators—"racemic epinephrine" by way of a nebulizer—to relax smooth muscles and relieve stridor; a nebulizer has a quicker effect for bronchodilation of the larger airways
      (2) Corticosteroids for anti-inflammatory effect (controversial)
      (3) Antibiotics if secondary bacterial infection is present
   b. Treatments
      (1) Humidified oxygen or high humidity by way of a vaporizer or tent. The cool mist helps moisten and decrease swelling of the mucous membranes.
      (2) IV fluid therapy for dehydration
      (3) Intubation or tracheostomy if necessary

TABLE 15-2   Comparison of Croup Syndromes

Factors	Acute Epiglottitis (Supraglottitis)	Acute Laryngotracheobronchitis (LTB)	Acute Spasmodic Laryngitis (Spasmodic Croup)	Acute Tracheitis
Age group affected	1-8 yr	3 mo–8 yr	3 mo–3 yr	1 mo–6 yr
Etiologic agent	Bacterial, usually *H. influenzae*	Viral	Viral with allergic component	Bacterial, usually *S. aureus*
Onset	Rapidly progressive	Slowly progressive	Sudden; at night	Moderately progressive
Major symptoms	*Dysphagia or avoidance of swallowing Stridor aggravated when supine *Drooling High fever Toxic Rapid pulse and respirations *Chin thrust forward to open airway	URI Stridor Brassy cough Hoarseness Dyspnea Restlessness Irritability Low-grade fever Nontoxic	URI Croupy cough Stridor Hoarseness Dyspnea Restlessness Symptoms waken child Symptoms disappear during day Tends to recur	URI Croupy cough Stridor Purulent secretions High fever No response to LTB therapy
Treatment	Airway protection Antibiotics	Humidity Racemic epinephrine	Humidity	Antibiotics

From Wong, DL, et al: *Whaley and Wong's Nursing care of infants and children,* ed 6, St Louis, 1999, Mosby.

*Classic findings

Box 15-1
Progression of Symptoms in Laryngotracheobronchitis

Stage I

Fear
Hoarseness
Croupy cough
Inspiratory stridor when disturbed

Stage II

Continuous respiratory stridor
Lower rib retraction
Retraction of the soft tissue of the neck
Use of accessory muscles of respiration
Labored respiration

Stage III

Signs of anoxia and carbon dioxide retention
Restlessness
Anxiety
Pallor
Sweating
Rapid respiration

Stage IV

Intermittent cyanosis
Permanent cyanosis
Cessation of breathing

As described by Forbes. From Krugman S, et al: *Infectious diseases of children,* ed 9, St. Louis, 1992, Mosby.

6. Nursing management: see Nursing Management of Epiglottitis, p. 436
   a. Acute care interventions
      (1) Observe for inspiratory stridor, and characteristic barking cough
      (2) Administer medications, as ordered, including bronchodilators (racemic epinephrine), and antibiotics
      (3) Use a secured car seat or elevate head of bed—may need to put the bed on blocks—to the comfort level of the child; reposition every 2 hours
      (4) Provide humidification with mist tent or vaporizer
      (5) Encourage oral intake of clear fluids
      (6) Encourage parents to stay to keep the child calm, which conserves energy for respiratory effort
      (7) Provide rest periods between procedures

III. Infections of the lower respiratory system

A. Bronchiolitis

1. Description: inflammation of the smaller bronchioles; caused by a virus and characterized by thick mucus
2. Etiology and incidence
   a. Virus most frequently involved is a respiratory syncytial virus (RSV); others include adenovirus, rhinovirus, and parainfluenza
   b. Transmission is by respiratory droplets
   c. Frequent cause of hospitalization for infants under 1 year of age; peak incidence at 2 to 5 months of age. Premature infants are at greater risk.
   d. Occurs most frequently in the winter and early spring
3. Pathophysiology
   a. RSV affects the epithelial cells of respiratory tract to cause fusion with cell membranes of adjacent epithelial cells, resulting in mutinucleated masses: "syncytia"
   b. Mucous membranes that line the bronchioles become edematous, along with cellular infiltrates, and cause obstruction of the smaller airways
   c. Obstruction of affected airways results in hyperinflation, and air trapping occurs
   d. Hypoxemia is the end result of the hyperinflation of alveoli
4. Assessment
   a. Early findings: rhinorrhea and pharyngitis; hacking, harsh cough; ear or eye infection; rhonchi and expiratory wheezes; and low-grade fever, with a rectal temperature of 100° to 102° F
   b. Findings with progression: increased coughing and wheezing; air hunger depicted by nasal flaring, grunting, and intercostal or sternal retractions; tachypnea; and cyanosis
5. Diagnostic procedures
   a. Laboratory studies
      (1) Nasal or nasopharyngeal cultures reveal the RS virus
      (2) CBC—elevated WBC is consistent with infection
      (3) Arterial blood gases—decreased pH; PaO_2 less than 60 mm Hg; $PaCO_2$ over 45 mm Hg
      (4) Immunofluorescent antibody (IFA) study or ELISA—used for RSV antigen detection
   b. Diagnostic studies: chest x-ray film—reveals hyperinflation, atelectasis, areas of consolidation, and fluid
6. Therapeutic management: medications
   a. Antivirals—ribavirin (Virazole) via aerosol during initial days of illness

⚠ Warning!

Pregnant health care providers should not be assigned to infants who receive ribavirin because of possible teratogenic effects.

    b. Antipyretics—to reduce fever

    c. Bronchodilators—to relax the smooth muscles of the bronchi and bronchioles

    d. Preventive measure: RSV immune globulin RSV-IGIV or RespiGam used prophylactically during RSV epidemic season in high-risk infant populations

  7. Other treatments: high humidity, supplemental oxygen, and adequate fluids

  8. Nursing management

    a. Nursing diagnosis: social isolation related to infection

    b. Expected outcome: child will maintain social contacts

    c. Interventions

      (1) Employ consistent hand washing, and avoid contact with nasal mucosa and conjunctiva

      (2) Group child with other children infected with the RS virus or assign a private room

      (3) Administer antiviral agents and bronchodilators, as ordered

      (4) Provide activities for diversion

    d. Other nursing diagnoses

      (1) Ineffective breathing pattern

      (2) Ineffective airway clearance

      (3) Fatigue

  9. Interventions, expected outcomes, and evaluation: refer to pneumonia on p. 445

B. Pneumonia

  1. Description: inflammation or infection of the pulmonary parenchyma, the alveoli

  2. Etiology and incidence

    a. Causative agents that serve as classifications for pneumonia: viruses, bacteria, mycoplasmas, and aspiration of foreign substances

    b. Viral pneumonia occurs more frequently than bacterial pneumonia

    c. Pneumonia occurs more frequently in infancy and early childhood than in the school-aged children and adolescents

  3. Pathophysiology

    a. Pattern of the illness depends on the child's age, causative agent, extent of infection, and systemic reaction to the infection (Table 15-3)

    b. May occur as a primary infection or be secondary to another illness or infection

  4. Assessment findings and therapeutic management (see Table 15-3)

  5. Nursing management

    a. Nursing diagnoses

      (1) Ineffective breathing pattern; impaired gas exchange

      (2) Hyperthermia

Text continued on p. 445

TABLE 15-3	Comparison of Types of Pneumonia in Children Based on Etiologic Agents			
Type of Pneumonia and Age Group Affected	**Etiologic Agents**	**Assessment Findings**	**Diagnostic Tests**	**Treatments**
Viral Pneumonia Affects all age groups	RSV Influenza Parainfluenza Rhinovirus Adenovirus	Mild to high fever Slight cough Wheezes, fine crackles	Chest x-ray film: diffuse or patchy infiltration	Symptomatic: fluids if dehydration present; measures to promote oxygenation
Bacterial Pneumonia All age groups 3 mo–5 yr: Staphylococcus pneumonia and H. Influenza >5 yr: Mycoplasma pneumonia	Streptococcus pneumoniae, Group A streptococcus, H. influenza (hib), Staphylococcus aureus, Mycoplasma pneumoniae	Abdominal pain Chest pain Cough Adventitious breath sounds Irritability Poor feeding Spike in temperature Headache, chills	Chest X-ray film: lobar consolidation and pleural effusion Gram stain and culture of organism Increased antistreptolysin O titer	Antibiotic therapy Bed rest Antipyretics for fever Oral or IV fluids Mist or tent Oxygen if in respiratory distress Pneumococcal vaccine for at-risk infants and children

Continued

Modified from Wong D: *Whaley and Wong's Nursing care of infants and children,* ed 5, St. Louis: Mosby, 1995.

TABLE 15-3 Comparison of Types of Pneumonia in Children Based on Etiologic Agents—cont'd				
Type of Pneumonia and Age Group Affected	Etiologic Agents	Assessment Findings	Diagnostic Tests	Treatments
Primary Atypical Pneumonia 5-12 yr	Mycoplasma pneumonia	Fever, chills Headache, malaise, anorexia Sore throat Dry, hacking cough Myalgia—aching muscles	Chest x-ray film: areas of consolidation and emphysema	Symptomatic
Aspiration Pneumonia Infants, young children	Food, fluids Vitamins Nasopharyngeal secretions Talcum powder Hydrocarbons	Coughing Choking Dyspnea Fever Typically found in right middle lobe, because right bronchus is most vertical	Chest x-ray film: radiopaque foreign bodies Bronchoscopy: diagnoses object in larynx or trachea	Oxygen therapy Hydration Treatment of secondary infection **WARNING!** Vomiting is contraindicated in hydrocarbon pneumonia

Modified from Wong D: *Whaley and Wong's Nursing care of infants and children,* ed 5, St. Louis: Mosby, 1995.

        (3) Risk for fluid volume deficit

        (4) Pain and discomfort

    b. Expected outcomes

        (1) Child recovers without pulmonary complications

        (2) Child's respiratory status returns to normal parameters

    c. Interventions

        (1) Assess vital signs and auscultate lungs every 2 to 4 hours and as required

        (2) Report signs of complications: increased dyspnea, pain with breathing, cyanosis, abdominal distention, and sudden temperature increase

        (3) Ensure chest physiotherapy every 4 hours as ordered

        (4) Provide cool mist environment

        (5) Administer antipyretics and antibiotics as ordered

        (6) Encourage the child to cough and breathe deeply every 2 hours; turn child every 2 hours

        (7) Assess oral fluid intake; encourage oral fluid intake every 2 hours

        (8) Provide play activities that encourage deep breathing and fluid intake

  6. Evaluation

    a. Questions to ask parents

        (1) What are your concerns about the acute care of your child?

        (2) Which actions might prevent recurrence of a pulmonary infection?

    b. Behaviors to observe

        (1) Child's respirations return to within 10% of baseline parameters

        (2) Parents and family members take precautions to prevent the spread of infection

    c. Evaluation of expected outcomes

        (1) Child recovers without pulmonary complications

        (2) Child's temperature remains within one degree of 99.6° F rectally for 24 to 48 hours before discharge

IV. Chronic respiratory conditions of childhood

A. Asthma

  1. Description: reversible "reactive" airway disease, characterized by a narrowing of the bronchi and bronchioles; results in lung obstruction and hyperinflation; a chronic condition with acute exacerbations

  2. Classification (Box 15-2)

  3. Etiology and incidence

    a. Asthma attacks are triggered by allergens such as dust mites, pollen, and food; other causes are strenuous exercise; weather changes, especially with increased humidity; cigarette or other types of smoke; viral infections; and cockroaches

Box 15-2
Asthma Severity Classification in Children 5 Years of Age and Older: Clinical Features*

Step 4: Severe Persistent Asthma

Continual symptoms
Frequent exacerbations
Frequent nighttime symptoms
Limited physical activity
Peak expiratory flow (PEF) or forced expiratory volume in one second (FEV_1) is 60% or less of the predicted value
PEF variability is more than 30%

Step 3: Moderate Persistent Asthma

Daily symptoms
Daily use of inhaled short-acting $beta_2$-agonists
Exacerbations affect activity
Exacerbations twice a week or more
Exacerbations may last days
Nighttime symptoms more than once a week
PEF/FEV_1 is over 60% to under 80% of the predicted value
PEF variability is over 30%

Step 2: Mild Persistent Asthma

Symptoms more than twice a week but less than once a day
Exacerbations may affect activity
Nighttime symptoms more than twice a month
PEF/FEV_1 is 80% or more of the predicted value
PEF variability is 20% to 30%

Step 1: Mild Intermittent Asthma

Symptoms twice a week or less
Exacerbations are brief (from a few hours to a few days); intensity may vary
Nighttime symptoms twice a month or less
Asymptomatic and normal PEF between exacerbations
PEF or FEV_1 is 80% or more of the predicted value
PEF variability is less than 20%

*The presence of one clinical feature of severity is sufficient to place a client in that category. A client should be assigned to the most severe grade in which any feature occurs. The characteristics in this table are general and may overlap because asthma is highly variable. A client's classification may change over time.
From National Asthma Education and Prevention Program: *Expert Panel Report II: Guidelines for the Diagnosis and Management of Asthma,* Bethesda, 1997, National Heart, Lung and Blood Institute.

b. The leading chronic lung disorder in children; primary cause of school absences

c. Most children have a first attack before 5 years of age

d. Increased prevalence, morbidity, and mortality in the United States

4. Pathophysiology

  a. Three factors contribute to the findings of obstruction

   (1) Inflammation and edema of the mucous membranes

   (2) Accumulation of tenacious secretions from the mucous glands

   (3) Smooth muscle spasm of the bronchi and bronchioles

  b. Some children also experience a hypersensitivity component to an asthma attack, which is mediated by immunoglobulin E

  c. Balance, normally maintained between vagal and sympathetic nerves for smooth muscle tone, is upset by irritants such as dust or cigarette smoke

  d. A chronic problem with acute exacerbations

5. Assessment

  a. Findings of an asthma attack—may occur in any sequence or grouping of signs and symptoms

   (1) Audible expiratory wheeze

> ⚠️ **Warning!**
>
> An inspiratory wheeze places the client at a higher risk of respiratory and cardiac arrest.

   (2) Diaphoresis

   (3) Paroxysmal, hacking, and nonproductive cough at onset; becomes rattling and productive of clear sputum

   (4) Restlessness and apprehension

   (5) Dyspnea and prolonged expiration

   (6) Nasal flaring

   (7) Intercostal retractions

   (8) Circumoral cyanosis and cyanosis of the nail beds

   (9) Coarse rhonchi

> ⚠️ **Warning!**
>
> In an acute asthma attack, the sudden cessation of wheezing can be an ominous sign that the airways are totally collapsed and constricted. Respiratory arrest is imminent.

  b. Diagnostic procedures

   (1) Laboratory studies

    (a) Arterial blood gases—reveals decreased pH and PaO_2; increased $PaCO_2$ as the attack progresses

    (b) Sputum culture—reveals the presence of eosinophils

    (c) CBC—reveals increased eosinophils in the differential

      (2) Diagnostic studies

         (a) Pulmonary function study—reveals a decreased tidal volume and vital capacity

         (b) **Peak expiratory flow rate (PEFR)** monitoring—reveals severity of an exacerbation

         (c) Skin tests—identify specific allergen

         (d) Chest x-ray film—reveals hyperinflation, pulmonary infiltrates, and atelectasis

  c. Complications

      (1) Status asthmaticus

      (2) Chronic emphysema

      (3) *Cor pulmonale*—enlargement of the right side of the heart from primary lung disease such as pulmonary fibrosis with pulmonary hypertension

      (4) Pneumothorax

6. Therapeutic management

  a. Medications (see Table 15-1, p. 431). Stepwise approach recommended based on the severity of symptoms; classified as

      (1) Long-term control to achieve and maintain inflammation for prevention of an asthma attack

         (a) Inhaled or oral corticosteroids: short-course dosing in "bursts" is used to manage persistent symptoms

         (b) Mast-cell stabilizers medications: such as cromolyn (Intal) (by a nebulizer or metered dose inhaler [MDI]) and nedocromil (Tilade) (by MDI) work by inhibiting the cell activation phase of inflammation. These are not to be used in acute asthma attacks.

         (c) Long-acting beta$_2$-agonists: inhaled [salmeterol (Serevent)] or given orally (albuterol). They relax the smooth muscles to open the airways.

         (d) Methylxanthines (theophylline): given orally relax the smooth muscles to open the airways

         (e) Leukotriene modifiers: zafirlukast (Accolate) and zileuton (Zyflo) given orally; not for use in children under 12 years of age because these drugs may induce smooth muscle bronchoconstriction. They increase vascular permeability and mucus secretion.

         (f) PEFR monitoring: as directed by the physician for evaluation of the daily respiratory status

      (2) Quick relief ("rescue") to treat acute symptoms during any exacerbation

         (a) Inhaled: short-acting beta$_2$-agonists (albuterol)

         (b) Systemic (SQ) beta$_2$-agonists (epinephrine, terbutaline)

         (c) Anticholinergics: ipratropium bomide (Atrovent) by nebulizer or MDI; used as a bronchodilator; reduces stimulation of the vagus nerve that causes smooth muscle contractions

    (d) Corticosteroids: oral prednisone

> ⚠️ **Warning!**
>
> Observe the child for refractoriness to therapy, which is no change in findings or findings that become worse. Expect that findings should diminish within 10 to 30 minutes after the initiation of therapy.

  b. Newer delivery devices available for use in asthma control

    (1) Spacer attached to MDI: allows better delivery because medication particles get into the airways instead of on the back of the throat

    (2) Dry powder turbahaler: spins a powder form of medication into the airways; is free of chlorofluorocarbons

  c. Treatments include oxygen therapy by mask; chest physiotherapy; injection therapy for hyposensitization of allergies; heliox, a helium-oxygen mixture used in treatment of status asthmaticus; and PEFR use at home for daily long-term monitoring

7. Nursing management

  a. Nursing diagnoses

    (1) Risk for suffocation; ineffective airway clearance

    (2) Impaired gas exchange

    (3) Anxiety

    (4) Activity intolerance

  b. Expected outcomes

    (1) Child breathes easily with less or a normal respiratory effort

    (2) Child's breath sounds are clear with optimal airflow

    (3) Child will be able to cough up mucous secretions at least every 1 to 2 hours

    (4) Child will demonstrate improved gas exchange: pink skin color, capillary refill between 3 to 5 seconds, and decreased restlessness

    (5) Child engages in age-appropriate activities

  c. Interventions

    (1) Assess respiratory status as indicated by the findings

    (2) Auscultate lungs for the presence of adventitious breath sounds

    (3) Assess cough: onset, duration, viscosity, frequency, productivity, and color of sputum

    (4) Position with head of bed elevated to child's comfort level for breathing: semi-Fowler's or upright position; use a secured car seat for infants and toddlers

    (5) Monitor the PEFR

    (6) Administer pulmonary medications as ordered

(7) Assess and monitor for signs of theophylline toxicity; serum levels over 20 μg/ml

⚠ Warning!

The initial toxic finding is nausea; a later finding is tremors. Note that tachycardia is an expected side effect. A decrease in the IV drip rate or dosage usually decreases the HR.

(8) Administer humidified oxygen as ordered
(9) Assess blood gases for changes
(10) Administer IV fluids, as ordered
(11) Encourage parents to stay with the child; place child in quiet environment

8. Evaluation
   a. Questions to ask parents
      (1) How is this attack different from the others? Is it more or less severe than usual? More or less frequent than usual?
      (2) Which concerns or needs do you have about long-term care?
   b. Behaviors to observe
      (1) Child participates in self-care to the degree expected for age-appropriate actions
      (2) Parents ask questions or offer actions to make the child more comfortable
   c. Evaluation of expected outcomes
      (1) Child avoids exposure to known allergens
      (2) Family and the child follow the prescribed medication regimen
      (3) Family and the child verbalize understanding of the disease process, importance for control of precipitating factors, symptoms of an attack, and findings that require immediate medical attention

B. **Cystic fibrosis (CF)**
   1. Description: *autosomal recessive disorder* involving the exocrine glands; characterized by thick, tenacious secretions that affect multiple organs, which are most commonly the lungs, pancreas, liver, and small intestine
   2. Although the disease is ultimately fatal, the median life expectancy has increased to 40 years of age
   3. Etiology and incidence
      a. CF affects 1 in 3500 white infants each year
      b. CF is caused by a biochemical defect
      c. The responsible mutated gene is located on chromosome 7, along with protein product CF transmembrane regulator (CFTR)
      d. When both parents carry the CF gene, 25% of offspring will have CF, 50% will be carriers, and 25% will not have the disease

4. Pathophysiology
   a. Characteristics of the disease process
      (1) Increased viscosity of mucous gland secretions
      (2) Marked elevation of sweat electrolytes: sodium and chloride
      (3) Increased organic and enzymatic constituents of saliva
      (4) Abnormal autonomic nervous system function: overactivity stimulates the cholinergic glands and innervates all exocrine glands to become overactive
   b. Primary factor responsible for many symptoms of the disease is the mechanical obstruction caused by the increased viscosity of mucous secretions; when stagnated in the lung, bacterial colonization of the mucus leads to lung tissue destruction
   c. Exocrine gland dysfunction affects multiple organ systems (Figure 15-1)

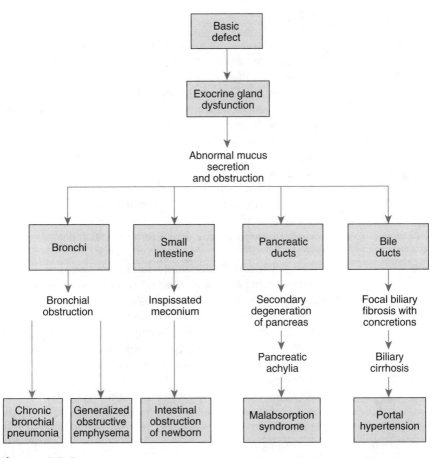

Figure 15-1 Various effects of exocrine gland dysfunction in cystic fibrosis. (From Wong DL, et al: *Whaley and Wong's nursing care of infants and children,* ed 6, St. Louis, 1999, Mosby)

5. Assessment
   a. Assessment findings
      (1) Meconium ileus (infants)
      (2) Salty-tasting skin—usually found by parents when they kiss the child
      (3) Profuse sweating in warm weather
      (4) Frequent infections
      (5) Dry, nonproductive cough
      (6) Increase in the amount and thickness of secretions
      (7) Wheezing and cyanosis
      (8) Digital clubbing from chronic hypoxia
      (9) Increased anterior-posterior diameter of the chest
      (10) **Steatorrhea,** fatty stools; **azotorrhea,** excessive loss of nitrogen in the stool
      (11) Thin extremities and muscle wasting
      (12) Failure to thrive
   b. Diagnostic procedures
      (1) Laboratory studies
         (a) Sweat test—iontophoresis of pilocarpine: a sweat chloride content of over 60 mEq is positive for CF; two tests are done to ensure reliability
         (b) Stool for fecal fat—reveals impaired fat absorption from pancreatic and liver dysfunction; stool is collected in the same container for 72 hours
      (2) Diagnostic studies
         (a) Pulmonary function study—indicates degree of impaired lung function
         (b) Chest x-ray film—findings consistent with CF are patchy atelectasis, areas of infiltrates, and bronchopneumonia
         (c) Screening for gene defect for at-risk families
   c. Complications
      (1) Heat prostration (exhaustion)—findings of weakness, vertigo, nausea, muscle cramps, loss of consciousness; caused by the depletion of body fluids/electrolytes from exposure to intense heat or inability to acclimatize to heat
      (2) Respiratory: bronchiectasis; hemoptysis; nasal polyps; emphysema; pneumonia, specifically *Pseudomonas aeruginosa* and *Burkholderia cepacia;* pneumothorax; and cor pulmonale
      (3) GI: bowel obstruction, gallstones, cirrhosis of the liver, and portal hypertension
      (4) Endocrine: diabetes mellitus
6. Therapeutic management
   a. Medications
      (1) Bronchodilators and adrenergic agonists: relieve bronchospasms; enable the removal of thick secretions; may

be given by a hand-held nebulizer and before chest physiotherapy

(2) Mucolytics: dornase alfa (Pulmozyme), acetylcysteine (Mucomyst)—decrease mucus viscosity

(3) Pancreatic enzymes: pancreatin (Viokase) treats pancreatic deficiency; must be given with meals

(4) Vitamins: water-miscible forms of vitamins A, D, E, and K

(5) Antibiotics: aerosolized for prophylactic or infection therapy

(6) Salt replacement: in warm weather, during febrile episodes, and during increased activity or play

(7) Anti-inflammatory drug: ibuprofen (Motrin, Advil) to decrease lung disease progression

b. Treatments

(1) Chest physiotherapy—includes postural drainage, chest percussion, vibration, and coughing

(2) Oxygen therapy—usually for respiratory distress

(3) Dietary supplementation—usually sodium

(4) Flutter Mucus Clearance Device—hand-held plastic pipe to facilitate mucus removal

⚠ Warning!

Store the Flutter Mucus Clearance Device away from children because it contains a stainless steel ball that poses a choking hazard.

(5) Preventive actions—yearly pneumonia vaccines and routine vaccinations

(6) ThAIRapy vest—loosens secretions by high-frequency chest wall oscillation

c. Surgical interventions

(1) Nasal polyp removal

(2) Lung transplantation

7. Nursing management

a. Nursing diagnoses

(1) Ineffective airway clearance

(2) Impaired gas exchange

b. Expected outcomes

(1) Child expectorates mucus with minimal effort

(2) Child's respiratory status is maintained within 10% of baseline parameters for child

c. Interventions

(1) Assess for changes in breathing pattern, tenacity of mucus and color, diminished breath sounds, and ability to cough and expectorate secretions every 2 to 4 hours

(2) Perform chest physiotherapy before meals, every 4 hours, at bedtime, and as needed

      (3) Assist child in coughing, or suction every 2 hours to promote airway clearance

      (4) Administer mucolytics and bronchodilators as ordered or indicated by findings

      (5) Place child in high Fowler's position as much as possible

  d. Nursing diagnosis: altered nutrition (less than body requirements)

  e. Expected outcomes

      (1) Child demonstrates weight gain or no loss of weight; child maintains appetite

      (2) Child has no more than 2 to 3 stools per day

  f. Interventions

      (1) Assess child's nutritional status, including height and weight

      (2) Administer pancreatic enzymes immediately before meals and snacks

      (3) Provide a high-calorie, high-protein, high-carbohydrate diet

      (4) Provide salt, especially during hot weather or excessive play

      (5) Administer water-miscible forms of vitamins A, D, E, and K, as ordered

      (6) Monitor number of daily stools

  g. Nursing diagnoses: high risk for infection

  h. Expected outcome: child will remain free of infection

  i. Interventions

⚠ Warning!

Because of the high risk of *B. cepacia* transmission in the hospital, place the child with positive cultures on room isolation with the door closed. This extremely virulent organism causes *cepacia* bacteremia, which is associated with pulmonary deterioration and death.

      (1) Assess for signs of infection; monitor WBC count for an increase with infection and a decrease with effective therapy

      (2) Monitor and provide frequent skin care to prevent irritation and breakdown

⚠ Warning!

Careful hand washing by all who care for CF clients is essential.

      (3) Carefully wash the respiratory equipment after each use and rinse under running water

      (4) Provide oral hygiene

8. Evaluation
   a. Questions to ask parents
      (1) What needs do you have for home care?
      (2) How are you coping with the stress of the daily care needed by your child?
      (3) What kind of help will decrease your stress or help your child's physical or emotional status?
   b. Behaviors to observe
      (1) Family adheres to prescribed medical regimen and follow-up care
      (2) Family seeks support from appropriate agencies
   c. Evaluation of expected outcomes
      (1) Child maintains respiratory status within 10% of baseline parameters
      (2) Child is able to cough up thick mucous secretions
      (3) Child remains free of infection
      (4) Child maintains weight above the 25th percentile for stature

V. Home care: family education topics and referrals

A. **Otitis media**
   1. Medication: emphasize the need to follow the prescribed antibiotic regimen
   2. Tube care: instruct parents to maintain the patency of tympanoplasty tubes: keep ears dry—earplugs should be worn during bathing, shampooing hair, and swimming; diving or submerging under water is not allowed; call the physician if the grommet falls out of the ear
   3. Follow-up: teach parents to observe for signs of hearing impairment
   4. Prevention techniques: eliminate tobacco smoke from child's environment, feed infants in an upright position and encourage the older child to play blowing games and chew gum; eliminate tobacco smoke and known allergens; explain ways to decrease ear discomfort during air travel, such as offering a pacifier to infants during take-off and descent or having older children chew gum or eat small snacks

B. **Epiglottitis, LTB, and pneumonia**
   1. Disease process: inform parents to report changes in sputum—thickness and color, breathing effort, respirations, and the child's level of comfort
   2. Medications: instruct parents in the correct method of antibiotic administration
   3. Treatments: chest physiotherapy; provide humidified environment with a cool mist humidifier; encourage increased fluid intake

C. **Asthma**
   1. Disease process: physiology of disorder; prevention of asthma

attacks and secondary infections; correct method and when to measure PEFR; symptoms of infection and attack; methods to remove allergens from the home; encourage installation of an air filter

2. Safety: removal of known allergens; actions to deal with an attack; breathing exercises with evaluation for effectiveness; findings indicating the need for immediate medical attention

3. Diet: need to eliminate allergenic foods

4. Medications: proper administration of bronchodilators and anti-inflammatory drugs; correct technique for the use of an inhaler, a spacer, or nebulizer

5. Activity: avoid excessive activity and stress

6. Referrals to the Asthma and Allergy Foundation of America and the American Lung Association

D. CF

1. Medications: administration of prophylactic antibiotics, water-miscible vitamins, and pancreatic enzymes (avoid crushing or chewing; take with meals or snacks; can mix oral enzyme with pureed apple sauce and administer with a spoon); need for routine immunizations and yearly pneumococcal and influenza vaccinations

2. Diet: need to supplement sodium intake in periods of salt depletion

3. Safety: need for yearly influenza vaccine; proper hand washing; aseptic technique when handling respiratory equipment

4. Referrals: genetic counseling; counseling services; local support agencies for CF; the Cystic Fibrosis Foundation

WEB Resources

www.vch.vh.org
   Virtual children's hospital sponsored by the Children's Hospital of Iowa to meet the informational needs of health care providers, clients, and families. Information and case studies on pediatric airway disease, including croup syndromes and epiglottitis are provided.

www.CFF.org
   Official site of the Cystic Fibrosis Foundation, which provides local chapter and family support groups and family information, research updates, and related literature.

www.aafa.org
   Allergy and Asthma Foundation of America website, which provides educational materials, local chapters, and support group information. Also provides professional education for nurses and other health professionals.

REVIEW QUESTIONS

1. The parents of a 10-year-old boy bring him to the emergency room with a severe asthma attack. Considering the child's diagnosis, the nurse expects to assess for which of these findings?
    1. A hacking, nonproductive cough
    2. Itching at the base of the neck or upper back
    3. Shortness of breath while sitting, with a prolonged expiratory phase
    4. Mild, expiratory wheezing

2. An 8-year-old child is admitted to the pediatric unit with a respiratory infection. The child was diagnosed with cystic fibrosis as an infant. The physician orders medications that fall into these classifications. Which one should the nurse question?
    1. Bronchodilator
    2. Antitussive
    3. Mucolytic agent
    4. Pancreatic enzyme

3. After a myringotomy, which action would facilitate drainage from the ear?
    1. Apply a gauze pack tightly to the affected ear
    2. Apply a warm pack to the affected ear
    3. Position the child to be on the affected side
    4. Put the child in a prone position

4. After a tonsillectomy, a child grows increasingly restless. The nurse assesses the child to find a pulse rate of 120 and frequent swallowing. Based on these findings, the nurse should suspect the client has which of these conditions?
    1. Airway obstruction
    2. Hemorrhage
    3. Infection
    4. Usual signs after this surgery

5. A 3-year-old is brought to the emergency department with these symptoms: fever, restlessness, and drooling. No coughing is observed. Based on these findings, the nurse should institute which action?
    1. Continuously monitor airway status
    2. Examine the throat with a tongue depressor
    3. Take a throat culture
    4. Prepare antibiotics for infusion

6. A mother states that her child experienced SOB after lunch at a local fast food restaurant. She states that these foods were eaten. Which is most likely to have caused an allergic reaction?
1. Chocolate shake
2. Salad
3. Turkey sandwich
4. Baked potato

ANSWERS, RATIONALES, AND TEST-TAKING TIPS

Rationales	Test-Taking Tips

1. Correct answer: 3

A child with a severe asthma attack is short of breath and tries to breathe more deeply. The expiratory phase becomes prolonged and is accompanied by audible wheezing (heard without a stethoscope). Asthma attacks begin with a hacking, nonproductive cough. Itching at the base of the neck or over the upper back is observed in the prodromal stage. Wheezing can occur on inspiration or expiration. However, in severe asthma, wheezing would be more than "mild."

The clues in the stem is the term "severe asthma attack." The descriptions in options 1, 2, and 4 do not correspond to a severe condition. Thus, option 3 is the correct answer.

2. Correct answer: 2

The medication group that inhibits coughing should be questioned. The increased viscosity of respiratory secretions in CF contributes to the risk of infection. Coughing moves secretions for expectoration and therefore decreases the risk of infection. The medications in options 1, 3, and 4 would not be questioned.

Bronchodilators usually are ordered to be given with a nebulizer to open the bronchi for easier breathing and expectoration. CF affects the body systems with exocrine secretions—lungs, liver, GI tract, and pancreas. Mucolytic agents are used to decrease the viscosity of mucous secretions or relieve meconium ileus. The secretions become very thick and tend to result in obstructions. Pancreatic enzymes are administered with meals and snacks so that digestive enzymes are mixed with the food to prevent stomach irritation and to ensure the chyme in the duodenum has enzymes to break down the food particles further.

3. Correct answer: 3

Lying on the affected side facilitates drainage of the

The terms that make two options incorrect are in option 1, "tightly,"

Rationales	Test-Taking Tips

exudate from the affected ear. A gauze pack should be applied loosely to allow accumulated drainage to flow out of the ear and onto the gauze. Local dry heat such as a hot water bottle may decrease the pain but does not help the flow of drainage. Warm soaks are contraindicated because the moisture may flow into the ear and cause further infection. The prone position is not an effective action to facilitate ear drainage.

and in option 2, "warm pad." Between options 3 and 4, use common sense. To drain something is to have it flow downward. Select option 3.

4. Correct answer: 2

The most obvious early sign of bleeding after internal throat surgery is frequent swallowing caused by blood trickling down the throat. Airway obstruction after a tonsillectomy is indicated by findings such as inspiratory stridor or sternal retractions from the increased effort required to pull air through an edematous upper airway. The findings in option 3 are not consistent with infection. Option 4 is a false statement.

Discomfort in swallowing is expected after this surgery. Remember that a first sign of bleeding is an increased HR, usually defined as a sustained increase in HR of 20 beats per minute over the client's baseline rate. However, in this question the HR is simply a distracter because the client is a child of unknown age. The normal range cannot be established. Also, the clue in the stem that "the child grows increasingly restless" guides you to disregard the HR. Restlessness can also cause the HR to increase. Restlessness is a first sign of tissue hypoxia in the brain.

5. Correct answer: 1

Three clinical observations have been known to predict epiglottitis: absence of a spontaneous cough, presence of drooling from a difficulty in swallowing as a result of airway edema, and agitation from hypoxia. Continuous monitoring of the respiratory status is a

Given the choices, use the principles of basic life support: airway, breathing and circulation (ABCs) to select option 1, an intervention related to airway and breathing. Go with what you know rather than an action you may be unsure of. Another approach is to cluster options 2, 3, and 4 under the theme

priority. When epiglottitis is suspected, no attempts are to be made to visualize the epiglottis or to obtain a throat culture. In option 4, there is not enough information in the stem to support a selection of this option.

6. Correct answer: 1

Chocolate is a hyperallergenic food source. Some foods can cause asthma-type reactions. Parents need to be advised to eliminate foods known to provoke symptoms. The foods in options 2, 3, and 4 are not known to cause allergic reactions. Turkey sandwiches, especially with mayonnaise, are more likely to cause food poisoning.

of "specific actions." Option 1 is an action to gather more information—to do further assessment. Do not forget to use the steps of the nursing process. If a child has a problem, further assessment is indicated rather than specific actions associated with the problem.

Milk and chocolate products more commonly cause allergic reactions in children and adults. Pulmonary, GI, and neurologic (headache) findings are reported as common reactions to these substances.

16

Nursing Care of Children with Gastrointestinal Disorders

FAST FACTS

1. Infants and children are more vulnerable to fluid volume deficits because they have a greater amount of fluid in the extracellular fluid compartment. Also, the organs that conserve water are immature in infants and children.
2. The sudden relief of pain in clients with appendicitis indicates perforation of the appendix. If the appendix ruptures, place the client into a right side-lying or low- to semi-Fowler's position to promote comfort or to localize the abscess.
3. After appendix rupture, antibiotics are administered to treat peritonitis.
4. Metabolic alkalosis and severe dehydration may more quickly develop in children with severe, prolonged vomiting.
5. Diet therapy in *celiac disease,* which is a problem of a gluten sensitivity, requires elimination of products made with wheat, rye, barley and oats.

CONTENT REVIEW

I. The gastrointestinal (GI) system
   A. **Structure and function**
      1. Anatomy
         a. GI development
            (1) In embryonic development the branchial arches, foregut, midgut, and hindgut give rise to the GI tract

      (2) At 4 weeks' gestation, the foregut, midgut, and hindgut are formed when the dorsal portion of the yolk sac is incorporated into the embryo

      (3) The oral cavity, developed from the branchial arches, develops early at 4 weeks' gestation

  2. Major physiologic functions of the GI system

    a. Assists in maintaining fluid and electrolyte balance and acid-base balance

    b. Processes and absorbs nutrients to maintain metabolism and support normal growth and development

    c. Excretes waste products from the digestive processes

  3. Pediatric considerations

    a. Stomach capacity is 1 ounce in newborns; therefore, they require small and frequent feedings every 1 to 2 hours for at least 2 to 4 weeks

    b. An increased peristalsis results in increased frequency and decreased solid consistency of stools

    c. A deficiency in pancreatic enzymes amylase, lipase, and trypsin that are present until 4 to 6 months of age.

    d. The liver cannot conjugate bilirubin and excrete bile during the neonatal period. Therefore, physiologic jaundice is expected 48 to 72 hours after birth. When jaundice occurs within the first day of birth, it is considered pathologic jaundice.

    e. Maturation of the digestive processes occurs by the end of the second year of life

B. Assessment

  1. Health history

    a. General

      (1) Diet

        (a) Typical 24-hour food intake

        (b) Food preferences and dislikes

        (c) Food intolerance

        (d) Religious and cultural food preferences

        (e) Weight gain or loss; over what period of time

        (f) **Pica** (see p. 478)

      (2) Medications: use and frequency

        (a) Laxatives, stool softeners, and antidiarrheal agents

        (b) Antiemetics and antacids

        (c) Aspirin, acetaminophen, and NSAIDs

        (d) Antibiotics

      (3) Activity

        (a) Recent stressful events

        (b) Exposure to infectious diseases

        (c) Recent travel history

b. Present condition
(1) Abdominal discomfort, distention, indigestion, and nausea
(2) Vomiting: describe character, amount, and frequency
(3) Diarrhea: describe character, amount, and frequency
(4) Constipation: describe toilet-training methods; describe the characteristics of the stool: shape, size, and color
c. History
(1) GI disorder: intestinal obstruction or inflammation
(2) Abdominal injury or surgery, especially if the appendix has not been removed
d. Family history
(1) Colon cancer
(2) Malabsorption syndrome
(3) Hirschprung disease
2. Physical examination
a. Abdomen—follow listed sequence of assessment
(1) Inspection
(a) Surface characteristics
(b) Presence of umbilical hernia
(c) Contour—expected finding in the infant or toddler: rounded "pot belly"
(d) Surface motion—peristalsis is not usually visible
(e) Distention
(2) Auscultation
(a) Presence of bowel sounds; number per minute; normal is 18 to 28 per minute
(b) Vascular sounds—venous hums or bruits should not be heard
(3) Percussion
(a) Tone—the abdomen of a child sounds louder in tympanic tones
(b) Liver span
(i) 6-month-old: 2.4 to 2.8 cm
(ii) 5-year-old: 7 cm
(iii) 12-year-old: 9 cm
(iv) 16-year-old: 6 to 12 cm
(4) Palpation
(a) Tenderness, firmness, and softness
(b) All four quadrants are assessed
(c) Organs: spleen, kidney, and bladder
(d) If suspicion of a neoplasm exists, especially near the kidney, limit the manipulation of the mass and the frequency of palpation
b. Anal-rectal area: surface characteristics and tenderness
3. Related laboratory and diagnostic studies (Table 16-1, p. 466)
C. **Commonly used GI medications in children** (Table 16-2, p. 467)

Text continued on p. 470

TABLE 16-1 Major Gastrointestinal Diagnostic Procedures in Pediatrics

Procedure	Function	Indications	Nursing Considerations
Stool Examination			
Ova and parasites	Examination of stool for presence of parasites and their eggs	Parasite infestation	Requires fresh, warm specimen Preservative required
Fat	Aids in diagnosis of pancreatic insufficiency	Cystic fibrosis Celiac disease Malabsorption syndrome	Child's stool needs to be collected for 72 hr in one container. No special preservatives are used. If collected at home, container is kept in the freezer. Instructions may be given regarding appropriate diet (high fat) and a diet diary might be required.
Occult blood, guiac	Detects presence of blood in stool	Infection Inflammation Ulcerative colitis	Requires stool collection usually × 3, each specimen sent to lab individually
Endoscopy			
Upper GI-esophagogastro-duodenoscopy; flexible sigmoidoscopy	Use of fiber-optic endoscope Allows visualization of mucosal lining of esophagus, stomach, and duodenum	Foreign body removal Inflammatory disorders Vomiting of blood	Upper GI: Child must be NPO 4 to 8 hours before the procedure Post-procedure: Withhold fluids until child is alert and swallow (gag) reflex returns, usually 2-4 hr Lower GI: Requires bowel cleansing with mag citrate or Go-LYTELY and clear liquid diet 48 hours before the procedure Positions during the procedure may be the left lateral decubitus, knee-chest, or lithotomy

Modified from Wong, DL, et al: *Whaley and Wong's nursing care of infants and children*, ed 6, St Louis, 1999, Mosby.

TABLE 16-2 Commonly Used Gastrointestinal Medications for Children

Medication and Indications	Route and Dosage	Side Effects	Nursing Implications
Antacid			
Aluminum hydroxide (Basaljel, Alu-cap) Gastritis	Oral 2-15 ml/dose q 4 to 6 hr	GI: constipation, anorexia, intestinal obstruction, fecal impaction Other: dementia (aluminum toxicity)	Shake well before administration Assess for constipation Maintain fluid intake Parent teaching: Monitor for constipation Do not take over-the-counter medication without physician consultation
Peptic ulcers Gastroesophageal reflux Aluminum and magnesium hydroxide Magaldrate (Riopan)			
Peptic ulcer Gastroesophageal reflux Hiatal hernia	Oral Peptic ulcer: 5-15 ml/dose q 3-6 hr Other: dosage depends on indication	GI: constipation, diarrhea Other: hypermagnesemia, especially in presence of impaired renal function	Shake well before administration Give with small amount of water Assess stool consistency and pattern Maintain fluid intake Parent teaching: Administer according to prescribed dosage Do not give over-the-counter medication without physician consultation

Continued

TABLE 16-2 Commonly Used Gastrointestinal Medications for Children—cont'd

Medication and Indications	Route and Dosage	Side Effects	Nursing Implications
Anticholinergic			
Propantheline bromide (Pro-Banthine)	Oral	CNS: dizziness, headache, insomnia	Obtain baseline vital signs
	Child:	CV: palpitations, tachycardia	Parent teaching:
Controls diarrhea associated with inflammatory bowel disease by decreasing peristalsis	0.375 mg/kg/day in 4 divided doses	GI: dry mouth, paralytic ileus	Monitor CNS symptoms for indication of overdose, mainly decreased LOC
		Genitourinary: urinary retention	Crush tablet and mix with small amount of food or fluid
		Skin: urticaria, pruritus	Sugarless gum or candy will relieve dry mouth
		Sensory: blurred vision	Drug may cause blurred vision
		Other: anaphylaxis	
Glycopyrrolate (Robinul)	Oral	CNS: drowsiness, weakness, headache	Monitor vital signs
Peptic ulcer	>12 yrs: 1 mg tid	CV: palpitations, tachycardia	Monitor input and output
Other GI diseases associated with hypermotility, hyperacidity, and spasm		GI: constipation	Parent teaching:
		Genitourinary: urinary hesitancy	Avoid high environmental temperature
		Sensory: blurred vision, photophobia	Monitor for rash, blurred vision
		Skin: rash	Advise use of sunglasses

Histamine H₂ Receptor Antagonist

Cimetidine (Tagamet)
Gastroesophageal reflux
Peptic ulcer disease
	Oral
	20-40 mg/kg/day
	in doses qid
		CNS: dizziness, headache
		CV: bradycardia
		GI: diarrhea
		Genitourinary: increased
		  BUN
		Hematology: neutropenia
		Skin: rash, dermatitis
		Other: muscular pain
			Monitor blood counts, renal and hepatic function during
			  treatment
			Assess mental and neurologic status
			Parent teaching:
			  Administer 30 min before or with meals
			  Tablet may be crushed
			  Do not stop medication or give over-the-counter
			    medications without physician consultation	

Ranitidine (Zantac)
Gastroesophageal reflux
Peptic ulcer
	Oral
	>12 yr 100 to 150 mg
	bid
		CNS: dizziness, malaise
		CV: bradycardia
		GI: nausea, constipation
		Skin: rash, urticaria
			Parent teaching:
			  May administer 30 min before or with meals
			  Tablets may be crushed and mixed with food
			  Notify physician if side effects occur
			  Do not give over-the-counter medication without
			    physician consultation	

II. Major concepts of fluid and electrolyte balance

A. **Distribution of body fluids**
1. Total body water comprises 65% to 85% of body weight in infants and children
2. Body water is divided into two major fluid compartments
   a. Extracellular fluid (ECF)—contained outside of cell walls; infants and children have a greater proportion of water here; subdivided into:
      (1) Interstitial—between cells
      (2) Intravascular—plasma in the vascular bed or the blood vessels
   b. Intracellular fluid (ICF)—contained within cell walls; therefore, fluid is more protected within this less-exposed environment
3. Infants and children are more vulnerable to fluid volume deficit because:
   a. A greater amount of their body water is in the ECF compartment, which offers less protection against fluid losses
   b. Organs that conserve water are immature, especially the kidneys
4. Children and infants have a greater free-water turnover than adults from:
   a. Increased basal metabolic rate with increased evaporative losses
   b. Elevated resting RR that adds to fluid losses

B. **Daily maintenance fluid requirements** (Table 16-3)

C. **Dehydration in infants and children is the most common fluid and electrolyte imbalance**
1. Losses of extracellular fluid and electrolytes caused by:
   a. Vomiting and diarrhea
   b. Burns
   c. Malnutrition
   d. Diaphoresis
   e. Decreased fluid intake
   f. Increased RR
2. Classification of dehydration (Table 16-4)

TABLE 16-3   **Fluid Requirements for Daily Maintenance**

Body Weight	Amount of Fluid per Day/Body Weight
1-10 kg	100 ml/kg
11-20 kg	1000 ml plus 50 ml/kg for each kg >10 kg
>20 kg	1500 ml plus 20 ml/kg for each kg >20 kg

From Wong DL, et al: *Whaley and Wong's nursing care of infants and children*, ed 6, St. Louis, 1999, Mosby.

TABLE 16-4 Clinical Manifestations of Dehydration in Children

	Isotonic (Loss of Water and Salt)	Hypotonic (Loss of Salt in Excess of Water)	Hypertonic (Loss of Water in Excess of Salt)
Skin			
Color	Gray	Gray	Gray
Temperature	Cold	Cold	Cold or hot
Turgor	Poor	Very poor	Fair
Feel	Dry	Clammy	Thickened, doughy
Mucous membranes	Dry	Slightly moist	Parched
Tearing and salivation	Absent	Absent	Absent
Eyeball	Sunken	Sunken	Sunken
Fontanel	Sunken	Sunken	Sunken
Body temperature	Subnormal or elevated	Subnormal or elevated	Subnormal or elevated
Pulse	Rapid	Very rapid	Moderately rapid
Respirations	Rapid	Rapid	Rapid
Behavior	Irritable to lethargic	Lethargic to comatose; convulsions	Marked lethargy with extreme hyperirritability on stimulation

From Wong DL, et al: *Whaley and Wong's nursing care of infants and children,* ed 6, St Louis, 1999, Mosby.

3. More accurate classification involves the loss of milliliters per kilogram of body weight over 48 hours or less
   a. Mild: less than 50 ml/kg
   b. Moderate: 50 to 90 ml/kg
   c. Severe: more than 100 ml/kg
4. Signs of dehydration
   a. Weight loss
   b. Decreased urine output, increased specific gravity
   c. Dry mucous membranes
   d. Sunken anterior fontanel in infants
   e. Prolonged capillary refill time
   f. Absence of tears, sunken look to the eyes
   g. Tachycardia
   h. Hemoconcentration: increased H&H
   i. Decrease in skin turgor; determined mainly in older children
   j. Lethargy, decrease in usual play activities

III. Gastrointestinal conditions that result in fluid and electrolyte imbalance

A. **Vomiting**
   1. Description: forceful expulsion of stomach contents
   2. Common findings of childhood are associated with these conditions:
      a. Allergic reaction or toxin exposure
      b. Overfeeding
      c. Infection: urinary and respiratory tracts
      d. CNS disorders
      e. Side effect of drugs
      f. Obstructive disorders such as pyloric stenosis and intussusception
   3. These findings often accompany vomiting:
      a. Nausea and retching
      b. Abdominal cramping, pain, and diarrhea
      c. Headache
   4. Careful assessment of these findings is useful in evaluating the cause of vomiting:
      a. Character of vomitus
      b. Frequency and persistence
      c. Amount
      d. Force—projectile vomiting is typical of pyloric stenosis or increased ICP
   5. Metabolic alkalosis and dehydration may develop with prolonged, severe vomiting
   6. The BRAT diet—bananas, rice cereal, applesauce, and toast—is used at home until nausea and vomiting subside for the treatment of short-term vomiting in older children

7. Hospitalization is necessary when the signs of dehydration, blood in the vomitus, more forceful or projectile vomiting, or abdominal pain are present

⚠ Warning!

Position the child who is vomiting, or resting, in such a way as to prevent the aspiration of emesis into the lungs.

8. Nursing diagnoses
   a. Fluid volume deficit
   b. Altered nutrition: less than body requirements

B. Diarrhea
1. Definition: the accelerated excretion of the intestinal contents; may be acute or chronic
2. Acute diarrhea is associated with:
   a. Gastroenteritis
   b. Dietary indiscretions: overfeeding, excess sugar or fat in formula; sensitivities to cow's milk, eggs, wheat, nuts, shellfish, and glutens
   c. Antibiotic use: medications such as ampicillin, erythromycin, and tetracycline cause decreased glucose absorption and disaccharidase activity; repeated or prolonged antibiotic use allows for the overgrowth of the anaerobic spore-forming toxin producing Clostridium difficile, that can cause pseudomembranous colitis
   d. Other illnesses: urinary or respiratory tract infections
   e. Note that infants may have episodes of diarrhea during teething, which is an expected normal finding
3. Chronic nonspecific diarrhea (CNSD) is the most common cause of protracted diarrhea in young children, especially in the toddler age group
   a. Caused by decreased transit time in the alimentary tract
   b. Factors associated with CNSD:
      (1) Food intolerance
      (2) Excessive fluid intake
      (3) Protein or carbohydrate intolerance
      (4) Drug ingestion
4. Other conditions associated with chronic diarrhea are cystic fibrosis and parasitic infections
5. Because a wide variety of stooling patterns occur in infants and children, the following criteria must be present to identify diarrhea: increased frequency of stools, watery consistency, and green stool
6. Complications of acute and chronic diarrhea are dehydration, metabolic acidosis, and malnutrition

7. Treatment for diarrhea:
   a. Placing the bowel at rest by keeping the child NPO or on a light diet of clear liquids and dry foods such as crackers or toast
   b. Fluid and electrolyte replacement

> ⚠️ **Warning!**
>
> No potassium should be added to the IV solution until the child has voided, which indicates adequate renal function.

   c. Elimination of underlying cause
8. Nursing diagnoses
   a. Fluid volume deficit
   b. Altered nutrition: less than body requirements
C. **Acute gastroenteritis** (Table 16-5)
   1. Definition: inflammation of the stomach and intestines, which may be acute or chronic
   2. Caused by various organisms, allergies, disease processes, and contaminated foods
   3. Infectious gastroenteritis is a term used when the diarrhea is caused by bacteria or virus

IV. Congenital defects: cleft lip and palate

A. **Description: failure of the soft tissue or bony structure to fuse during embryonic development; may occur separately or in combination; may involve one or both sides of the midline of the palate**
B. **Etiology and incidence**
   1. Caused by fetal insult; teratogenic factors include drugs, exposure to radiation or the rubella virus, chromosomal abnormalities, or maternal smoking or nicotine use in the first trimester
   2. Cleft lip has an incidence of 1 in 800 live births, with a male predominance
   3. Cleft lip occurs mostly in Native American and Asian populations
   4. Cleft palate occurs in 1 in 2000 live births and is more common in females
C. **Pathophysiology**
   1. Lip: maxillary prominence fails to fuse with medial nasal prominence between 7 and 8 weeks' gestation
   2. Palate: maxillary bone plate fails to close during 7 to 12 weeks' gestation
   3. Cleft lip and palate may occur as an isolated defect or in combination
D. **Assessment**
   1. Cleft lip: unilateral or bilateral; extent varies from a slight notch in the vermillion border to a complete separation from the floor of the nose

Text continued on p. 477

TABLE 16-5   Acute Pediatric Gastroenteritis: Causes, Findings, Transmission, Peak Incidence

Organism/Treatment	Age Affected	Assessment Findings	Pathology	Transmission	Peak Incidence
Viral Agents					
Rotavirus Prevent dehydration	6-24 mo	Fever Vomiting Diarrhea	Mucosal atrophy Inflammation	Person-to-person	Winter
Norwalk virus Prevent dehydration	All	Fever Anorexia Vomiting Abdominal pain	Inflammation of mucosa Villi damage Decreased enzymes	Person-to-person	Winter
Bacterial Agents					
Escherichia coli Antibiotics Prevent dehydration Antispasmodics	0-18 mo	Green liquid stools Fever Vomiting	Enterotoxin production Invasion of GI epithelium	Person-to-person Ingestion of contaminated food, water, inanimate objects	All year, especially summer

Salmonella
 No specific treatment
 Major goal:
   Prevent dehydration
 Antibiotics:
   Typically not indicated
	0-2 yr	6-48 hr after eating contaminated food, sudden onset of diarrhea, watery stools containing blood, pus, or mucus
		 Colicky abdominal pain
		 Vomiting
		 Fever
			Inflammation and necrosis of GI mucosa
			 Symptoms may last 7 days
				Contaminated food and drink from animal sources—eggs, poultry, milk
				 Pets (especially turtles)
					All year, especially July–October

Continued

Modified from Wong DL, et al: *Whaley and Wong's nursing care of infants and children*, ed 6, St Louis, 1999, Mosby.

TABLE 16-5 **Acute Pediatric Gastroenteritis: Causes, Findings, Transmission, Peak Incidence—cont'd**

Organism/Treatment	Age Affected	Assessment Findings	Pathology	Transmission	Peak Incidence
Bacterial Agents—cont'd					
Shigella Preferred treatment: Supportive Likelihood of encountering antibiotic-resistant organisms is high Major goal: Prevent dehydration	0-10 yr	Diarrhea, stools contain pus Fever Abdominal pain *Tenesmus*—persistent, ineffective spasms of rectum accompanied by a desire to empty bowel; may be painful	Enterotoxin production	Person-to-person Isolation and strict hand-washing precautions essential	Late summer Must be reported to public health department
Food Poisoning					
Staphylococcus Prevent dehydration Bed rest Analgesics	All	Nausea Vomiting Severe abdominal cramping Occurs 6-12 hr after ingestion of contaminated food	Enterotoxin production	Contaminated food sources—inadequately cooled or refrigerated (e.g., custards, mayonnaise)	All year

Modified from Wong DL, et al: *Whaley and Wong's nursing care of infants and children*, ed 6, St Louis, 1999, Mosby.

    2. Cleft palate: unilateral or bilateral; varying degree for the extent of palate involvement evident on visual inspection

E. Therapeutic management

    1. Surgery: reconstructive surgery is performed for cleft lip during the first weeks of life; palate correction is done at either 12 or 18 months before speech habits are established; corrections often require several stages and surgeries

    2. Medications: analgesics (narcotic or nonnarcotic) to control postoperative pain

    3. Feeding devices: before surgery use of a soft, elongated lamb's nipple; a Brecht feeder (asepto syringe with rubber tubing attached) is useful for infants with a large cleft palate

    4. Speech therapy: ongoing until school age or as indicated

F. Nursing management

    1. Preoperative care

      a. Nursing diagnosis: altered nutrition (less than body requirements) related to altered feeding

      b. Expected outcome: parents demonstrate effective feeding techniques

      c. Interventions

        (1) Assess the infant's feeding requirements

        (2) Assess the nature of the defect and its impact on feeding

        (3) Monitor the infant's respiratory status and ability to suck during feeding

        (4) Encourage breast feeding if appropriate

        (5) Initiate feeding with special devices, as required: Brecht feeder, elongated lamb's nipple

        (6) Feed small amounts gradually; place the infant in an upright or a semi-sitting position

        (7) Burp the infant frequently, every 15 to 30 ml; offer 5 to 10 ml of water after each feeding

        (8) Remove crusted formula or milk with a cotton-tipped applicator moistened with water

        (9) Demonstrate special feeding or suctioning techniques to parents

    2. Postoperative care

      a. Nursing diagnoses: risk for injury, risk for infection

      b. Expected outcome: suture line remains clean and free of trauma and infection

      c. Interventions

        (1) Assess suture line for drainage, crusting, and signs of infection

        (2) Cleft lip repair: cleanse lip suture line after feeding and as ordered; use cotton-tipped applicator moistened with sterile saline or other solution as preferred by the surgeon

(3) Position the infant on the back or side, or use a secured car seat; avoid positioning the infant on the abdomen (prone) to prevent rubbing of the surgical site against the mattress

(4) Maintain a lip protective device—a Logan bow or a butterfly bandage strip on the operative site

(5) Restrain the infant with soft elbow or jacket restraints; remove—one at a time—periodically or at least every 3 to 4 hours to perform range-of-motion exercises

(6) Avoid contact with sharp objects, straws, or forks near the surgical site

(7) Anticipate the child's needs to prevent crying

(8) Feed the infant with a cup, wide bowl, or soup spoon—not a regular spoon; if the palate is repaired: avoid putting a spoon into the mouth because this action may disrupt the sutures; a full liquid diet as ordered in the immediate postoperative period

(9) Avoid oral suction or placing objects into the mouth such as a tongue depressor or oral thermometer

(10) Prevent sucking to prevent strain on the suture lines: no pacifiers or use of straws for oral fluid intake

3. Additional nursing diagnoses
   a. Ineffective airway clearance
   b. Anxiety
   c. Ineffective family coping

G. **Evaluation**
   1. Child exhibits an absence of trauma and infection at the incision site
   2. Child maintains a patent airway without pulmonary aspiration
   3. Parents provide appropriate feeding techniques and incision care

V. Gastric ingestion of foreign substances

A. *Pica:* **craving and purposeful act of ingesting nonfood substances such as dirt, chalk, clay, starch, paint chips, glue, ice, hair, and crayons**
   1. Certain forms of pica are associated with a mineral deficiency, for example, eating chalk is linked to a calcium deficiency
   2. Sometimes pica is a factor in lead poisoning; however, most cases of lead poisoning are associated with a child's instinctual behavior to explore with the mouth

B. **Poisonings—common accidental ingestions are given in Table 16-6**

VI. Gastric motility disorders

A. **Hirschsprung disease (congenital aganglionic megacolon)**
   1. Description: a congenital defect that results in a mechanical obstruction from inadequate motility of an intestinal segment, usually the descending or sigmoid colon (Figure 16-1, p. 480)

TABLE 16-6   Common Accidental Ingestions: Findings, Treatment, Interventions

Ingestion	Assessment Findings	Treatment	Priority Nursing Interventions
Acetaminophen (Tylenol)	Nausea, vomiting Pallor Liver involvement—jaundice, stupor, coagulation abnormalities	Induce emesis Mucomyst, PO, usually QID × 3-4 days Activated charcoal	Monitor tests for liver function—ALT, AST Teach parents proper administration and dosage of acetaminophen
Salicylate (aspirin)	Tinnitus Hyperventilation Initially: Respiratory alkalosis Metabolic acidosis	Induce emesis or gastric lavage IV fluids and electrolytes IV sodium bicarbonate if pH <7.2 Vitamin K if bleeding	Assess for bleeding Monitor renal function—serum creatinine Caution parents to avoid giving aspirin to children with a suspected viral infection to prevent Reye syndrome
Hydrocarbons (e.g., gasoline, kerosene)	Nausea, vomiting Altered sensorium Weakness Pulmonary involvement—cyanosis, tachypnea, sternal retractions	Administer oxygen Treatment controversial; depends on agent ingested	Remove clothing and wash skin in contact with poison Monitor vital signs Support ventilation Support parents
Corrosives (e.g., strong acids or alkalis as found in household cleaning products and drain cleaner)	Mouth, throat, stomach burning Edema of lips, tongue, pharynx Drooling Signs of shock Anxiety Vomiting, hemoptysis	Vomiting contraindicated Dilute agents with water Analgesics for pain NPO May insert gastric tube	Ensure patent airway Monitor vital signs, LOC Monitor acid-base status Support parents

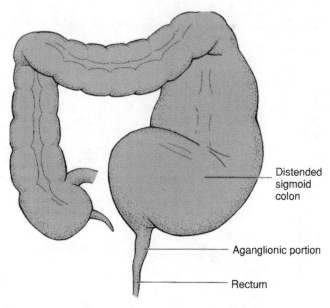

Distended
sigmoid
colon

Aganglionic portion

Rectum

Figure 16-1   Hirschprung disease. (From Wong DL, et al: *Whaley and Wong's nursing care of infants and children,* ed 6, St. Louis, 1999, Mosby.)

2. Etiology and incidence
   a. May be accompanied by other GI and genitourinary anomalies
   b. Increased incidence in children with Down syndrome
   c. Follows a familial pattern of inheritance in some cases
3. Pathophysiology
   a. Absence of ganglion cells in one or more intestinal segments that results in a lack of peristalsis
   b. Bowel proximal to the defect dilates because of a lack of peristalsis
   c. Failure of the anal sphincter to relax; fecal matter accumulates in the aganglionic segment
4. Assessment
   a. Assessment findings
      (1) Neonatal period, the first 4 weeks of life
         (a) Failure to pass meconium within 24 to 48 hours after birth
         (b) Bile-stained (yellow-brown) vomitus
         (c) Abdominal distention
      (2) Infancy
         (a) Inadequate weight gain
         (b) Altered bowel elimination that ranges from constipation to bloody diarrhea
         (c) Foul-smelling stools; visible peristalsis

       (3) Childhood
          (a) Ribbonlike, foul-smelling stools
          (b) Poor growth
          (c) Palpable fecal masses
   b. Diagnostic procedures
       (1) Barium enema—reveals narrowed segment of bowel
       (2) Rectal biopsy—reveals absence of aganglion cells
       (3) Abdominal X-ray film—reveals dilated loops of intestine proximal to the narrowed bowel segment
       (4) Rectal manometry—reveals failure of the internal sphincter to relax
5. Therapeutic management
   a. Medications: preoperative antibiotics to sterilize the bowel to minimize the risk of infection
   b. Treatments: enema therapy and nasogastric (NG) tube placement
   c. Surgery: two-stage process
       (1) Temporary colostomy construction
       (2) Resection of aganglionic segment; anastomosis of the intact ganglion segment to the rectum is performed during a "pull-through" procedure
   d. Colostomy closure usually occurs 3 months after the pull-through procedure
6. Nursing management
   a. Acute care: preoperative
       (1) Nursing diagnoses
          (a) Altered nutrition: less than body requirements
          (b) Fluid volume deficit related to nausea and vomiting
          (c) Constipation related to the absence of ganglion cells
       (2) Expected outcome: nutritional status is promoted before surgery and fluid volume is restored
       (3) Interventions
          (a) Assess daily the child's weight and abdominal girth; fluid and electrolyte status with input and output measurements every 8 hours
          (b) Assess bowel sounds every 4 hours
          (c) Assess for signs of bowel perforation: a sudden boardlike abdomen, fever, or increased abdominal distention
          (d) Offer a diet high in calories and protein, low in residue; administer TPN in extreme situations, as ordered
          (e) Administer enemas, as ordered

⚠ Warning!

Tap water enemas should never be used in a child with Hirschprung disease; isotonic solution should be used. Colonic irrigations with antibiotic solution are often ordered prior to "pull through" procedure.

b. Acute care: postoperative
   (1) Nursing diagnoses: same as the preoperative phase; impaired skin integrity related to the presence of an ostomy
   (2) Expected outcomes: nutritional status is maintained without dehydration or negative nitrogen balance; electrolyte balance is maintained; skin breakdown is prevented
   (3) Interventions
       (a) Monitor child's hydration status, including NG, colostomy, and indwelling urinary catheter drainage; monitor IV, NG, and oral intake
       (b) Assess skin condition at the surgical site; provide ostomy care as ordered
       (c) Maintain patency of NG tube
       (d) Monitor return of bowel sounds, usually within 48 to 72 hours after surgery before initiation of oral feedings
7. Evaluation
   a. Parents provide colostomy care and use the proper technique
   b. Child exhibits adequate hydration and any dehydration is prevented or treated effectively
   c. Child has restored nutritional status

B. Gastroesophageal reflux (GER)
1. Description: presence of stomach contents in the esophagus
2. Etiology and incidence
   a. Exact cause unknown
   b. Incidence: predisposing factor is delayed maturation of esophageal neuromuscular control
3. Pathophysiology
   a. Gastric-content reflux into the lower esophagus results in tissue inflammation, scarring, and formation of a **stricture**—an abnormal temporary or permanent narrowing of a hollow organ
   b. The cause is an incompetent cardiac sphincter at the esophageal-gastric junction
   c. These effects occur as a result of GER:
       (1) Esophagitis—esophageal stricture or carcinoma
       (2) Aspiration of gastric contents—can cause aspiration pneumonia or apnea with cyanosis, especially in infants
4. Assessment
   a. Assessment findings
       (1) Chronic vomiting
       (2) Failure to thrive
       (3) Esophageal bleeding manifested by hematemesis or melena

  b. Diagnostic procedures
    (1) Esophageal manometry—reveals abnormal lower esophageal sphincter pressure
    (2) Barium swallow and upper GI series—reveals reflux after swallowing and excludes other anatomic obstructions
    (3) Intraesophageal pH monitoring—reveals abnormal pH of the distal esophagus with reflux contents
    (4) Endoscopy—assesses for the presence of esophogitis
5. Therapeutic management
  a. Medications (see Table 16-2, p. 467)
    (1) Cholinergics
      (a) Increase esophageal tone and peristaltic activity
      (b) Decrease esophageal pressure by relaxing pyloric and duodenal segments
      (c) Increase peristalsis without the stimulation of increased gastric secretions
    (2) Histamine H_2 receptor antagonists: decrease gastric acidity and pepsin secretion
    (3) Antacids: neutralize gastric acid between feedings
    (4) Antisecretory agent: omeprazole (Prilosec)—characterized as a gastric acid pump inhibitor, since it blocks the final step of acid production
    (5) Prokinetics: metoclopramide hydrochloride (Reglan) decreases reflux
  b. Feedings: Thicken feedings and put the child into a high- or mid-Fowler's position during and for 1 to 2 hours after feedings
  c. Surgery: for severe complications of GER, *Nissen fundoplication* is performed, which is the creation of a valve mechanism by wrapping the greater curvature of the stomach (fundus) around the distal esophagus to restore competence of the lower esophageal sphincter
6. Nursing management
  a. Nursing diagnoses
    (1) Ineffective airway clearance related to vomiting
    (2) Altered nutrition: less than body requirements
  b. Expected outcomes
    (1) Child maintains patent airway
    (2) Child reestablishes adequate nutrient and fluid intake
  c. Interventions
    (1) Assess airway status and lung sounds
    (2) Assess feeding patterns, routines, and environment
    (3) Record vomitus: amount, characteristics, and frequency
    (4) Assess for signs of dehydration or aspiration pneumonia
    (5) Thicken formula with baby rice cereal to minimize reflux: 1 tablespoon of cereal to every 6 ounces of formula

   (6) Feed slowly; burp often after each ounce

   (7) Handle child minimally after feedings

   (8) Position child as ordered; sleeping position is usually prone with head of mattress at a 30-degree angle to prevent aspiration; may be accomplished with the use of a wedge under the mattress or a commercially available harness

 7. Evaluation

  a. Child exhibits minimal reflux activity as the family adheres to preventive actions

  b. Family exhibits decreased anxiety about the illness and child care

  c. Family demonstrates the proper technique for feeding and assessment techniques for complications

  d. Infant gains or maintains weight

VII. Obstructive disorders

A. Hypertrophic pyloric stenosis (HPS)

 1. Description: hypertrophy of the circular muscle of the pylorus, which causes a narrowing of the pyloric canal between the stomach and duodenum

 2. Etiology and incidence

  a. Cause of pyloric muscle hypertrophy is unknown

  b. Most commonly seen between 1 and 6 months of age

  c. Occurs mainly in term male infants; genetic predisposition exists; therefore, siblings are at risk

 3. Pathophysiology

  a. Narrowed pyloric canal gradually becomes obstructed; inflammation and edema result in a complete obstruction (Figure 16-2)

  b. Pyloric muscle enlarges to twice normal size; the stomach dilates

  c. Clinical picture develops gradually; in the early stage of hypertrophy the infant appears and eats well

  d. Vomiting progresses from mild regurgitation to projectile vomiting

 4. Assessment

  a. Assessment findings

   (1) Vomiting: usually shortly after feeding; child will then appear hungry and accept more food

   (2) Emesis of a greenish color contains gastric contents, is nonbilous (no yellow-brown color), and is possibly blood-tinged

   (3) Failure to gain weight or weight loss

   (4) Upper abdominal distention: palpable olive-shaped mass in epigastrium to the right of the umbilicus

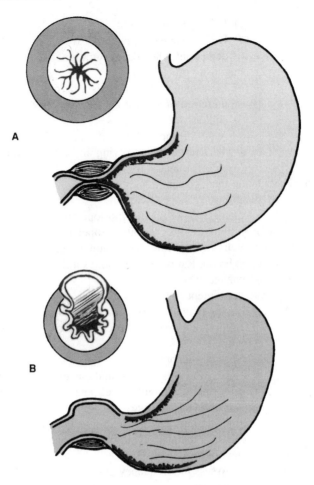

Figure 16-2 Hypertrophic pyloric stenosis. **A,** Enlarged muscular tumor nearly obliterates pyloric channel. **B,** Longitudinal surgical division of muscle down to submucosa establishes adequate passageway. (From Wong DL, et al: *Whaley and Wong's nursing care of infants and children,* ed 6, St. Louis, 1999, Mosby.)

        (5) Peristaltic waves are visible from left to right across the epigastrium

        (6) Signs of dehydration are apparent as vomiting increases in frequency and amount

    b. Diagnostic procedures

        (1) Laboratory studies

            (a) Serum electrolytes—increased sodium and potassium if dehydrated, and decreased chloride

            (b) Arterial blood gases (ABGs)—increased pH and bicarbonate, indicating metabolic alkalosis from the loss of hydrochloric stomach acid

(c) Urine pH—increased
(d) H&H—increased, resulting from extracellular fluid depletion; a hemoconcentration
(2) Diagnostic procedures
(a) Ultrasonography—reveals a narrowed pyloric canal; preferred procedure because less risk for aspiration of contrast medium exists
(b) X-ray of upper abdomen with barium—reveals delayed gastric emptying and elongation of the pyloric canal
5. Therapeutic management
a. Medications
(1) Analgesics—to manage postoperative pain
(2) Antibiotics—to prevent postoperative infection
b. Surgery: **pyloromyotomy**—incision through muscle fibers of the pylorus: Fredet-Ramstedt operation; surgical laporoscopy is used
6. Nursing management
a. Acute care: preoperative
(1) Nursing diagnoses: risk for fluid volume deficit related to dehydration; see also altered nutrition (postoperative care below)
(2) Expected outcomes
(a) Child maintains fluid and electrolyte balance, with normal urine output and potassium within the normal parameters for age
(b) Child has dehydration prevented or treated effectively
(c) Child maintains acid-base balance
(3) Interventions
(a) Assess the frequency and volume of vomiting after feedings
(b) Assess the hydration status: daily weights along with input and output every 8 hours; urine specific gravity as needed
(c) Monitor for signs of dehydration: grayish skin color, depressed fontanels, dry skin, and sunken eyes
(d) Monitor serum electrolytes and ABGs
(e) Administer IV fluids of glucose and electrolytes as ordered
(f) Maintain patency of gastric tube (if present)
b. Postoperative care
(1) Nursing diagnosis: altered nutrition: less than body requirements
(2) Expected outcomes
(a) The child consumes adequate amount of nourishment
(b) Parents verbalize correct feeding technique and follow-up care

(3) Interventions
   (a) Begin small, frequent feedings postoperatively: begin with glucose water, advance to diluted formula, then full-strength formula
   (b) Feed in upright position and burp frequently
   (c) Handle minimally after feedings
   (d) After feedings, position the child with head elevated and on the right side, which helps the normal flow of fluid from the stomach to the intestine
c. Additional nursing diagnoses
   (1) Risk for injury
   (2) Anxiety
   (3) Alteration in comfort
7. Evaluation
a. Child maintains weight, acid-base balance, and fluid balance
b. Parents provide appropriate care and feeding and incision care before hospital discharge

B. Intussusception
1. Description: telescoping of one portion of the bowel into another portion, resulting in obstruction of the passage of intestinal contents (Figure 16-3, p. 488)
2. Etiology and incidence
a. Cause unknown
b. Most common cause of intestinal obstruction between 3 months and 2 years of life
c. Children at risk are those diagnosed with cystic fibrosis, celiac disease, and gastroenteritis
3. Pathophysiology
a. Inflammation and ischemia occur in the intestinal wall as portions press against one another
b. Eventual tissue necrosis, perforation, and peritonitis may occur
c. Most common site involved is the ileocecal valve (see Figure 16-3, p. 488)
4. Assessment
a. Assessment findings
   (1) Paroxysmal acute pain in abdomen with distention
   (2) Vomiting
   (3) "Currant-jellylike" stools, a reddish-purple color, indicated a mixture of blood and mucus
   (4) Cylindrical mass above the affected area
b. Diagnostic procedures—abdominal X-ray film and barium enema reveal the affected area of the intestine
5. Therapeutic management
a. Treatment: hydrostatic reduction using water-soluble contrast and air pressure

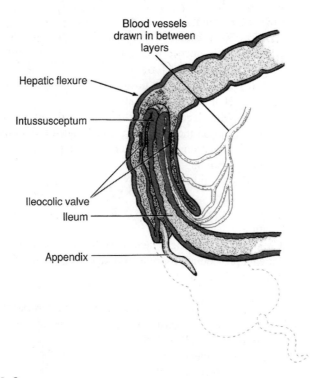

Blood vessels
drawn in between
layers

Hepatic flexure

Intussusceptum

Ileocolic valve
Ileum

Appendix

Figure 16-3 Ileocolic intussusception. (From Wong DL, et al: *Whaley and Wong's nursing care of infants and children,* ed 6, St. Louis, 1999, Mosby.)

        b. Surgery: performed if reduction by barium enema is not successful or tissue necrosis is present

        c. Medications:

            (1) Antibiotics to treat peritonitis

            (2) Analgesics to manage postoperative pain

    6. Nursing management

        a. Acute care: preoperative

            (1) Nursing diagnoses

                (a) Risk for injury related to necrosis and peritonitis

                (b) Pain related to invagination of the bowel

            (2) Expected outcomes

                (a) The child demonstrates minimum discomfort

                (b) The child has minimal or no necrosis and peritonitis

            (3) Interventions

                (a) Assess child for findings of intussusception

                (b) Maintain patency of NG tube

                (c) Administer IV fluids as ordered

                (d) Inform parents of rationale for NG tube and NPO status, which is to rest the bowel

(e) NG tube size depends on child's size, weight, and fluid to be infused

Age	Catheter Size
Newborns, infants	5-6, 8 F
>6 yr	8-10 F
Adolescent	12-16 F

(f) Inform parents of the possible need for surgery if hydrostatic reduction is not successful or intussusception recurs

b. Postoperative care
(1) Nursing diagnosis: alteration in bowel elimination
(2) Expected outcome: child demonstrates normal bowel pattern
(3) Interventions
(a) Assess the child for the return of bowel sounds
(b) Monitor the child for passage of stool and barium (barium stool will be whitish-clay-colored)
(c) Inform parents that the passage of brown stools indicates that invagination has been corrected
(d) Encourage fluids to prevent impaction from the barium

7. Evaluation
a. Family verbalizes information about therapies, procedures, and findings to report to the physician
b. Child displays absence of complications and absence of recurrence of invagination

VIII. Malabsorption: celiac disease (gluten-sensitive enteropathy)

A. Description: intolerance to *gluten,* the protein component of wheat, barley, rye, and oats; causes impairment of the absorptive processes

B. Etiology and incidence
1. Symptoms occur 3 to 6 months after introduction of gluten-containing grains into the diet; usually before 2 years of age
2. Evidence supports a genetic link in the occurrence of the disorder
3. Mainly found in the white population

C. Pathophysiology
1. Gliadin fraction of gluten causes damage to mucosal cells; the villi atrophy, causing malabsorption (Figure 16-4, p. 490)
2. Initially, fat absorption is impaired; later, protein and carbohydrate absorption are also impaired

D. Assessment
1. Assessment findings
a. Early signs
(1) Diarrhea; failure to regain weight after the diarrheal episode

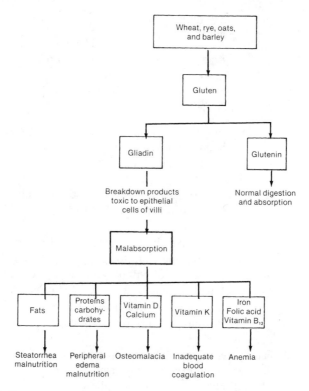

Figure 16-4 Malabsorptive defect in celiac disease. (From Wong DL, et al: *Whaley and Wong's nursing care of infants and children,* ed 5, St. Louis, 1995, Mosby.)

        (2) Constipation
        (3) Vomiting
        (4) Abdominal pain
        (5) **Steatorrhea**—foul smelling, pale, fatty stools
    b. Later signs
        (1) Behavioral changes: irritability and apathy
        (2) Muscle wasting, with loss of subcutaneous fat
    c. Celiac crisis—a rare event that requires immediate medical intervention
        (1) Severe dehydration
        (2) Metabolic acidosis
  2. Diagnostic procedures
        (1) Laboratory studies: stool analysis—reveals steatorrhea
        (2) Diagnostic studies
            (a) Jejunal biopsy—reveals an atrophy of the mucosal cells
            (b) Serum antigliadin and antireticulin antibodies—presence of these is indicative of the disorder
            (c) Sweat test—rules out CF

E. **Therapeutic management**
1. Medications
   a. Vitamin supplements—the fat-soluble vitamins A, D, E, and K *supplied in a water-miscible form*
   b. Mineral supplements
   c. Steroids—used in a celiac crisis to decrease bowel inflammation
2. Treatments: dietary management
   a. Gluten-free diet: substitute corn, rice, or millet for grain
   b. Lifelong elimination of gluten sources: wheat, rye, oats, and barley
   c. Strict adherence to gluten-free diet decreases the risk of developing lymphoma of the small intestine, a complication of the disease
F. **Nursing management**
1. Acute care
   a. Nursing diagnosis: altered nutrition (less than body requirements) related to dietary intolerances, malabsorption
   b. Expected outcomes
      (1) Child adheres to a prescribed diet with no signs of bowel inflammation
      (2) Child's growth and development are adequate with height and weight within the norms for age
   c. Interventions
      (1) Assess for findings of celiac disease, assess daily weights, and monitor stools
      (2) Provide a gluten-free diet
      (3) Administer corticosteroids and water-miscible vitamins, as ordered
2. Additional nursing diagnoses
   a. Risk for fluid volume deficit
   b. Diarrhea
   c. Noncompliance
G. **Evaluation**
1. Family identifies acceptable and unacceptable foods in the gluten-free diet
2. Child maintains a symptom-free state
3. Parents exhibit less anxiety and effective coping resources

IX. Inflammatory disorder: appendicitis

A. **Description: inflammation of the *appendix*, a blind sac connected to the end of the cecum; may lead to perforation, peritonitis, and sepsis if left untreated**
B. **Etiology and incidence**
1. Caused by obstruction of the lumen of the appendix; most commonly a result of a fecalith or hardened feces
2. Other causes are lymphoid hyperplasia, tumors, and fibrotic stenosis; other factors possibly implicated are worms and a low-fiber diet

3. Rapid progression to peritonitis is a characteristic process in infants and young children
4. Occurs mainly in school-aged children and adolescents

C. Pathophysiology
1. Lumen obstruction causes blockage of mucous secretion, blood vessels become compressed, and ischemia results
2. Bacterial invasion and necrosis subsequently occur
3. Acute inflammation rapidly progresses to bowel perforation and peritonitis if left undiagnosed

D. Assessment
1. Assessment findings
   a. Appendicitis
      (1) Pain and cramping initially located in periumbilical area; descends to the right lower quadrant; most intense at **McBurney's point**—located midway between the anterior superior iliac crest and the umbilicus; occasionally severe suprapubic pain occurs
      (2) Rebound tenderness and abdominal rigidity
      (3) Low-grade fever under 100° F orally
      (4) Vomiting and nausea
      (5) Constipation or diarrhea
      (6) Side-lying position with abdominal guarding; legs flexed
   b. Peritonitis
      (1) Fever increases to 102° F or higher, pallor, restlessness, and chills
      (2) Progressive abdominal distention and a severe increase in abdominal pain, with rigid guarding of the abdomen
      (3) Tachycardia; tachypnea

 Warning!

The nurse must carefully monitor for a sudden cessation of pain, which indicates rupture of the appendix. The client has a boardlike abdomen, findings of shock, and a greater risk of sepsis.

2. Diagnostic procedures
   a. Laboratory studies
      (1) CBC—WBC count increases to 15,000 to 20,000/mm^3 usually with polymorphonuclear leukocytosis. An increased percentage of bands or immature WBCs greater than the sigs—this is called a "shift to the left" and indicates an infection. If the segs or mature WBCs percentage increase is greater than the bands—this is called a "shift to the right" and indicates liver disease.
      (2) Urinalysis—reveals pyuria

b. Diagnostic studies
  (1) Abdominal x-ray film—reveals the presence of fecalith in the appendix
  (2) Ultrasonography—reveals abscess location before surgery

E. Therapeutic management
  1. Surgery: *appendectomy*—surgical removal of the appendix using laporoscopy before perforation; if rupture occurs, laporatomy is performed using a Penrose drain or an open incision, which requires more intense postoperative care
  2. Medications
    a. Analgesics—narcotic and nonnarcotic for pain control
    b. Antibiotics—systemic; usually only given to prevent or treat peritonitis if rupture of the appendix has occurred or if the appendix was abscessed
  3. Treatments after rupture of the appendix
    a. Immediately preoperative: IV fluids and electrolytes, IV antibiotics, NG suction, urinary urethral catheter insertion
    b. Postoperative: promote external drainage with a Penrose drain; wound irrigations because the incision may be left open to heal from the inside out

F. Nursing management
  1. Acute care: preoperative
    a. Nursing diagnoses: pain related to inflammation; risk for infection
    b. Expected outcomes
      (1) The child's pain is reduced or eliminated
      (2) The complications of peritonitis are prevented in the child
    c. Interventions
      (1) Assess pain: onset, duration, location, severity, and character; check for rebound tenderness
      (2) Assess vital signs every 2 to 4 hours; report a sustained HR for increases of 20 or more from the baseline; report shallow, fast respirations and a temperature of over 100° F
      (3) Maintain NPO status
      (4) Monitor closely for signs of peritonitis
      (5) Provide comfort interventions
        (a) Analgesics
        (b) Antipyretics—will be minimally effective if the appendix is abscessed
        (c) Right side-lying or low- to semi-Fowler's position to promote comfort or to localize the abscess if the appendix ruptures
      (6) Apply ice packs to abdomen for 20 to 30 minutes every hour; avoid any heat applications

(7) Report any changes in type, level, or location of pain; if the appendix ruptures, pain typically stops or significantly decreases

(8) Provide activities for quiet play

⚠ Warning!

Avoid the use of laxatives and enemas because they stimulate bowel motility and increase the risk of perforation.

2. Postoperative
   a. Nursing diagnosis: risk for infection
   b. Expected outcome: child has an incision that remains free of infection, with a soft abdomen
   c. Interventions
      (1) Assess the incision for signs of infection: redness, swelling, pain, and character of drainage
      (2) Assess the incision for the presence of a Penrose drain; if present, drainage may be profuse for the first 12 hours; maintain NG suction and patency, NG usually is present if the appendix ruptured
      (3) Position in right side-lying or low- to semi-Fowler's position with legs flexed to facilitate drainage
      (4) Change dressing as ordered or reinforce as necessary; record type and amount of drainage
      (5) Administer antibiotics and analgesics as ordered
      (6) If an open incision exists, teach parents sterile wound care, irrigation, and packing techniques. Wet or dry dressings may be ordered.
      (7) Monitor temperature for elevations every 2 to 4 hours
      (8) Assist the child in turning and deep breathing every 2 hours; splint the operative site with a pillow
      (9) Assist the child with the use of an incentive spirometry
3. Additional nursing diagnoses
   a. Anxiety
   b. Risk for fluid volume deficit
   c. Diarrhea or constipation
   d. Hyperthermia
   e. Altered nutrition: less than body requirements
G. Evaluation
1. Child's incision heals without infection
2. Child has relief from or controlled pain with the ordered medications
3. With an open incision, parents can perform correct sterile technique during the process of wound irrigation, packing, and dressing
4. Parents state findings to report to the physician

X. Home care: family education topics and referrals

A. **Hirschprung disease**

1. Elimination: enema therapy or care of the ostomy; colostomy care: the use and care of equipment, skin care, and colostomy irrigation
2. Nutrition: provide information about dietary management, which includes a high-residue or normal diet, and adequate fluid intake
3. Referrals: enterostomal therapist; dietician

B. **GER**

1. Nutrition: instruct parents about proper feeding techniques; positioning of the child; avoidance of fatty foods, chocolate, tomato products, carbonated liquids, full-strength fruit juices, and spicy foods; avoidance of vigorous play after feeding; and avoidance of feeding before bedtime. If surgery was performed, teach care of the gastrostomy tube and prepare for the possibility of postsurgical problems such as gas bloating, choking on solids, and delayed gastric emptying.
2. Medication: teach proper administration of omeprazole (Prilosec) or other enteric-coated capsules

C. **Pyloric stenosis; intussusception; appendicitis**

1. Incision: dressing changes—use of aseptic or sterile technique with procedures; review the list of necessary equipment
2. Medication: administration and side effects
3. Diet: demonstrate feeding procedure and incision care

D. **Celiac disease**

1. Diet: gluten-free diet: lifetime elimination of oats, wheat, barley, and rye; stress hidden sources of gluten in, for example, hydrolyzed vegetable protein and pizza dough; stress acceptable substitutes: rice, corn, and millet
2. Medications: proper administration of vitamins and mineral supplements
3. Referrals: dietician, public health nurse, and support group

WEB Resources

www.csaceliacs.org

Website provides information on the diagnosis and treatment of celiac disease. Also includes dietary basics, recipes, and pharmaceutical information.

www.uog.org

United Ostomy Society website provides client self-help information, support groups, and chapter news. Ostomy equipment suppliers are listed.

REVIEW QUESTIONS

1. After a pyloromyotomy, an infant needs to be positioned in which manner?
    1. On the right side in a low-Fowler's position all the time
    2. In a prone position on a pillow only at night
    3. After feedings, slightly on the right side in an infant car seat
    4. After feedings, slightly on the left side with the head of the bed elevated by using a wedge under the mattress

2. An infant is admitted to the hospital with a sudden episode of acute abdominal pain. To help establish a diagnosis of intussusception, the nurse should ask which of these questions?
    1. "Did the infant have a recent infection?"
    2. "Has the infant had projectile vomiting?"
    3. "Does the infant's stool look reddish-purple?"
    4. "Do you burp the infant frequently while feeding?"

3. A toddler is admitted to the hospital with acute gastroenteritis. An IV infusion has been ordered. Before adding potassium to the IV solution, which of these actions should the nurse take?
    1. Check the order with the physician
    2. Determine whether the child has voided
    3. Retake the child's vital signs
    4. Weigh the child

4. A staff member includes all of these interventions for an infant who has had cleft lip repair surgery. Which action indicates that the staff member needs additional instruction?
    1. Elbow restraints were placed on the infant
    2. The infant was placed in prone position
    3. The infant's suture line was gently cleansed after feedings, as ordered
    4. Restraints were removed periodically

5. After instructions about a celiac crisis, which comment by parents would indicate a correct understanding of the instructions?
    1. "Celiac crisis is not a serious complication."
    2. "My child must avoid exposure to infections."
    3. "Antihistamines are recommended."
    4. "Skipping a meal such as breakfast is not a problem."

ANSWERS, RATIONALES, AND TEST-TAKING TIPS

Rationales	Test-Taking Tips

1. Correct answer: 3

The infant is positioned in this manner to facilitate gastric emptying. A semi- to high-Fowler's position is preferred after feeding (not constantly) to decrease the possibility of vomiting and help gastric emptying. Option 2 may be a position for an infant with gastroesophageal reflux. The position in option 4 hinders gastric emptying.

After reading the question and options, take time to recall the normal anatomy and physiology of the upper GI tract. The pyloric valve, which divides the stomach from the duodenum, is located in the upper right quadrant of the abdomen. Therefore, to facilitate gastric emptying, select the option in which the infant is turned to the right side and somewhat upright. Gravity will help move the food downward into the duodenum.

2. Correct answer: 3

As intussusception progresses, the infant demonstrates increased vomiting, apathy, and passage of stools mixed with blood and mucus, which look like currant jelly—a reddish-purple color. An antecedent infection is not part of the disease process. Projectile vomiting is a classic finding in pyloric stenosis. The disease process is not linked to feeding techniques. It is a structural abnormality of the intestine in the lower GI tract. Feeding difficulties such as with burping tend to be associated with upper GI findings.

One approach is to eliminate options 1, 2, and 4 from your basic knowledge of GI diagnoses and findings. Also, note the key timeframe is "sudden," "acute." Options 1 and 4 would not indicate an acute problem. Projectile vomiting may lessen any pain because it decreases pressure in the stomach. A last approach for this question is to eliminate the options you know are incorrect. Thus, option 3 may be the only option left to select. This is a situation to select the option you do not know about after you have eliminated the other three options based on what you do know.

3. Correct answer: 2

If the child has voided, it establishes that adequate renal function is present. The actions in options 1 and 3 are not necessary before adding potassium to an IV fluid. A child with a history of acute

Reread the options and summarize each in this manner to clarify the information with a theme: option 1, communication with physician; option 2, renal function; option 3, arterial circulation; and option 4, hydration status. The priority

Rationales	Test-Taking Tips

gastroenteritis should be weighed at admission and daily. Weight would not influence a decision to give or hold a potassium administration.

information to associate with potassium administration is renal function, option 2. Recall that in renal failure, serum potassium and phosphate levels become elevated.

4. Correct answer: 2

Infants who have had cleft lip repair must be prevented from lying on the abdomen, which allows rubbing of their face on the sheet. In options 1, 3, and 4, the actions are correct with no need for further instruction. The use of elbow restraints is recommended to prevent infants from rubbing the incisions. Cleansing after feedings prevents infection and enhances healing. The suture line is cleansed of formula as needed. Removal of the restraints one at a time with supervision allows for exercise of the arms and for stimulation and body contact. Removal of these restraints is similar to other restraints, that is, every 2 to 3 hours with supervised range-of-motion exercises done at the time of removal.

The process to select the correct answer is to make sure you read the question again after initially reading through the options. This sharpens your focus to look for an incorrect action as you read the options through. You may also want to close your eyes after each option to picture the action in your mind's eye.

5. Correct answer: 2

Exacerbation of celiac disease, also called a crisis, can be prevented by adherence to a gluten-free diet and a prevention of the child's contact with persons who have infections. Celiac crisis, although rare, is a serious complication that requires prompt medical intervention to correct dehydration and metabolic acidosis. Drugs with

If you have no idea of the correct answer, select the option that pertains to infections rather than the other options that are aimed at more specific content. Recall that children and adults with chronic diseases are more susceptible to getting infections, since the immune system may be suppressed from the stress response to the disease. Celiac disease is characterized by an intolerance for a gliadin faction of

anticholinergic effects such as antihistamines that may precipitate a celiac crisis must be avoided. Meals should be eaten on a regular basis.

gluten, a protein found in wheat, barley, rye, and oats. Corn, rice, and millet are substitute grains. Foods such as pizza, brownies, spaghetti, pies, and sandwiches contain some degree of wheat, barley, rye, or oats. Recall tip--remember the little story of B.O. from R.W. and stay away from both: B, barley; O, oats; R, rye not rice; and W, wheat.

17

Nursing Care of Children with Genitourinary and Renal Disorders

FAST FACTS

1. With either a suspected or confirmed diagnosis of Wilms tumor, avoid palpation of the abdomen to prevent spread of the tumor cells.
2. *Orchiopexy* is surgical correction of *cryptorchidism,* undescended testicle(s), that is performed when a child is about 3 years old.
3. Children with undescended testicles often receive human gonadotropins as a first approach to therapy.
4. Therapeutic management of UTI is aimed at elimination of infection, identification and correction of anatomic or functional abnormalities, prevention of recurrence, and preservation of renal function.
5. A child exhibiting the following findings should be evaluated for possible glomerulonephritis: periorbital edema, anorexia, decreased urinary output, dark-colored urine, and a history of a streptococcal infection within the past 3 to 6 months.

CONTENT REVIEW

I. Renal system overview
A. Renal structure and function
1. Kidneys are the major organs of the renal system
   a. Cortex—outermost section; contains 85% of nephrons and their

surrounding blood supply; is responsible for the secretion of androgens, steroids, and aldosterone

b. Medulla—innermost section; contains portions of the collecting system and renal pyramids; is responsible for epinephrine and norepinephrine secretion

c. Pelvis—collects and transports urine from the kidney to the ureter

2. Nephrons are the functional units of the kidney; responsible for urine production, they consist of two parts

a. Glomeruli—clusters of capillaries surrounded by Bowman's capsule

b. Tubules—proximal, loop of Henle, distal, and collecting

3. The newborn's renal function is immature; the system continues to mature throughout childhood

4. Functions of the renal system:

a. Fluid regulation

b. Electrolyte balance

c. Excretion of metabolic wastes

d. Acid-base balance

e. Hormonal function: production and control of vitamin D, renin, erythropoietin, and prostaglandins

B. **Renal development**

1. Kidney development begins within the first weeks of embryonic life

2. Kidneys develop from the mesoderm, the primary germ layer of the embryo

3. Embryonic development of the kidneys occurs in three stages; the kidney is able to form urine at 10 to 12 weeks' gestation

4. Fetal urine provides a major source of amniotic fluid, especially in the third trimester of pregnancy

C. **Assessment of the renal system**

1. Health history

a. General considerations

(1) Medications: use of antihypertensives, diuretics

(2) Urinary characteristics: frequency, color, volume consistent with fluid intake, ease of starting and force of the stream, ability or inability to empty the bladder, incontinence, urgency

b. Present problem

(1) **Dysuria**—painful urination

(2) Urinary frequency

(a) Change in usual pattern

(b) Change in volume, color, or amount

(c) Incontinence

(d) Change in urinary stream

(e) *Nocturnal enuresis*—voiding during sleep

(3) Hematuria

(a) Color—bright red, pinkish, rusty brown, cola- or tea-colored; cloudy, or whitish characteristics may be indicative of infection with microscopic blood

(b) Associated symptoms—pain on voiding, that is, burning at the meatus; bladder spasms; suprapubic pain or costovertebral or flank pain

(4) Bleeding

    (a) Parental suspicion of insertion of a foreign object; sexual abuse, with sexually transmitted diseases

    (b) Associated symptoms—pain and bladder spasms

(5) Pain

    (a) Character, location, and frequency

    (b) Contributory factors: use of bubble bath, use of irritating soaps or detergents, tight clothing in the perineal area

(6) Vaginal discharge

    (a) Relationship to diapers: frequency of changing diapers; type of diaper material—cloth or disposable

    (b) Use of lotions and powders; lack of cleansing with diaper changes

    (c) Possible sexual abuse

(7) Undescended testicles; testicular mass or pain

(8) Inguinal area enlargement

    (a) Ability to reduce mass

    (b) Pain in the groin

c. Medical history

(1) Urinary tract: surgery or injury; congenital anomalies

    (a) Undescended testicles

    (b) Hypospadias; epispadias

    (c) Hydrocele; varicocele

    (d) Ambiguous genitalia

(2) Major illness

    (a) Kidney disease

    (b) Cardiac disease

    (c) Diabetes mellitus

(3) Vaginal infections

(4) Sexually transmitted diseases

d. Family history

(1) Kidney disease

(2) Infertility in siblings

(3) Hernias

(4) Congenital anomalies

2. Related laboratory and diagnostic studies (Table 17-1, p. 504)

3. Physical examination

a. General approach

(1) Examination of genitalia after assessment of the abdomen while the child is still in a supine position

    (a) In adolescents, inspection of genitalia may be done last

    (b) Use a matter-of-fact approach to decrease anxiety

TABLE 17-1 Major Diagnostic Genitourinary and Renal Tests for Children

Procedure	Purpose	Indications	Developmental Considerations/ Nursing Responsibilities
IV pyelogram (IVP)	Outlines complete renal anatomy Identifies masses Provides information regarding renal integrity	Renal cysts, calculi Kidney stones Difficulty voiding Possible tumors	Preparation: <2: no solid food, omit one bottle on the morning of the procedure >2: give cathartic the evening before the procedure, NPO after midnight, enema the morning of the procedure Sedation for agitated child—chloral hydrate
Renal/bladder ultrasonography	Determines kidney/bladder size and shape	Hydronephrosis Cystic kidney disease Neurogenic bladder	
Scout film Kidney, ureters, bladder (KUB)	Evaluates kidney size Identifies presence of foreign bodies Provides one-dimensional view of renal system	Difficulty voiding Increased BUN, creatinine	Provide an explanation as for a routine X-ray film
Voiding cystoure-thography	Visualization of bladder, urethra Reveals reflux of urine or bladder emptying problems	Voiding problems Urinary tract infections	
Cystoscopy	Provides direct visualization of bladder and lower urinary tract by means of scope inserted via urethra	Bladder and lower-tract lesions	Prepare child for urethral catheterization Child must remain NPO after midnight
Radioisotope imaging studies	Reveals vascularization and function of kidneys by injection of DTPA radioactive isotope	Glomerulonephritis Intrarenal masses	Provide an explanation of procedure and use of low-dose radiation Insertion of IV line Sedation—age appropriate NPO 4-6 hr before test
Renal biopsy	Identifies renal histology by removal of kidney tissue	Distinguishes between types of nephrotic syndromes Hematuris Nephritis	Sedation—age appropriate Post-procedure: Bedrest for 24 hours Monitor child for abdominal pain Position supine for 4 to 6 hours with a back roll over the biopsy site Quiet activities

(Modified from Wong, DL, et al: *Whaley and Wong's nursing care of infants and children*, ed 6, St Louis, 1999, Mosby.)

(c) Inspection of female genitalia is usually limited to the external structures for children up to and including the teens, unless specific information requires an internal examination

b. Inspection
   (1) Pubic region
      (a) Hair distribution and configuration
      (b) Surface characteristics of region or external genitalia—breaks in the skin, sores, or bruises
   (2) Presence of inguinal hernia
   (3) Location of urinary meatus
   (4) Vaginal or urethral discharge
c. Palpation: external genitalia
   (1) Presence of testes with each scrotal sac
   (2) Presence of lesions or growths

E. **Common pediatric medications related to renal and genitourinary (GU) function (Table 17-2, p. 506)**

II. Genitourinary (GU) tract disorders

A. **Urinary tract infection (UTI)**
   1. Description: presence of infection of the upper (ureters, renal pelvis, renal parenchyma) or lower portion (urethra, bladder) of the urinary tract
   2. Etiology and incidence
      a. *Escherichia coli* and other gram-negative organisms are most often implicated
      b. Peak incidence for nonstructural UTI is between 2 and 6 years of age
      c. At all ages, except neonatal, females have a much greater risk of UTI because of a shorter urethra
   3. Pathophysiology
      a. By location the urinary meatus is in close proximity to the rectum; thus, stool easily contaminates the meatus and bacteria ascend into the urethra and then up into the bladder; the most common organism is *E. coli* in females
      b. Frequent, prolonged bubble baths may contribute to infections in toddlers, preschoolers, and school-aged children
      c. Urinary stasis is the most critical host factor in development of UTI in older children; urine that remains in the bladder is an excellent medium for bacterial growth
   4. Assessment
      a. Assessment findings—in all populations a temperature of over 101° F
         (1) Infancy period: dehydration and failure to thrive; vomiting and diarrhea; irritability; and strong-smelling urine and persistent diaper rash

Medication and Indications	Route and Dosage	Side Effects	Nursing Implications
Loop Diuretic Furosemide (Lasix) Edema in renal failure Nephrotic syndrome	Oral: 2 mg/kg q day Child: may increase by 1 mg/kg day IV: 1 mg/kg/day q day or bid; may increase by 1 mg/kg q 2 hr, not to exceed 6 mg/kg/day	CNS: vertigo, tinnitus, headache, confusion CV: orthostatic hypotension GI: nausea, vomiting, anorexia Hepatic: jaundice, increased liver enzymes GU: profound diuresis, fluid and electrolyte imbalances Hematologic: agranulocytosis Skin: rash, urticaria	Assess baseline vital signs Monitor input and output every hour, as necessary; weigh daily Monitor serum electrolytes: sodium, potassium, chloride Monitor blood glucose creatinine, creatinine clearance Assess for hearing loss Monitor BP standing and lying down Parent teaching: Administer same time daily with food. Do not administer after 3:00 PM to prevent bed wetting Caution child to rise slowly to avoid fainting, dizziness Eat potassium-rich foods
Thiazide Diuretic Chlorothiazide (Diuril) Edema associated with renal dysfunction Mild to moderate hypertension	10-20 mg/kg/day	CNS: dizziness, weakness CU: hypotension GI: nausea, vomiting Skin: photosensitivity, rashes GU: hypokalemia, dehydration MS: muscle cramps Hematologic: blood dyscrasias	Monitor BP, I & O, weight Assess for edema Monitor serum electrolytes (especially potassium) *Parent teaching:* Administer medication at same time each day Teach dietary potassium requirements
Anticholinergic Propantheline bromide (Pro-Banthine) Bladder control Vesicoureteral reflux	See Table 16-2, p. 467	See Table 16-2, p. 467	See Table 16-2, p. 467

Antibiotic, Sulfonamide

Drug	Dosage	Side Effects	Nursing/Parent Teaching
Trimethoprim (TMP)/ sulfamethoxazole (SMZ) (Bactrim, Septra, Co-Trimoxazole) UTI	Oral: TMP/SMZ 8-10 mg/kg/day in divided doses q 12 hr	CNS: lethargy, nervousness GI: nausea, vomiting GU: increased BUN Hematology: neutropenia, leukopenia Skin: rash, urticaria Other: **Stevens-Johnson syndrome***	*Parent teaching:* Shake suspension well before administration Tablet may be mixed with small amount of food Give on an empty stomach Administer full course of therapy Maintain hydration Protect child from sun

Antihypertensive, vasodilator

Drug	Dosage	Side Effects	Nursing/Parent Teaching
Hydralazine (Apresoline) Glomerulonephritis Chronic renal failure	Oral: Child: 0.75 mg/kg/day in 2-4 doses (initial dose not to exceed 20 mg) IV: 1.7-3.5 mg/kg/day in 4-6 divided doses (initial dose not to exceed 20 mg)	CNS: headache, nervousness CV: palpitations, tachycardia GI: nausea, vomiting GU: dysuria Hematology: agranulocytosis Integumentary: rash, flushing F & E: sodium retention	Monitor BP closely (q15 minutes during IV administration) Assess daily weight, I&O Monitor CBC, electrolytes *Parent teaching:* Administer same time daily Have child: Avoid quick position change Avoid high-sodium foods Avoid OTC products such as cold and allergy medications

Antihypertensive Beta Adrenergic Blocking Agent

Drug	Dosage	Side Effects	Nursing/Parent Teaching
Propranolol (Inderal) Glomerulonephritis	See Table 13-1, p. 378	See Table 13-1, p. 378	See Table 13-1, p. 378

Warning: Stevens-Johnson is a serious, sometimes fatal, inflammatory disease presumed to be an allergic reaction to certain drugs. The disease is characterized by acute onset of fever, bullae on the skin, and ulcers on the mucous membranes. Pneumonia, joint pain, and prostration are common. Treatment includes bed rest, antibiotics for pneumonia, steroids, analgesics, mouthwashes, and sedatives.

    (2) Preschool period: vomiting; weak urinary stream; increased frequency; burning on urination; and abdominal pain, which usually is suprapubic

    (3) School-aged period: dysuria, frequency, urgency, and change in urinary odor

    (4) Adolescent period: dysuria, frequency, urgency, and hematuria

  b. Diagnostic studies

    (1) Urine culture—identifies the type of bacterial infection

    (2) IV pyelography—allows visualization of abnormalities in renal structures

    (3) Voiding cystourethrography—reveals the anatomic abnormalities that predispose the child to UTI

    (4) Dimercaptosuccinic (DSMA) scan—performed after the infection subsides to determine anatomic abnormalities

5. Therapeutic management

  a. Medications: antibiotics—penicillins and sulfonamides, ciprofloxacin hydrochloride (Cipro) for 10 to 14 days

  b. Surgical correction of anatomic defect, if present

6. Nursing management

  a. Nursing diagnoses

    (1) Altered urinary elimination related to dysuria

    (2) Hyperthermia related to the infectious process

    (3) Risk for fluid volume deficit related to fever; decreased fluid intake for a fear of pain with voiding

  b. Expected outcomes

    (1) Child's body temperature returns to baseline parameters

    (2) Child's urine cultures are negative for an infectious agent after the course of treatment

    (3) Child drinks adequate amount of fluid (see Table 16-3, p. 470)

  c. Interventions

    (1) Observe urinary stream when possible; collect a clean-catch specimen for a culture and sensitivity to identify causative organism

    (2) Initiate antibiotic administration, as ordered

    (3) Assess temperature with the use of age-appropriate routes every 1 to 2 hours for sudden elevations and during the initial 24 to 48 hours of the therapy

    (4) Administer antipyretic, as ordered, for temperatures over 102° F

    (5) Provide lightweight clothing and bed linens

    (6) Use tepid sponge bath for 30 minutes; to prevent chilling, dry each body part after sponging while keeping the child covered except for part being bathed

    (7) Encourage oral fluid intake every 2 hours for a total of 150 ml/kg/day

    (8) Encourage frequent voiding to minimize urinary stasis

    (9) Use a cooling blanket, if appropriate

7. Evaluation
   a. UTI is eliminated
   b. Child has no fever
   c. Child resumes usual pattern of urinary elimination, which is normally 1 ml/kg/hr

B. **Vesicoureteral reflux (VUR)**
   1. Description: condition caused by the back flow of urine from the bladder into the ureters and sometimes the kidneys
      a. Primary reflux occurs as a result of a congenital anomaly that affects ureterovesical junction
      b. Secondary reflux occurs as a result of an acquired condition
   2. Etiology and incidence
      a. Causative factors: infection, congenital malformation, obstruction, and neurologic dysfunction
         (1) Occurs most often in children under 5 years of age, before growth alters the renal structures
         (2) Renal scarring is present in 30% to 60% of children with VUR
   3. Pathophysiology
      a. Two processes are responsible for the increased risk of VUR
         (1) Ureterovesical junction dysfunction
         (2) Voiding dysfunction
      b. Defect graded according to the degree of the upper urinary tract and the effect on the lower ureter
   4. Assessment
      a. Assessment findings
         (1) Frequency, urgency, and dysuria
         (2) *Nocturia,* excessive urination at night; *nocturnal enuresis,* involuntary urination while asleep at night
         (3) Flank pain, unilateral or bilateral; pain found on the side of involvement
         (4) Colic
      b. Diagnostic studies
         (1) IV pyelography—determines the presence of the defect
         (2) Voiding cystourethrography—reveals the anatomic location of the abnormality
         (3) Renal ultrasonography—assesses for urethral obstruction after surgical correction
         (4) Urine C&S—indicate the presence of an infectious agent and the specific type of antibiotic therapy required
   5. Therapeutic intervention
      a. Medications
         (1) Antibiotics to treat the organism identified in the urine culture
         (2) Analgesics to control postoperative pain

(3) Antispasmodics to relax the smooth muscle of the bladder and decrease any discomfort associated with bladder spasm; for example, oxybutynin chloride (Ditropan)

(4) Anticholinergics for bladder control; for example, propantheline (Pro-Banthine)

b. Surgery—ureteral re-implanation for correction of reflux in severe cases

6. Nursing management

a. Acute care

(1) Nursing diagnoses

(a) Altered urinary elimination related to backflow of urine into ureters

(b) Risk for injury or infection

(2) Expected outcome: child establishes a normal pattern of elimination

(3) Interventions

(a) Assess urine output from the indwelling urinary catheter: amount, presence of blood, clots, odor, and color

(b) Assess indwelling catheter site for presence of redness, swelling, and drainage

(c) Use sterile technique to change the dressings or perform catheter care

(d) Maintain urinary collection bag below the level of the bladder or the tube insertion site; assess tube often to prevent kinking

(e) Secure catheter to groin or upper thigh to avoid placing tension on the catheter

(f) Note the time and amount of the first voiding after an indwelling catheter is removed; maximum time usually is 12 hours and a sufficient amount of urine is about 30 ml/hr in older children and 1 ml/kg/hr in younger children

b. Additional nursing diagnoses

(1) Pain

(2) Hyperthermia

(3) Altered renal tissue perfusion

7. Evaluation

a. Family complies with administration of the antibiotic regimen

b. Child remains free of UTIs

c. Child reestablishes a normal urinary elimination pattern

III. Glomerular disease

A. Acute poststreptococcal glomerulonephritis (APSGN)

1. Description: an acute autoimmune disorder characterized by an inflammation of the glomeruli that follows an antecedent group A beta-hemolytic streptococcal infection

2. Etiology and incidence
   a. Occurs 10 to 14 days after an upper respiratory infection, streptococcal pharyngitis or otitis media
   b. Age of onset is between 4 and 7 years of age; peak seasons are winter and spring
3. Pathophysiology
   a. Antigen-antibody complexes damage glomeruli in the basement membrane
   b. Inflammation of the glomeruli occurs, and glomeruli become infiltrated with polymorphonuclear leukocytes
   c. Plasma filtration decreases; excess water accumulates and sodium is retained
4. Assessment
   a. Assessment findings
      (1) Puffiness of face—especially around the eyes *(periorbital);* facial edema is more prominent in the morning
      (2) Anorexia
      (3) Decreased urine output; urine is cloudy and often described as the color of tea or cola
      (4) Irritability, lethargy, and headaches
      (5) Abdominal discomfort or vomiting
      (6) Elevated BP, with the diastolic BP over 90 mg Hg
   b. Laboratory studies
      (1) Urinalysis—reveals the presence of protein, hematuria, and casts; RBCs and WBCs
      (2) Creatinine clearance—most specific test of glomerular dysfunction; serum creatinine is increased with impaired renal function
      (3) Serum electrolytes—increased levels of potassium and phosphate if renal failure occurs
      (4) BUN—increased with impaired renal function
      (5) Antistreptolysin O (ASO) titer—reveals previous streptococcal infection (250 Todd units or higher)
      (6) ASKase and ADNase-B titers—increased; ASKase, ADNase-B antistreptokinase, antideoxyribonuclease-B reveal previous streptococcal skin infection
      (7) Erythrocyte sedimentation rate—increased in the presence of any acute inflammatory process
      (8) Throat culture—positive for streptococcal infection at the time of throat inflammation
   c. Complications
      (1) Acute renal failure
      (2) Hypertension
      (3) Hematuria and proteinuria
      (4) Hypertensive encephalopathy and seizures
      (5) Nephrotic syndrome

5. Therapeutic management
   a. Medications
      (1) Antibiotics—specific to identified microorganism for 10 to 14 days of therapy
      (2) Antihypertensives (beta blockers, ACE inhibitors)—with diuretics to treat mild hypertension until resolved
   b. Treatments
      (1) Low-sodium diet for children with edema or hypertension
      (2) Restricted potassium and phosphate in the diet if renal failure occurs
6. Nursing management: acute care (Table 17-3)
   a. Nursing diagnoses
      (1) Fluid volume excess related to oliguria
      (2) Altered nutrition (less than body requirements) related to anorexia
      (3) Activity intolerance related to fatigue and the infectious process
      (4) Risk for infection related to renal impairment
   b. Expected outcomes
      (1) Child's dietary requirements are maintained with adequate fluid balance
      (2) Family verbalizes an understanding of the disease process and follow-up care
7. Evaluation
   a. Child demonstrates stable weight and improved urine output
   b. Family complies with treatment plan, which includes medication, diet regimen, and follow-up care

B. **Nephrotic syndrome**
   1. Description: clinical condition caused by damage to the glomerular structure of the kidneys, resulting in proteinuria and hypoalbuminemia
   2. Etiology and incidence
      a. Classified according to the duration and extent of kidney damage:
         (1) Minimal change nephrotic syndrome (MCNS)—cause unknown
         (2) Secondary nephrotic syndrome—occurs in conjunction with or follows glomerular damage caused by APSGN, collagen diseases, or drug toxicity
         (3) Congenital nephrotic syndrome—caused by a recessive gene
      b. MCNS accounts for 80% of diagnosed cases; predominant type of nephrotic syndrome in the preschool child
      c. In the congenital type, death occurs within the first 2 years of life if dialysis or kidney transplantation is not performed
   3. Pathophysiology
      a. In MCNS, a nonspecific illness such as a viral upper

TABLE 17-3 Comparison of Acute Glomerulonephritis and Nephrotic Syndrome (Minimal Change)

Renal Disorder	Causative Factor	Assessment Findings	Treatment	Priority Nursing Interventions	Age of Onset
Minimal change nephrotic syndrome (primary)	Infections	Generalized severe edema (anasarca) Massive proteinuria Microscopic or no hematuria Serum protein: decreased Serum lipid: elevated Fatigue Normal or low BP	Prednisone Lasix Immunosuppressant therapy	Edema: Skin care Bed rest Infection: Antibiotics Diet: Low sodium High protein High potassium	2-3 yr
Acute poststreptococcal glomerulonephritis (ASPGN)	Immune complex formation	Primary periorbital and peripheral edema Moderate proteinuria Gross or microscopic hematuria Serum potassium: elevated Fatigue Elevated BP	Antibiotics Antihypertensives Dialysis	Hypertension: Loop diuretics, antihypertensives Fluid restriction Monitor BP, neurologic status Diet: Low sodium and potassium diet according to disease stage Fluid balance: Daily weights	5-7 yr

respiratory disorder precedes the symptoms of MCNS by 4 to 8 days

b. The membrane of glomeruli, usually impermeable to albumin and large proteins, now becomes permeable especially to albumin

c. Decreased serum albumin causes fluid to accumulate in the interstitial spaces and the body cavities

d. The result is hypovolemia, which stimulates the renin-angiotensin mechanism and increases the secretion of antidiuretic hormone and aldosterone

e. Serum cholesterol, phospholipids, and triglycerides all are elevated

4. Assessment

a. Assessment findings

(1) Generalized edema: periorbital edema present in the morning; abdominal swelling or dependent edema is more evident in afternoon

(2) Proteinuria

(3) Lethargy and irritability

(4) Abdominal ascites

(5) Pallor

(6) Decreased urine volume; urine is opalescent and frothy

b. Diagnostic procedures

(1) Laboratory studies

(a) Urinalysis—reveals massive proteinuria, presence of hyaline casts, increased RBCs, and increased specific gravity

(b) Serum albumin—decreased

(c) Serum cholesterol—increased to 450 to 1500 mg/dl

(d) Serum phospholipids and triglycerides—elevated

(e) CBC—reveals increased H&H and increased platelet count from the hemoconcentration

(2) Diagnostic studies: renal biopsy—reveals the type of nephrotic syndrome and the presence of edema from the renal abnormality

5. Therapeutic management

a. Medications

(1) Corticosteroids: prednisone—suppresses clinical manifestations of inflammation; induces remission (see Table 18-2, p. 529)

(2) Immunosuppressants: cyclophosphamide (Cytoxan)—for use in children who do not respond to steroid therapy or have frequent relapses

(3) Diuretics: furosemide (Lasix) in combination with metolazone—used in children with edema that interferes with respiration or causes hypertension

b. Treatments—diet: no added salt during periods of severe edema;
high-protein diet throughout life
6. Nursing management: acute care
a. Nursing diagnoses
(1) Fluid volume excess, especially in the interstitial spaces
related to sodium and water retention
(2) Risk for impaired skin integrity related to edema
(3) Altered nutrition (less than body requirements) related to
anorexia
(4) Activity intolerance related to fatigue
(5) Body image disturbance related to body appearance changes
b. Expected outcomes
(1) Child is receptive and adheres to the therapy
(2) Child demonstrates no evidence of skin breakdown
(3) Child gradually resumes normal activities for age as edema
subsides
(4) Parents exhibit knowledge about the disease, actions for
follow-up procedures, and proper technique of medication
administration
7. Interventions (see Table 17-3, p. 513)
8. Evaluation
a. Parents implement therapies and follow-up care
b. Child exhibits decreased edema with resumption of
age-appropriate activities and no evidence of skin breakdown

IV. Miscellaneous GU disorders
A. **Hypospadias and epispadias**
1. Description: congenital defects that involve the abnormal placement
of the urethral orifice of the penis
2. Etiology and incidence
a. Cause theorized to be a multifactorial genetic defect; occurs
during intrauterine development, with a failure of fusion that
involves the folds that close the urethra in the penis or results
from a failure of urethral folds to fuse completely over the
urethral groove
b. Epispadias is far less common and occurs in varying degrees of
severity
c. Hypospadias occurs in 1 out of 300 children; incidence is
greatest in families with a history of the defect
3. Pathophysiology
a. Hypospadias—in mild cases the meatus is just below the tip of
the penis; severe cases involve the meatus placement on the
perineal surface between the halves of the scrotum
b. Severe cases of hypospadias also involve a ventral curvature caused
by the replacement of normal skin with a fibrous band of tissue
c. Epispadias is often associated with exstrophy of the bladder

   4. Assessment
      a. Hypospadias—orifice located below glans penis along the ventral surface; may be associated with chordee
      b. Epispadias—urethral orifice located on dorsal (top) surface of the penis
   5. Therapeutic management: surgical correction for both defects
      a. Hypospadias: urethral lengthening; construction of meatal orifice; chordee release
      b. Epispadias: penile and urethral lengthening; bladder neck reconstruction to establish urinary continence
   6. Nursing management: postoperative
      a. Nursing diagnosis: altered pattern of urinary elimination related to the indwelling urinary catheter
      b. Expected outcome: child remains free of postoperative complications such as urinary retention or infection after the indwelling urinary catheter is removed
      c. Interventions
         (1) Assess urinary output and urine characteristics
         (2) Apply restraints, if necessary, to protect urinary diversion
         (3) Provide support and privacy for the child during catheter removal and afterward during attempts to void
         (4) Assess for pain, inability to void, and abdominal distention after urinary catheter removal; maximum time allowed is 10 to 12 hours after the urinary catheter is removed
         (5) Encourage increased fluid intake (a minimum of 30 ml/hr)
         (6) Use aseptic technique when handling urinary catheter tubing or bag
         (7) Administer prophylactic antibiotics, as ordered
      d. Additional nursing diagnosis: pain related to surgery
   7. Evaluation
      a. Child exhibits return of a normal urinary elimination pattern after catheter removal
      b. Parents verbalize the positive effects of surgical correction with minimal anxiety
      c. Child expresses positive behaviors to cope with the effects of surgery
B. **Wilms tumor or nephroblastoma**
   1. Description: an encapsulated tumor of the kidney
   2. Etiology and incidence
      a. Peak incidence is 3 years of age; the most common intra-abdominal tumor in childhood
      b. Prognosis depends on the stage of the disease on diagnosis
      c. Often associated with other congenital anomalies
      d. Evidence of genetic transmission exists; increased incidence among siblings and twins

3. Pathophysiology
   a. The tumor originates from the renoblast cells that originate in the renal parenchyma and extend into the surrounding tissues
   b. Metastasis occurs two ways: through the blood stream to the lungs, liver, and bone, and by way of the lymphatic system into the lymph nodes
   c. A rapidly growing tumor may cause obstruction of the inferior vena cava or intestine
4. Staging of Wilms tumor
   a. Stage 1: tumor is limited to one kidney and is surgically excised
   b. Stage 2: tumor extends beyond the kidney and is completely excised
   c. Stage 3: tumor has residual nonhematogenous tumor cells confined to the abdomen
   d. Stage 4: tumor metastasis to a distant site: the liver, lung, bone, or brain
   e. Stage 5: tumor involvement occurs in both kidneys at the time of diagnosis
5. Assessment
   a. Assessment findings
      (1) Firm, nontender mass located in the abdomen, deep within the flank
      (2) Anemia
      (3) Hematuria
      (4) Hypertension
      (5) Fever
   b. Diagnostic procedures
      (1) Laboratory studies
         (a) Liver enzymes—elevated ALT, SGOT, and LDH with metastasis
         (b) Urinalysis determines the presence of hematuria
         (c) CBC reveals increased RBCs, or polycythemia, as the tumor secretes more erythropoietin, which stimulates the bone marrow to produce RBCs
      (2) Diagnostic studies
         (a) CT scan and abdominal ultrasonography—detect the mass and its size
         (b) Renal angiography—reveals the extent of renal involvement
         (c) Bone marrow aspiration—reveals whether involvement extends to the bone marrow
6. Therapeutic management
   a. Medications: chemotherapeutic agents—dactinomycin (actinomycin-D) and vincristine for Stage 1 tumors; doxorubicin (Adriamycin) combination for other stages
   b. Treatments: radiation therapy—may be preoperative or postoperative; for all stages except Stage 1

    c. Surgery: tumor removal or resection; total, partial, or bilateral nephrectomy depending on the clinical situation

    d. Regional lymph node biopsy

7. Nursing management: acute care

    a. Nursing diagnosis: risk for injury related to the procedure and treatments to detect and excise the abdominal tumor

    b. Expected outcome: child remains free of injury

    c. Interventions

      (1) Assess vital signs preoperatively and postoperatively (BP may be elevated due to excess renin production)

      (2) Bathe and handle the child carefully with minimal or no pressure on the abdomen

> **⚠ Warning!**
>
> Avoid unnecessary palpation of abdominal mass. Post a sign at the bedside. Palpation tends to spread tumor cells. Diapers are to be fastened loosely.

      (3) Monitor the bowel sounds postoperatively for a return within 48 to 72 hours

      (4) Assess the incision for signs of infection

      (5) Assess the mucous membranes for signs of breakdown or dehydration

      (6) Provide meticulous oral and anal care to prevent UTIs

      (7) Maintain reverse isolation if leukopenia is present; limit visitors

      (8) Monitor for signs of altered renal function: irritability, elevated BP, headache, weight gain; first sign of renal failure—a decrease in the amount and frequency of voiding, less than 1 ml/kg/hr for young children; less than 30 ml/kg/hr in adolescents

    d. Nursing diagnosis: anxiety

    e. Expected outcomes

      (1) Parents express decreased anxiety as they become aware of the disease, treatment, and prognosis

      (2) Child exhibits minimal anxious behaviors

    f. Interventions

      (1) Assess psychological impact on parents after the physician's discussion of the diagnosis and therapy

      (2) Provide parents with opportunities to express feelings related to the diagnosis

      (3) Provide age-appropriate activities for the child to decrease anxiety

      (4) Discuss coping mechanisms with parents for effectiveness or ineffectiveness

      (5) Assign a consistent caregiver with the provision of opportunities for parents to participate in the child's care

    (6) Provide parents with information about community agencies and support groups

  g. Additional nursing diagnoses

    (1) Altered tissue perfusion

    (2) Ineffective family coping

    (3) During chemotherapy and radiation

      (a) Altered bowel elimination

      (b) Altered nutrition: less than body requirements

      (c) Body image disturbance

8. Evaluation

  a. Parents express reduction in anxiety and a positive attitude about the effects of therapy

  b. Child remains free of complications related to surgery, radiation, and chemotherapy

  c. Child uses opportunities and play activities to express or to work through anxiety and other negative feelings

V. Home care: family education topics and referrals

A. UTI

1. Disease process: discuss with the parents the cause of the infection, contributing factors, and actions for prevention
2. Medications: administration of antibiotics for the full course of therapy, 10 to 14 days
3. Follow-up care: instruct the parents how to collect a urine specimen for a culture before and after antibiotic therapy, then usually at monthly intervals for 3 months, and ending with 3-month intervals for 6 months
4. Preventive interventions for recurrence: avoid use of frequent, prolonged bubble and tub baths; avoid tight-fitting nonabsorbable clothing; teach proper feminine hygiene—wiping perineal area from front to back; encourage fluid intake; encourage child to void every 2 to 3 hours and to completely empty the bladder with each urination; suggest the use of cotton underwear, especially under pantyhose for teenaged girls; avoid long periods between voidings; void every 3 to 4 hours at the maximum

B. Vesicoureteral reflux

1. Medications: instruct parents to administer antibiotics and which side effects to report to the physician, including diarrhea; the findings for superinfections; skin rash
2. Elimination: proper technique to obtain a urine specimen for a culture by clean-catch midstream technique; Instruct parents on the care of an indwelling urinary catheter, if child is discharged with one in place
3. Follow-up: notify physician if there is a change in the pattern of urinary elimination until voiding cystourethrography reveals the absence of VUR; or if the child has signs of infection—cloudy

urine, spike in temperature, increased frequency of bladder spasms, which may indicate a bladder infection

C. **Acute poststreptococcal glomerulonephritis**
   1. Disease process and follow-up care: teach parents how to take BP and to test for albumin; recommend family members be screened for streptococcal infections
   2. Diet: review "no salt added" restriction
   3. Medications: proper administration of diuretics, antihypertensives, and antibiotics
   4. Activity: return to normal routines with an allowance for rest periods

D. **Nephrotic syndrome**
   1. Medications: teach safe administration of corticosteroids
   2. Diet and activity: see APSGN
   3. Follow-up: teach how to test the urine for protein daily; avoid contact with persons who have an infectious disease; contact the physician for signs of fever recurrence, chest pain, dyspnea, or respiratory distress

E. **Hypospadias and epispadias**
   1. Urinary elimination: teach the signs of urinary tract infection and infection of the incision; urinary diversion device (such as a silicone stent) if child goes home with such
   2. Activity: avoid straddling bicycle or similar toys until healing is complete
   3. Medications: administration of antibiotics or other medications such as antispasmodics to control bladder spasm

F. **Nephroblastoma: refer to Leukemia** (see Chapter 14, p. 412)

WEB Resources

www.kidney.org/

Site sponsored by the Council of Nephrology Nurses and technicians of the National Kidney Foundation.

Provides information about publications, research, and programs. Also has news and information for the general public on kidney-related topics such as nephrotic syndrome.

REVIEW QUESTIONS

1. A child has been diagnosed with a UTI. Which statement about appropriate dietary choices should be given to the parents?
   1. The child should drink adequate amounts of water and juices
   2. Carbonated beverages and those with caffeine can be given in small, frequent quantities
   3. Citrus juices are highly effective in the elimination of UTIs
   4. Fluids of any type are to be taken every 1 to 2 hours

2. A 6-year-old has been diagnosed with acute poststreptococcal glomerulonephritis (APSGN). During the admission process the nurse expects the child to most likely to have which of these findings?
   1. Normal blood pressure and reports of diarrhea
   2. Periorbital edema and grossly bloody urine in the urinalysis report
   3. Severe generalized edema and ascites
   4. Severe suprapubic pain and reports of vomiting

3. A 2-month-old infant who was born 8 weeks prematurely is seen at a local health clinic. The parent is concerned that one of the child's testicles is missing. Which information should the nurse provide?
   1. Explain that the testes do not descend until 8 months of age
   2. Infants born before the seventh month of gestation have an increased incidence of undescended testes
   3. The testes should have been present in the scrotal sac at birth
   4. Surgical correction will be necessary to descend the testicle after the child is 1 year old

4. During physical assessment of an infant with hypospadias with chordee, the nurse should expect which of these findings?
   1. The bladder is exposed with a visible urethral opening
   2. A bulge in the scrotal sac is observed
   3. The urethra opens on the dorsal aspect of the penis
   4. The urethra opens on the ventral side of the penis

5. After surgical correction for hypospadias, the postoperative care plan for a 1-year-old should include which of these interventions?
   1. The collection of frequent urine samples
   2. The use of a nonnarcotic medication for pain control
   3. Transillumination of the scrotal sac
   4. The use of restraints to prevent catheter disruption

ANSWERS, RATIONALES, AND TEST-TAKING TIPS

Rationales	Test-Taking Tips

1. Correct answer: 1

Increased fluid intake will dilute concentrated urine. Juices and vitamin C will acidify the urine, and bacterial growth is minimized in acidic urine. Beverages with caffeine act as a diuretic and are not a recommended dietary choice. Option 3 is a false statement. Juices acidify the urine but are not "highly" effective in the elimination of UTIs. Option 4 is a false statement since it would include caffeinated drinks.

Of the given options, option 1 is the best to select even though the word "adequate" may have distracted you. Adequate in this case may be defined as forcing fluids to the normal intake of 2 L/day. The clue in option 3, "highly effective in the elimination," is incorrect information. The clue is "any type" that makes option 4 an incorrect answer.

2. Correct answer: 2

In APSGN, decreased plasma filtration results in an excessive accumulation of water and sodium retention within the vascular space. Initial signs unique to children are puffiness of the face, especially around the eyes, and the passage of dark-colored urine, which typically indicates that blood is present. In APSGN, the BP is mildly to moderately increased and anorexia is the major GI finding. The findings in option 3 are consistent with nephrotic syndrome. The findings in option 4 are associated with acute UTIs.

In a disease ending in "itis," think inflammation and malfunction. The kidney is inflamed and therefore not filtering appropriately. Thus, blood in the urine and fluid retention are expected. Select option 2.

3. Correct answer: 2

Normally the testes develop in the abdomen, from which they descend into the scrotum during the seventh to ninth month of gestation. *Therefore, infants born prematurely usually demonstrate undescended testes.* Option 3 is

If you have no idea of the correct option, match the clue in the stem with the clue in the option. Match the clue in the stem, "premature birth," with the clue in option 2, "infants born before the seventh month of gestation are premature."

only a true statement for most
term infants. The majority of
cryptorchid testes will descend
spontaneously without need for
surgery. If undescended by the
age of 1 year, hormonal
injections may be given. If no
success is achieved with
hormonal therapy,
surgery—called orchioplexy—is
done. Cryptorchidism is a
developmental defect
characterized by undescended
testes in the scrotum.

4. Correct answer: 4

Hypospadias is a condition in
which the urethral opening is
located on the underside of the
glans penis or anywhere along
the ventral surface of the penile
shaft. The sphincters are not
defective; thus, incontinence
does not occur. Option 1 is a
description of exstrophy of the
bladder. Hypospadias is a
urethral anomaly, and does not
describe problems located within
the scrotal sac. Option 3 is a
description of epispadias, in
which the sphincters are
defective and the child may
experience incontinence.

The clues are the key terms
"hypospadias" and "ventral,"
indicating the underside of a
structure. "Dorsal" indicates the top
side of a structure. Test recall tip:
think of the alphabetical order of
the words *dorsal* and *ventral*.
Dorsal comes at the top of the
alphabet. Associate dorsal with the
top of a body part. Ventral is at the
bottom of the alphabet. Associate
ventral with the bottom or underside
of a body part.

5. Correct answer: 4

Hypospadias repair may require
urinary diversion to promote
optimal healing and maintain
patency of the newly formed
urethra. In options 1 and 2, the
actions are not associated with
hypospadias correction. Option 3
is an assessment technique to
identify scrotal anomalies. It has
no purpose in the care of this
child.

Use a general knowledge to focus on
the care of this postoperative client
to select option 4. Also note that the
client is a 1 year old, who would
pull at the lines. Prevention for
accidental removal of tubes and
lines is especially important for
children.

18

Nursing Care of Children with Musculoskeletal Disorders

FAST FACTS

1. Bone growth and ossification adhere to a specific sequential process in childhood.
2. Bone growth is completed at about 20 years of age.
3. Persistent infantile reflexes and unilateral hand use at 6 months of age are findings associated with cerebral palsy.
4. Classic findings for scoliosis include asymmetric scapulae, shoulders, hips and breasts; and a lateral S-shaped curvature of the spine evident when the child leans forward at the waist.

CONTENT REVIEW

I. Musculoskeletal system overview

A. Structure and function

1. Skeletal system
   a. Skeleton is composed of 206 bones, which determine the framework and body size
      (1) Bones are classified according to shape: long, short, flat, and irregular
      (2) Bones have proximal and distal diaphyses that provide sites for muscle and ligament attachment and lend support to the bone

          (3) The site at which the bones are attached is called a joint, which provides mobility and stability to the skeleton

          (4) Ligaments are fibrous connective tissue that connect bones and provide support to the joints between the bones

    b. The skeleton lies within the muscles and soft tissues; it has two divisions

       (1) Axial skeleton—composed of bones that make up the longitudinal axis of the body

       (2) Appendicular skeleton—includes bones of the upper and lower extremities

    c. Functions of the skeletal system

    d. Support for the body

    e. Protection of the vital organs and spinal cord

    f. Movement: locomotion

    g. Storage for minerals

    h. Hematopoiesis in red bone marrow mainly found in the long bones

  2. Muscular system

    a. Makes up 25% of the infant's body weight

    b. Muscles are classified as voluntary or involuntary

       (1) Skeletal muscles are voluntary and controlled by conscious effort

       (2) Cardiac and smooth muscle such as blood vessels, intestines, and bladder are involuntary and contract independently of conscious effort

    c. Tendons are connective tissue between a muscle and the bone to which it is attached

    d. Functions of the muscular system include movement, posture, and heat production during contraction

B. Development of the musculoskeletal system

  1. The musculoskeletal system is derived from the mesoderm germ layer; it is developed after the third week of conception

  2. Throughout infancy and childhood, the long bones increase in length as a result of proliferation of cartilage at the epiphyses

  3. The timing of bone growth and ossification adheres to a specific sequence in childhood

  4. Bone growth is completed at about 20 years of age when the last epiphysis closes

C. Assessment of the musculoskeletal system

  1. Related laboratory and diagnostic studies (Table 18-1)

  2. Health history

    a. General considerations

       (1) Exercise: extent, type, frequency, stress on specific joints, participation in organized sports or the type of repetitive movements in selected occupations

       (2) Nutrition: amount of calcium, vitamin D, and protein

       (3) Medications: muscle relaxants and anti-inflammatory agents

TABLE 18-1   Major Musculoskeletal Diagnostic Procedures for Children

Procedures	Purpose	Indications	Developmental Considerations
X-ray film	Isolate and identify musculo-skeletal pathology	Suspected child abuse Bone fractures	Infants and young children may need sedation or restraints to be immobilized
Computerized tomography scan	Diagnose bone pathology Determine size and location of masses, tumors	Soft tissue masses or bone tumors	Sedation may be necessary for infants and young children Age-appropriate explanations should be provided before procedure
Magnetic resource imaging	Evaluate pathological changes in musculoskeletal system	Spinal or joint structural defects Bone deformities	Child and family need thorough instructions, including need for immobility and expected noises during procedure, loud clicking
Arthroscopy	Provide direct visualization of joints by means of endoscope	Joint damage Ligament damage Synovial disease	Child must be kept NPO after midnight Procedure done under general or spinal anesthesia
Bone scan	Detect pathology of musculo-skeletal system	Bone pain Osteomyelitis Metastatic bone disease	Explanation must be provided regarding injection of radioactive isotopes Sedation may be necessary to immobilize child Child must void before procedure

  b. Present problem

   (1) Joint, muscular, or skeletal complaints: character; precipitating factor(s); efforts to treat with specific actions, prescribed drugs, over-the-counter medications, or herbs; and a growth spurt

   (2) Injury: the date and mechanism of injury, pain, and swelling

   (3) Developmental milestones: fine and gross motor skills appropriate for age

  c. Medical history

   (1) Trauma to the nerves, soft tissue, bones, and joints

   (2) Surgery—skeletal or muscular

   (3) Skeletal deformities or congenital anomalies

  d. Family history: congenital anomalies; scoliosis; and rheumatoid, gouty, or osteoarthritis

 3. Physical examination

  a. Inspection

   (1) Skeleton and extremities: alignment, symmetry of body parts, and size

   (2) Skin and subcutaneous tissues over muscles and joints: color and ecchymosis, swelling and masses

   (3) Contralateral muscles: size, symmetry, and spasms

  b. Palpation of bones, joints, and muscles for muscle tone, heat, tenderness, swelling, pain, crepitus, nodules, and masses

  c. Test joint range of motion

  d. Test muscle strength

 D. Musculoskeletal medications (Table 18-2)

II. Musculoskeletal disorders

A. Congenital defects

 1. Developmental dysplasia of the hip (DDH)

  a. Description: variety of conditions in which the femoral head and acetablum are not properly aligned

  b. Etiology and incidence

   (1) Increased incidence with breech delivery; occurs in 1-2 of 1000 births, predominantly in females

   (2) Predisposing factors: fetal positioning; cerebral palsy, meningocele, arthritis, cultural infant care practices, large infant size, maternal estrogen

   (3) Left hip is more commonly involved

  c. Pathophysiology

   (1) Condition ranges from mild lateral hip displacement to complete dislocation of the femoral head from the acetabulum

   (2) *Subluxation,* or incomplete dislocation of the hip, is the most common type

Text continued on p. 532

TABLE 18-2 Commonly Used Musculoskeletal Medications for Children

Medication and Indications	Route and Dosage	Side Effects	Nursing Implications

NSAID
Ibuprofen (Motrin)
JRA
Mild to moderate pain
	Oral
	20-40 mg/kg/day in divided doses
		CNS: dizziness, headache
		CV: fluid retention, hypertension, palpitations
		GI: heartburn, nausea, vomiting, bleeding
		Respiratory: dyspnea
		Hepatic: jaundice
		GU: polyuria
		Sensory: blurred vision, tinnitus
		Misc: allergic reactions
			Assess prior allergy to this drug, aspirin, or other NSAID
			Monitor BUN, creatinine, ALT, and AST
			Assess for visual disturbances and bleeding disorders
			Administer with food
			Parent teaching:
			  Administer with food as directed
			  Avoid other over-the-counter medications, unless prescribed
			  Report rash, flulike symptoms, visual changes to physician

Anti-Inflammatory (Steroidal)
Prednisone (Meticorten, Deltasone)
JRA
Suppress inflammatory responses and reactions
	Oral
	0.14-2 mg/kg/day
		CNS: euphoria, psychotic behavior, ↑ICP
		CV: edema, hypertension, thromboembolism
		GI: nausea, vomiting, peptic ulcer
		Musculoskeletal: suppressed bone growth
		Hematologic: thrombocytopenia
		Endocrine: Cushing's syndrome
			Obtain baseline height and weight
			Monitor serum electrolytes
			Parent teaching:
			  Monitor input and output; weigh child daily
			  Administer with food

Continued

TABLE 18-2 Commonly Used Musculoskeletal Medications for Children

Medication and Indications	Route and Dosage	Side Effects	Nursing Implications
Anti-Inflammatory (Steroidal)—cont'd			
		Skin: impaired wound healing, facial redness, acne, hirsutism Sensory: increased intraocular pressure Misc: Cushingoid appearance (moon face, buffalo hump)	Do not withdraw or stop medication abruptly Child should wear medical alert bracelet Observe for signs of infection because child has an increased risk Report sudden weight gain to physician Inform all health care providers that child is on this medication
Antibiotic			
clindamycin (Cleocin) Used to treat gram-positive bacterial infections Osteomyelitis	Oral: >1 month 2-5 mg/kg q 6 IM, IV <1 month 3.75-5 mg q 6 >1 month 3.75-10 mg/kg q 6	GI: nausea, vomiting, diarrhea, pseudomembranous colitis CV: hypotension, cardiac arrest Hematology: leukopenia, eosinophilia, polyarthritis Integumentary: rash, pruritis, urticaria, anaphylaxis	Assess for previous allergies to this drug Administer orally on empty stomach Assess for signs of superimposed infection, especially yeast (vaginitis) Monitor liver studies (ALT, AST) and renal studies (creatinine, BUN) for elevations Parent teaching: Teach parents the importance of entire course of medications Teach the need to inform physician of any side effects, especially diarrhea

Antibiotic

Nafcillin (Nafcil)
Used to treat penicillinase-producing staphylococcus aureus
Osteomyelitis

Oral:
6.25-12.5 mg/kg q 6 hr
IM:
25 mg/kg q 12 hr
IV:
10-20 mg/kg q 4 hr

CNS: lethargy, anxiety, depression
GI: nausea, vomiting, pseudo membranous colitis
GU: vaginitis, hematuria, proteinuria
Integumentary: rash, pruritis
Hematology: thrombocytopenia, leukopenia
Misc: allergic reactions

Assess for previous allergies to this drug
Administer orally on an empty stomach
Dilute IV medication according to label instructions
IM injection painful—give Z-track if possible

Antibiotic

Penicillin G potassium, penicillin V
Gram-positive and gram-negative organisms
Osteomyelitis

Oral (Penicillin V):
Child
2.5-8.3 mg/kg q 4
IM, IV (Penicillin G):
Children
8333-16,667 units/kg q 4
Infants
30,000 units/kg q 12

CNS: seizures
GI: nausea, vomiting, pseudo membranous colitis
GU: vaginitis, moniliasis
Hematology: anemia, bone marrow depression
Integumentary: rash

Assess for previous allergies
Assess liver, blood, and renal studies
Administer orally on an empty stomach with a full glass of water
Stress importance of medication compliance
Notify MD if fever, fatigue, or diarrhea develop; may indicate a superinfection

  d. Assessment
    (1) Assessment findings
      (a) Asymmetry of the skin folds on the inner thigh of an infant or child in the prone position with legs extended
      (b) Shortening of the affected leg (Allis sign)
      (c) Positive **Ortolani's sign** in infants, which is a classic "click" as the hips are flexed when the infant is in the supine position
      (d) Waddling gait in older child
    (2) Diagnostic studies
      (a) Pelvic x-ray film—difficult to interpret in newborns because ossification of femoral head does not occur until 3 to 6 months of age. An x-ray usually is done at this time.
      (b) Pelvic ultrasonography—detects slight subluxations and dislocations
  e. Therapeutic management
    (1) If diagnosed early, the hip joint may be maintained with a **Pavlik harness** for infants up to 6 months of age
    (2) **Bryants' traction,** hip spica casting, or both are also used if adduction contracture is present
    (3) Closed reduction of the hip under anesthesia (age 6 to 18 months)
    (4) Operative reduction, traction, and tendonotomy in the older child
  f. Nursing management: acute care
    (1) Nursing diagnoses: Risk for impaired physical mobility related to immobility, traction, or cast application; risk for infection
    (2) Expected outcomes
      (a) Child has the correct position for the femur, and the acetabulum is maintained without skin breakdown
      (b) Child remains free of infection
    (3) Interventions
      (a) Assess infant for signs of hip dysplasia
      (b) Assess neurovascular status of the lower extremities
      (c) Apply prescribed actions such as a Pavlik harness or special diapering to maintain abduction of the legs

⚠ **Warning!**

With a Pavlik harness and because of the infant's growth rate, the straps should be checked every 2 weeks for adjustment needs. Vascular or nerve damage may occur if the harness is not properly adjusted.

       (d) Demonstrate for parents the correct application and removal of harness or other treatment devices along with skin inspection

   (4) Additional nursing diagnoses

       (a) Risk for injury (see Fractures, p. 545 and Box 18-3, p. 547)

       (b) Altered growth and development

       (c) Anxiety

       (d) Knowledge deficit

 g. Evaluation

   (1) Child regains appropriate hip position without injury, skin breakdown, or infection

   (2) Parents can demonstrate correct technique for application of Pavlik harness or other treatment devices

2. Congenital clubfoot (talipes equinovarus)

 a. Description: orthopedic condition involving an adducted forefoot, inwardly tilted heel, and plantar flexion of the ankle

 b. Etiology and incidence

   (1) Unilateral clubfoot is more common than bilateral clubfoot

   (2) Occurs as single defect or in association with other disorders or chromosomal anomalies

   (3) Cause unknown; boys more commonly affected; familial tendency

 c. Pathophysiology

   (1) Arrested fetal development of skeletal and soft tissue during weeks 9-10 gestation, when foot development occurs

   (2) Primary germ plasma defect possible contributor to ankle dysplasia

 d. Assessment

   (1) Assessment findings

       (a) Foot pointed inward and downward

       (b) Fixed position of the foot or ankle

       (c) Inability to return the foot and ankle into alignment

   (2) Diagnostic study—radiographic examination of the foot

 e. Therapeutic management

   (1) Serial casting to gradually manipulate the foot into a normal position; the cast is changed weekly after manual manipulation

   (2) Braces are employed to maintain alignment after serial casting

   (3) Surgery—tendonotomy for the more severe forms

 f. Nursing management: acute care

   (1) Nursing diagnoses

       (a) Risk for injury

       (b) Impaired physical mobility

       (c) Risk for altered skin integrity

        (2) Expected outcomes

            (a) Parents demonstrate the correct techniques for use of corrective devices

            (b) Child maintains correct positioning of the feet without circulatory complications

        (3) Interventions

            (a) Assess the type of deformity and related treatment; Refer to Cast Care under Fractures, p. 547

            (b) Assess the neurovascular status of the lower extremities

            (c) Inform parents of the stages of corrective treatment, as indicated by the physician

    g. Evaluation

        (1) Child attains maximum use of the affected foot and ankle without circulatory complications

        (2) Parents readily participate in the long-term medical regimen

B. Disorder related to musculoskeletal growth: scoliosis

  1. Description: lateral curvature of the spine that most commonly affects the thoracic area

  2. Etiology and incidence

    a. Classified as two basic types

        (1) Structural—results from congenital deformity of the spinal column

        (2) Functional—usually occurs secondarily to another preexisting problem such as unequal leg length or poor posture

    b. Most cases of structural scoliosis are *idiopathic,* unknown cause

    c. Other causes that may contribute

        (1) Trauma

        (2) Neuromuscular disorders: muscular dystrophy or cerebral palsy

    d. Most often occurs in adolescent girls during growth spurts, normally between the ages of 10 to 16 years

  3. Pathophysiology

    a. A rotary deformity caused by rotation of the vertebrae that results in physiologic changes in the spine, chest, and pelvis

    b. Curves progress quickly during periods of rapid growth; curves continue to progress until skeletal maturity is achieved

  4. Assessment

    a. Assessment findings

        (1) Asymmetric scapulae

        (2) Asymmetric shoulders, hips, and breasts

        (3) Lateral S-shaped curvature of the spine; localized lordosis

    b. Diagnostic studies

        (1) Anterioposterior and lateral x-ray films of spine—taken with child standing reveals curvature of the spine and the degree of curvature

        (2) Scoliometer—reveals the deformity while the child is in a forward-bending position with arms held above the head

        (3) MRI and CT scan—provide a more detailed picture of the deformity

5. Therapeutic management—based on the degree and location of the curvature

  a. Nonsurgical

        (1) Boston brace—for curvatures of 20 to 40 degrees; must be worn 23 hours a day; can be removed 1 hour for bathing

        (2) Exercises—to prevent atrophy of spinal and abdominal muscles in situations of 10- to -20 degree spinal curvature. The value of exercises is questionable.

        (3) Electrical stimulation—causes the muscles to contract at regular intervals, which causes the spine to straighten; used with mild to moderate curvatures

  b. Surgical: performed when the nonsurgical methods are unsuccessful to halt the progression of the spinal curvature

        (1) Traction is used before surgery in severe curvatures

        (2) Spinal fusion is performed to halt the progressive worsening of the curvature; various instrumentations are used to internally stabilize the spine

           (a) Harrington instrumentation

           (b) Luque segmental spinal instrumentation

           (c) Dwyer or Zielke (anterior approach) instrumentation

           (d) Cotrel-Dubousset instrumentation

6. Nursing management: acute care

  a. Nursing diagnoses

        (1) Risk for altered skin integrity related to the prescribed therapy

        (2) Risk for injury related to a brace

  b. Expected outcomes

        (1) Child demonstrates adaptation to corrective device

        (2) Child will have no or minimal skin breakdown

  c. Interventions

        (1) Nonsurgical management

           (a) Assess areas in contact with the brace for signs of irritation or skin breakdown

           (b) Massage the bony prominences

           (c) Assess environment for hazards: encourage the use of side rails, holding the stair rail when going up and down the steps, and avoidance of slippery surfaces

        (2) Postsurgical management

           (a) Promote adequate pulmonary function: encourage periodic deep breathing and keep the child well hydrated

           (b) Maintain child's body in alignment

Warning!

Instruct child to avoid twisting movements that may cause the indwelling instrumentation to twist the spine.

      (c) Place the child on a special bed; log roll from side to side every 2 hours with two pillows between the legs and one pillow under the head

      (d) Assist with range-of-motion exercises as directed by physician

      (e) Encourage participation by the child in activities of daily living (ADL) when possible

   d. Other nursing diagnoses

     (1) Pain

     (2) Altered growth and development

     (3) Impaired breathing pattern

     (4) Body image disturbance

  7. Evaluation

   a. Child actively participates in the orthopedic regimen

   b. Child participates in appropriate family and social activities within the given restrictions of the condition

III. Inflammatory and infectious disorders

A. Juvenile rheumatoid arthritis (JRA)

  1. Description: chronic inflammatory disease that affects the joints; juvenile onset is diagnosed before 16 years of age

  2. Etiology and incidence

   a. Cause unknown; familial tendency; occurs more frequently in females

   b. Two peak age periods for the onset: between 2 and 5 years of age and between ages 9 and 12 years

   c. Types and subtypes of JRA (Table 18-3)

     (1) Pauciarticular—involves less than five joints

     (2) Polyarticular—involves five or more joints

     (3) Systemic onset—involves arthritic symptoms, elevated temperature, rash, and dysfunction of other organs such as the heart, lungs, eyes, and any organs located within the abdominal cavity

  3. Pathophysiology

   a. Synovial inflammation results in joint effusion and erosion, then gradual destruction of joint cartilage

   b. Muscle spasm initially causes limited movement; later, ankylosis or contracture is the cause of limited movements

   c. Surgery, infection, and injury can cause exacerbation of JRA symptoms

  4. Assessment findings and diagnostic procedures (Table18-3)

TABLE 18-3 Juvenile Rheumatoid Arthritis Characteristics Related to Mode of Onset

	Systemic Onset	Pauciarticular (Two or Three Subtypes)	Polyarticular (Two Subtypes)
Percentage of patients	30%	45%	25%
Age at onset	Bimodal distribution 1-3 years of age 8-10 years of age	Type I: less than 10 years Type II: over 10 years	Throughout childhood and adolescence
Sex ratio (female-male)	1.5:1	Type I: almost all female Type II: 1:9	Mostly female
Joints involved	Any Only 20% have joint involvement at time of diagnosis	Usually confined to lower extremities—knees, ankles, and eventually sacroiliac; sometimes elbows	Any joints: usually symmetric involvement of small joints Hip involvement in 50% Spine involvement in 50%
Extra-articular manifestations	Fever, malaise, rash, pleuritis or pericarditis, adenomegaly, splenomegaly, hepatomegaly	Type I: chronic iridocyclitis; mucocutaneous lesions Type II: acute iridocyclitis; sacroiliitis common; eventual ankylosing spondylitis in many Type III: arthritis only	Systemic signs minimal Possible low-grade fever, malaise, weight loss, rheumatoid nodules, and/or vasculitis
Laboratory tests	Elevated ESR, RF negative; ANA rarely positive; anemia; leukocytosis	Elevated ESR; ANA positive Type I: HLA-DRW5 positive Type II: HLA-B27 positive Type III: HLA-TMo positive	Elevated ESR Type I: RF positive Type II: RF negative
Long-term prognosis	Mortality: 1%-2% of all JRA patients Joint destruction in 40%	Continuous disease; eventual remission in 60% Type I: ocular damage; functional blindness in 10% Type II: ankylosing spondylitis Type III: best outlook for recovery	Longer duration; more crippling; remission in 25% Type I: high incidence of disabling arthritis Type II: outlook good

ESR, Erythrocyte sedimentation rate; *RF,* rheumatoid factor; *ANA,* antinuclear antibody; *HLA,* human leukocyte antigen.
From Wong DL, et al: *Whaley & Wong's nursing care of infants and children,* ed 6, St. Louis, 1999, Mosby.

5. Therapeutic management: medications
   a. NSAIDs—naproxen (Naprosyn), ibuprofen (Advil, Motrin), and aspirin to relieve fever, inflammation, and pain
   b. Slow-acting antirheumatic drugs—gold salts and penicillamine inhibit collagen formation or prostaglandin synthesis
   c. Corticosteroids—prednisone to suppress inflammation; used sparingly for short periods of time because of the undesirable side effects
   d. Cytotoxic drugs—cyclophosphamide (Cytoxan), methotrexate—used when other anti-inflammatory agents have not been effective
6. Nursing management: acute care
   a. Nursing diagnoses
      (1) Pain related to inflamed joints
      (2) Impaired physical mobility related to joint discomfort
   b. Expected outcomes
      (1) Child verbalizes relief of pain, with a reduction of inflammation
      (2) Child exhibits signs of minimal and adequate joint function
   c. Interventions
      (1) Assess severity of joint pain, as well as quality, location, onset, and duration
      (2) Assess limitations of mobility imposed by the pain and degree of the deformity
      (3) Administer NSAIDs and aspirin as ordered; evaluate their effectiveness

> ⚠️ **Warning!**
>
> The child needs to be monitored closely for signs of aspirin toxicity, which can affect vision, hearing, clotting, and renal and liver functions.

      (4) Assist to a position of comfort: support the painful joints with movement
      (5) Provide warm baths or showers
      (6) Provide opportunities for the use of nonpharmacologic pain relief methods: imagery, diversional activities, and relaxation techniques
      (7) Apply splints and sandbags as ordered; place the child flat on the bed with a firm mattress
      (8) Apply warm compresses to affected areas; whirlpool and paraffin dips as ordered
      (9) Encourage swimming as a therapeutic activity
   d. Nursing diagnosis: self-care deficit
   e. Expected outcome: child demonstrates abilities to independently carry out ADL with adaptation to other activities as the disease permits

f. Interventions
  (1) Assess the current level of functioning with ADL
  (2) Provide opportunities for independent behavior; assist as necessary
  (3) Provide necessary equipment and assistance devices to perform ADL
  (4) Consult occupational therapy for adaptive equipment; reinforce self-care techniques
  (5) Inform parents of child's need for independence and progression in ADL
g. Additional nursing diagnoses
  (1) Altered growth and development
  (2) Fatigue
  (3) Ineffective family coping
7. Evaluation: child exhibits positive actions to maintain ADL with minimal help from parents and to adapt play activities to the condition

B. Osteomyelitis
1. Description: infection of the bone tissue; usually involves the long bones and is preceded by infection or trauma in another part of the body
2. Etiology and incidence
  a. Occurs more commonly in males aged 5 to 14 years
  b. Although any organism may cause this infection, staphylococci is the major cause in older children; *Haemophilus influenza* is the major causative agent in younger children
  c. Sources of infection
    (1) Exogenous—from an outside source, as a result of a wound, fracture, or surgical contamination
    (2) Hematogenous—preexisting focus of infection is a skin abrasion, impetigo, tooth abscess, infected burn, or otitis media
  d. Predisposing factors: poor nutrition, hygiene, and physical condition; unsanitary environment
3. Pathophysiology
  a. Organisms invade the bone metaphysis; the infectious process leads to bone destruction and abscess formation
  b. Pressure from the abscess causes a lift of the periosteum
  c. Infection spreads under the periosteum, and additional bony necrosis and granulation occur; sinus cavities form between the dead bone and skin surface
4. Assessment
  a. Assessment findings
    (1) History of trauma to the affected bone
    (2) Fever
    (3) Warmth and swelling over the area, pain and tenderness of the affected area

      (4) Irritability

      (5) Guarding or unwillingness to move the affected limb; maintains a limb position of semi-flexion

   b. Diagnostic procedures

      (1) Laboratory studies

         (a) Positive blood culture

         (b) CBC—indicates leukocytosis

         (c) Erythrocyte sedimentation rate—elevated

      (2) Diagnostic studies

         (a) X-ray films—reveal soft tissue swelling

         (b) CT scan—reveals bone changes

5. Therapeutic management

   a. Medications: long-term IV antibiotics (penicillin, clindamycin, nafcillin) may be required for a few months (see Table 18-2, p. 259)

   b. Treatments

      (1) Splint the affected limb; bed rest

      (2) Surgical incision and drainage of the area; drainage tube insertion such as a Penrose drain

      (3) Closed-tube antibiotic irrigation of the bone

6. Nursing management: acute care

   a. Nursing diagnoses

      (1) Pain related to inflammation and infection

      (2) Impaired physical mobility related to infection

      (3) Risk for infection related to the procedures and therapy

   b. Expected outcome: child verbalizes relief of pain and associated symptoms

   c. Interventions

      (1) Assess the site for pain with movement and guarding; monitor the site for drainage

      (2) Use age-appropriate pain-rating scale to assess discomfort level

      (3) Monitor vital signs every 4 hours for increased temperature, pulse, and respiration; monitor for a change in the WBC count, sedimentation rate, and blood cultures

      (4) Administer antibiotics as ordered by way of a venous access device

      (5) Immobilize the limb; support the affected extremities with pillows at a 30-degree elevation

      (6) Apply warm compresses to the affected area; administer analgesics, as ordered

      (7) Use sterile technique for dressing changes

   d. Additional nursing diagnoses

      (1) Risk for injury

      (2) Hyperthermia

7. Evaluation: child exhibits behaviors that the pain is minimized or controlled

IV. Neuromuscular dysfunction: cerebral palsy (CP)

A. **Description: nonprogressive motor function disorder characterized by impaired movement and posture; usually is associated with abnormal or premature birth and intrapartal asphyxia**

B. **Etiology and incidence**
   1. Most common permanent physical disability of childhood; occurrence rate is 1 in 1000
   2. Other factors associated with CP
      a. Congenital and perinatal infections
      b. Congenital brain anomalies
      c. Intrauterine ischemia
   3. Classification of CP is based on the nature and distribution of the neuromuscular dysfunction (Box 18-1)

C. **Pathophysiology**
   1. Caused by permanent neurologic lesions that range from gross brain malformations to vascular occlusion, neuron loss, and laminar degeneration

---

Box 18-1
Clinical Classification of Cerebral Palsy

Spastic: May Involve One or Both Sides

Hypertonicity with poor control of posture, balance, and coordinated motion
Impairment of fine and gross motor skills
Active attempts at motion increase abnormal postures and overflow of movement to other parts of the body

Dyskinetic, Athetoid: Abnormal Involuntary Movement

Athetosis, characterized by slow, wormlike, writhing movements that usually involve the extremities, trunk, neck facial muscles, and tongue
Involvement of the pharyngeal, laryngeal, and oral muscles causes drooling and dysarthria (imperfect speech articulation)
Involuntary movements may take on *choreoid* (involuntary, irregular, jerking movements) and *dystonic* (disordered muscle tone) manifestations that increase in intensity with emotional stress and around adolescence

Ataxic

Wide-based gait
Rapid, repetitive movements performed poorly
Disintegration of movements of the upper extremities when the child reaches for objects

Mixed type, Dystonic: Combination of Spasticity and Athetosis

From Wong DL, et al: *Whaley and Wong's nursing care of infants and children*, ed 6, St. Louis, 1999, Mosby.

2. Cerebral anoxia is the most significant factor in the brain damage
3. In the dyskinetic type, basal ganglia damage results in uncontrollable involuntary movement; dyskinetic CP is aggravated by stress

D. **Assessment** (Box 18-2)

 Warning!

Preterm and LBW infants or infants with a low Apgar score at 5 minutes should be carefully evaluated for CP.

1. Assessment findings (in a 2 year old)
   a. Delayed gross motor development
   b. Abnormal motor performance—unilateral instead of bilateral hand use at 6 months of age
   c. Abnormal posturing—evident with spastic CP
   d. Altered muscle tone: spasticity of the hip adductor muscle and lower extremities
   e. Persistence of primitive infantile reflexes and reflex hyperactivity beyond 4 months
2. Associated disabilities
   a. Mental retardation
   b. Seizures
   c. Attention Deficit-Hyperactivity Disorder (AD-HD)
   d. Sensory impairment: strabismus and hearing loss

Box 18-2
Warning Signs of Cerebral Palsy

Physical Signs

Poor head control after 3 months of age
Stiff or rigid arms or legs
Pushing away or arching of the back
Floppy or limp body posture
Inability to sit up without support by 8 months of age
Use of only one side of the body, or only the arms, when crawling

Behavioral Signs

Extreme irritability or crying
Failure to smile by 3 months of age
Feeding difficulties
Persistent gagging or choking when being fed
After 6 months of age, tongue pushes soft food out of the mouth
Note. These warning signs are not diagnostic of cerebral palsy

Data from Pathways Awareness Foundation, Chicago, 1991, The Foundation. Parents. . . If you see any of these warning signs. . . don't delay.

       3. Diagnostic procedures
         a. Detailed neurologic examination and history
         b. Laboratory studies: changes in serum electrolyte values
         c. Diagnostic procedures
            (1) Electroencephalogram (EEG)—aids in differential diagnosis—metabolic disorders, brain tumors
            (2) CT—visualizes brain abnormalities and brain damage, to rule out brain tumor

E. Therapeutic management
    1. Medications: diazepam and muscle relaxants for spasticity; antiepileptics for seizure activity
    2. Botulisum toxin type A (Botox) used for paralyzing specific muscles
    3. Assistive devices for mobility and communication
    4. Physical and occupational therapy
    5. Surgery—tenotomy of the adductors, with lengthening of the tendons and hamstring release, and correction of hip and adductor muscle spasticity
    6. Selective dorsal *rhizotomy* (nerve block)—to improve the ability to walk

F. Nursing management: acute care
    1. Nursing diagnosis: self-care deficit—feeding, hygiene, and toileting
    2. Expected outcome: child performs ADL, as tolerated
    3. Interventions
        a. Encourage the child to participate in ADL according to the condition with referral to occupational therapy
        b. Adapt clothing and grooming aids to enable the child to dress and groom independently
        c. Adapt feeding utensils (wide-bowled spoon) to allow self-feeding; provide finger foods
        d. Assist parents in toilet training according to the child's abilities
    4. Nursing diagnoses: risk for injury; impaired physical mobility
    5. Expected outcomes
        a. Child remains free of injury
        b. Child will acquire locomotion within capabilities
    6. Interventions
        a. Assess child's environment for potential risks
        b. Provide safety interventions: side rails up when in bed, safety helmet, padded furniture, and restraints when in chair or moving vehicles
        c. Adhere to seizure precautions if child has a history of seizures
        d. Provide adequate rest periods between activities
        e. Select toys appropriate for age: use to obtain desired behavior such as locomotion

    f. Participate in therapies that strengthen and improve muscle
       control; use range-of-motion exercises
    g. Correctly apply orthotic devices such as ankle-foot braces
7. Additional nursing diagnoses
    a. Altered growth and development
    b. Impaired verbal communication
G. **Evaluation**
    1. Child engages in self-care activities to maximum ability
    2. Child remains safe within the environment

V. Muscular dysfunction: pseudohypertrophic or Duchenne muscular dystrophy (DMD)

A. **Description: most severe and common form of muscular dystrophy (MD) a group of inherited disorders characterized by muscle fiber degeneration, resulting in muscle wasting and weakness**
B. **Etiology and incidence**
    1. Transmitted as sex-linked recessive gene
    2. Affects males, most commonly aged 3 to 5 years
    3. Life expectation is 15 to 25 years after the diagnosis, and death
       usually is due to respiratory complications
    4. Results from mutation of the gene that encodes *dystrophin,* a
       protein product in skeletal muscle
C. **Pathophysiology**
    1. Bilateral wasting of the voluntary muscles
    2. Hypertrophy of the muscles; replacement of muscle tissue with
       fatty deposits and connective tissue
D. **Assessment**
    1. Assessment findings
        a. Progressive muscle weakness, wasting, and contractures
        b. Calf muscle hypertrophy
        c. Waddling gait and lordosis
        d. Difficulty in rising from a sitting or supine position
        e. Frequent falls and clumsiness
        f. Developmental delays
    2. Complications include contractures, disuse atropy, infection,
       obesity, and cardiac failure
    3. Diagnostic procedures
        a. Laboratory studies—serum enzyme studies reveal markedly
           increased creatine phosphokinase (CPK) and asparate
           aminotransferase in the first 2 years of life; levels diminish
           with muscle deterioration
        b. Diagnostic studies
            (1) Electromyography—reveals decreased electrical activity in
                the affected muscles

        (2) Muscle biopsy—reveals muscle degeneration and replacement with fatty tissue

        (3) Prenatal diagnosis possible using polymerase chain reaction

E. Therapeutic management

  1. Medications: antibiotics for respiratory infection

  2. Treatments: physical therapy—range of motion, casting, bracing, and occupational therapy for ADL

  3. Surgery: release of contractures

F. Nursing management: acute care

  1. Nursing diagnoses

    a. Impaired gas exchange

    b. Ineffective airway clearance

  2. Expected outcome: child maintains optimal gas exchange with absence of infections

  3. Interventions

    a. Assess respiratory function and breathing pattern

    b. Evaluate respiratory muscle strength

    c. Reinforce diaphragmatic breathing techniques taught by respiratory therapist

    d. Position to ease respiratory effort; suction as needed

  4. Nursing diagnosis: impaired physical mobility

  5. Expected outcome: child maintains optimal physical mobility and independence

  6. Interventions

    a. Assess strength of muscles and mobility

    b. Assess body alignment, and provide good back support

    c. Monitor changes in CPK and AST as indicators of muscle deterioration

    d. Offer physical and occupational therapy to reinforce range-of-motion and ADL program

  7. Additional nursing diagnoses

    a. Risk for impaired skin integrity

    b. Impaired verbal communication

    c. Body image disturbance

G. Evaluation

  1. Child remains ambulatory as long as possible without skin breakdown

  2. Child remains free of respiratory infection

VI. Bone malfunction: fractures

A. Description: break in bone associated with a fall or other trauma; classified according to the tissue injury and the type of bone break

  1. Simple or closed fracture—has no open wound

  2. Compound or open fracture—the bone breaks through the skin and results in an open wound

  3. Comminuted fracture—the bone is splintered or crushed

  4. Complete fracture—fracture fragments are separate

    5. Incomplete fracture—fracture fragments remain attached; in a greenstick fracture, the bone is bent but is fractured only on the outer arc of the bend. Immobilization is usually effective and healing is rapid. Also called a hickory stick fracture.

B. Etiology and incidence

    1. Greenstick fracture is the most common type in children under 3 years of age

    2. Other fracture types occurring in childhood
       a. Open or closed
       b. Buckle (torus) impact injury—characterized by a projection near the metaphysis
       c. Complete fracture—involves the entire cross-section of the bone
       d. Bends—occur in ulna and fibula, often with fracture of radius and tibia

    3. Epiphyseal (growth) plate injuries are common in children

    4. Common fracture sites for children: forearm, clavicle, femur, tibia, and fibula

    5. Motor vehicle accidents are a frequent cause of bone injury at all ages, particularly between 4 and 7 years of age

C. Pathophysiology

    1. Growth in length occurs at the epiphyseal plate, which is the weakest point of the long bones

    2. Children's bones are more pliable and porous than those of adults, which allows children's bones to bend, buckle, or result in a greenstick fracture

    3. Fractures occur as a result of a direct or indirect force on the bone, repeated stress on a bone, or pathologic conditions

    4. Healing of bone is more rapid in children: bone healing takes 1 week for every year of life up to 10 years of age

D. Assessment

    1. Assessment findings
       a. Pain and tenderness; swelling and limited movement
       b. Abnormal positioning and guarding, crepitus

    2. Diagnostic procedures
       a. Laboratory studies
          (1) Serum enzymes—CPK, AST, and LDH, all elevated according to amount of muscle damage
          (2) H&H—decreased owing to destruction of RBCs
          (3) Bilirubin—increased
          (4) WBC count—elevated neutrophils

    3. Diagnostic study: X-ray film—reveals a fracture at an injury site; subsequent radiographic studies taken after fracture reduction and during healing process

E. Complications include circulatory impairment, nerve damage, compartment syndrome, Volkmann (ischemic) contracture, **damage to the epiphyseal plate, infection, pulmonary emboli, and kidney stones**

F. Therapeutic management

1. Medications: analgesic, narcotic, and nonnarcotic for pain control
2. Treatments: casting or traction—skin or skeletal—to immobilize and realign the affected area (Box 18-3 and Figure 18-1, p. 348)
3. Surgery: open reduction, with or without pinning

G. Nursing management: acute care

1. Nursing diagnosis: pain related to muscle spasm
2. Expected outcome: child verbalizes reduced pain
3. Interventions
   a. Assess child for pain and discomfort using age-appropriate pain scale
   b. Immobilize and elevate the affected extremity; reposition the unaffected parts for comfort; maintain body alignment
   c. Administer analgesic or muscle relaxant, as ordered

Box 18-3
Client Education Guide to Cast Care

Do Not

- Get cast wet*
- Remove any padding
- Insert any foreign object inside cast
- Bear weight on new cast for 48 hours (not all casts are made for weight bearing; check with health care provider when unsure)
- Cover cast with plastic for prolonged periods

Do

- Apply ice directly over fracture site for first 24 hr (avoid getting cast wet by keeping ice in plastic bag and protecting cast with cloth)
- Check with physician before getting cast wet†
- Dry cast thoroughly after exposure to water:
    Blot dry with towel
    Use hair dryer on low setting until cast is thoroughly dry
- Elevate extremity above level of heart for first 48 hours
- Move joints above and below cast regularly
- Report signs of possible problems to health care provider:
    Increasing pain
    Swelling associated with pain and discoloration of toes or fingers
    Pain during movement
    Burning or tingling under cast
    Sores or foul odor under cast
- Keep appointment to have fracture and cast checked

---

*Plaster of Paris cast.
†Synthetic cast.
From Lewis SM, Heitkemper MM, Dirksen SR: *Medical-surgical nursing: assessment and management of clinical problems*, ed 5, St. Louis, 2000, Mosby.

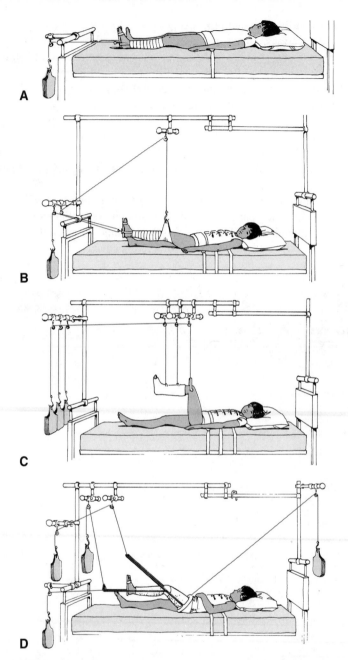

Figure 18-1   Examples of skin and skeletal traction. **A,** Buck extension traction, skin. **B,** Russell traction, skin. **C,** "90-90" traction, skeletal. **D,** Balance suspension traction shown with Thomas ring splint and Pearson attachment. May be used with or without skin or skeletal traction. (From Wong DL, et al: *Whaley and Wong's nursing care of infants and children,* ed 6, St. Louis, 1999, Mosby.)

       d. Apply cold to the site for the first 48 hours to decrease swelling, as ordered

       e. Encourage relaxation techniques and other nonpharmocologic methods of pain control

  4. Nursing diagnosis: altered peripheral tissue perfusion

  5. Expected outcome: child exhibits a reduced risk of neurovascular complications

  6. Interventions

       a. Assess the site distal to the fracture every 1 to 2 hours until stable to note color (pallor or cyanosis), sensation, capillary refill, movement without pain, pulse for equality to unaffected extremity, and temperature of cool not cold to the touch

⚠ Warning!

Signs of neurologic impairment include: numbness, tingling, a burning type of pain and loss of motion.

       b. If casted, allow cast to dry; turn child every 2 hours, handling the cast with the palms of the hand, not the fingers

       c. Elevate casted extremity on one to two pillows to above the level of the heart

       d. Remove articles with small parts from the area to prevent child from putting them into the cast

       e. Petal cast if rough edges exist

       f. Outline the area of drainage on the cast with a pen; place date and time near the drainage mark

       g. Clean plaster cast with vinegar and water; clean fiberglass cast with mild soap and water

       h. Provide quiet age-appropriate activities

       i. Provide range-of-motion exercises to the unaffected extremities

       j. Massage skin at the cast edges to prevent breakdown; do not use lotions or powder, which soften skin to increase breakdown risk

       k. Reinforce techniques of walking with crutches or the use of other assisting devices

  7. Additional nursing diagnoses

       a. Risk for injury

       b. Impaired physical mobility

       c. Risk for infection

H. Evaluation

  1. Child verbalizes decreased pain

  2. Parents and child demonstrate proper techniques of cast care and use of assisting devices

VII. Home care: family education topics and referrals

A. **Developmental dysplasia of the hip**
   1. Disease process: treatment, importance of follow-up care; application and maintenance of reduction device (Pavlik harness) or brace
   2. Cast care: teach parents the care of the infant in a cast (refer to Nursing Management, Fractures, pp. 547, 549) neurovascular assessment, and skin care

B. **Talipes equinovarus**
   1. Treatment program: importance of serial castings and manipulations; care of corrective appliance
   2. Cast care: refer to Nursing Management, Fractures, pp. 545 and 549, and Box 18-3, p. 547

C. **Scoliosis**
   1. Mobility: correct use and care of a Boston brace including: wearing for 23 hours per day; removal of the brace for 1 hour to allow for hygiene and skin care; importance of massaging the bony prominences and monitoring for areas of skin breakdown; recommend daily bath or shower schedule
   2. Referrals: *orthotist* (a person skilled in orthotics and practicing its application in individual cases); American Academy of Orthopedic Surgeons; physical therapists; and support groups

D. **Juvenile rheumatoid arthritis (JRA)**
   1. Treatment: purpose and use of pain medications, importance of regular exercise
   2. ADL: teach use of necessary equipment and assisting devices; inform parents of child's need for independence and progression in ADL
   3. Referrals: physical and occupational therapy, Juvenile Rheumatoid Arthritis Organization

E. **Osteomylitis**
   1. Disease process: pathophysiology of infectious process; signs of recurring infection
   2. Medications: administration of antibiotics, analgesics
   3. Treatment: use and care of splints or cast; importance of follow-up
   4. Referrals: physical and occupational therapist, home health nurse, support groups

F. **Cerebral palsy**
   1. ADL: adapt clothing and grooming aids to enable child to dress and groom independently; adapt feeding utensils (wide-bowled spoon) to allow self-feeding; provide finger foods
   2. Safety: provide safe home environment: pad furniture, bed side rails, avoid use of scatter rugs and floor polish, suggest age-appropriate and safe toys that improve motor function, encourage wearing of helmet and safety restraints

    3. Elimination: assist parents to toilet train the child

    4. Referrals: physical and occupational therapy to reinforce range-of-motion and ADL program; speech therapy; special education provider; dentist; parent support groups

  G. Duchenne muscular dystrophy (DMD)

    1. Oxygenation: teach diaphragmatic breathing exercises; avoid contact with known sources of infection

    2. Activity: need for exercise program to build muscle strength

    3. Referrals: genetic counseling, physical and occupational therapy, adaptive physical education classes, parent support groups

  H. Fractures

    1. Mobility: cast care and assessment of neurovascular status; reinforce techniques of walking with crutches; inform parents how to apply a sling; suggest age-appropriate activities

    2. Elimination: importance of drinking fluids and eating adequate dietary fiber

WEB Resources

www.aaos.org

American Academy of Orthopedic Surgeons website that provides client education, brochures, and research on orthopedic topics. Information related to fractures, scoliosis, and various foot problems is available.

www.arthritis.org

Site sponsored by the Arthritis Foundation. Of particular interest is the American Juvenile Arthritis Organization page for parents and teachers.

www.uscpaa.org

United Cerebral Palsy Athletic Association site that provides product information as well as links to the American Academy of Cerebral Palsy (AACP) and Developmental Medicine site for health professionals, parents, and persons with cerebral palsy.

www.mdausa.org

The Muscular Dystrophy Association home page provides research information, clinics and services, and community program updates. Also in Spanish.

REVIEW QUESTIONS

1. A parent has been given instructions about a Pavlik harness to be worn by the infant with congenital hip dysplasia. Which of these statements by the parent indicates that there is an understanding of the instructions?
   1. "We plan to remove the harness for 1 hour every day."
   2. "We'll make follow-up appointments for harness readjustment."
   3. "We must maintain the legs in an adducted position."
   4. "We can remove the harness for diaper changes."

2. During the physical assessment of a 12-year-old client, the nurse would expect which of these findings related to scoliosis?
   1. Asymmetry of the shoulders, back, and waist
   2. Convex angulation in thoracic area
   3. Concave curvature of the lumbar spine
   4. An S-shaped curvature of the lumbar spine with malformation of vertebrae

3. An 18-month-old boy is scheduled for application of a plaster cast to correct a clubfoot. The postoperative plan should include which of these interventions?
   1. Elevate the cast above the level of the heart
   2. Handle the cast with the hands
   3. Reposition the child every 2 hours
   4. Spray the cast with acrylic

4. A 9-year-old girl has been brought to the emergency department after an automobile accident and is diagnosed with a femoral fracture. Which of these goals should receive priority in the child's care?
   1. Adequate nutrition will be maintained
   2. Infection will be prevented
   3. Risk for bleeding will be reduced
   4. Pain will be reduced

5. An adolescent must wear a Boston brace. To promote the teen's optimal functioning, which of these actions should the nurse take?
   1. Discourage participation in activities of daily living (ADL)
   2. Inform the teen that the brace may be removed for several hours daily for comfort
   3. Teach appropriate application, removal, and care of the brace
   4. Teach non-weight-bearing techniques

ANSWERS, RATIONALES, AND TEST-TAKING TIPS

Rationale	Test-Taking Tips

1. Correct answer: 2

The practitioner should examine the infant before any adjustment is attempted. It is important to ensure that the hips are in correct placement before the harness is re-secured. Harnesses may or may not allow for removal during bathing. A Pavlik harness is used to maintain the hip in an abducted position. Diapering may be accomplished without the harness removal.

Eliminate option 1 because no reason for the removal is given. Eliminate option 3—to keep legs adducted—as you recall that the client has the abductor pillows to keep the proper hip placement after hip prostheses surgery. Eliminate option 4 because you most likely are not sure of it and option 2 is more likely to be an appropriate action. Go with what you know.

2. Correct answer: 1

This is a classic finding in scoliosis, which is identified when the client (facing away from the examiner) is asked to raise both arms and bend forward at the waist, allowing the arms to dangle. Another way to describe the findings is an unequal height of the hips or shoulders. Option 2 is a description of kyphosis, which is a more common finding in older women with osteoporosis. Option 3 is a description of lordosis, which may normally be found in children, usually toddlers, and middle-aged men who have gained weight in the abdominal area. Scoliosis involves spinal curvature of the thoracic not the lumbar section of the spinal column. Remember that scoliosis is an S-shaped curvature of the spine that results in asymmetry of the back structures.

Avoid knee jerk selections of options. Did you only see "S-shaped curvature" in option 4 and select it? If so, you need to note that when options have two parts, you have a tendency to read the first part, skim over the second part, and make a decision. You missed the location of the curvature in option 4, which is lumbar, and this makes the option incorrect. To avoid making this mistake in the future, read the second part of two-part options first. Then read the first part of that option. This test error of misreading 2-part options is easily corrected by this simple action.

Rationale	Test-Taking Tips

3. Correct answer: 3

Turning the child every 2 hours will help to dry the cast evenly. Drying can take up to 72 hours if traditional plaster cast materials are used. The extremity in a cast should be elevated on a pillow to increase venous return and will not, in all cases, be elevated above the heart, especially in an 18-month-old child. Another technique for appropriate extremity elevation is to raise the distal joint higher than the proximal joint of the extremity. The cast should be handled using the *palms of the hands* to prevent any indentations into the cast, which creates pressure areas. Option 4 is not a nursing responsibility.

If you narrowed the options to 1 and 3, reread the stem to note that the age of the child is 18 months. Therefore, option 3 is the better selection. At this age, the child is more active and would be quite difficult to keep in a position in which one leg is elevated above the heart. Also recall that a cast needs to be repositioned to facilitate drying, especially within the first 24 to 48 hours.

4. Correct answer: 4

Control of pain, hemorrhage, and edema are the priorities in caring for the child with a femur fracture. Option 1 is not an immediate priority for a child with a fracture. If a surgical incision were present, the goal in option 2 would likely be included in the child's plan of care. Option 3 is an action for a potential need—the risk for bleeding.

Both options 3 and 4 are correct answers. However, option 4 focuses on actual need and option 3 is a potential need. There is not enough information in the stem to support the focus of your actions on bleeding concerns.

5. Correct answer: 3

When a brace must be worn, the use and care of the orthopedic appliance is explained to facilitate correction of the defect. Repeat demonstrations should be done before the parents and

Eliminate options 1 and 4 because they are false statements. Reread the question and note the key words "to promote optimal functioning." Select option 3 because it more adequately answers the question.

adolescent go home. Adolescents should participate maximally in ADL to meet their physical developmental needs and tasks. The Boston brace may be removed for 1 hour daily for bathing and at no other time. The action in option 4 is not an appropriate intervention for an adolescent with a brace.

Option 2 presents only one aspect of optimal functioning.

19

Nursing Care of Children with Endocrine Disorders

FAST FACTS

1. The endocrine system controls four processes: growth, maturation, metabolism, and reproduction.
2. Pituitary dysfunction is manifested by a growth alteration in children.
3. Regular insulin, short-acting, is drawn into the syringe before intermediate-acting insulin, isophane insulin suspension [Neutral Protamine Hagedorn (NPH)]. Tip for recall: Go clear to cloudy, meaning regular insulin then NPH.
4. Growth hormones should be administered at bedtime for optimal stimulation of the pituitary gland.

CONTENT REVIEW

I. Endocrine system overview

A. Structure and function

1. Glands of the endocrine system are located throughout the body (Table 19-1, p. 558)
2. Endocrine glands produce and secrete hormones directly into the blood stream in response to specific signals

TABLE 19-1	Major Endocrine Hormones and their Actions

Gland/Hormone	Actions
Anterior Pituitary	
Growth hormone (GH)	Promotes bone and soft tissue growth and protein synthesis
	Facilitates fat mobilization for energy
Thyroid-stimulating hormone (TSH)	Promotes growth and secretory activity of thyroid
	Promotes growth and development
Adenocorticotropic hormone (ACTH)	Stimulates growth and secretory activity of adrenal cortex (cortisol, androgens)
Follicle-stimulating hormone (FSH)	Development of seminiferous tubules and spermatogenesis in males
	Follicle malleation and estrogen stimulation in females
Luteinizing hormone (LH)	Stimulates secretion of progesterone by corpus luteum in females
	Causes rupture of follicle and release of mature ova
Prolactin	Stimulates milk secretion
	Provides maintenance of corpus luteum during pregnancy
Posterior Pituitary	
Antidiuretic hormone (ADH)	Regulates osmolarity and water volume
	Increases permeability of collecting ducts of kidneys
Oxytocin	Stimulates uterine contraction
	Stimulates *let down reflex*—release and flow of breast milk
Thyroid Gland	
Thyroxine (T_4) and triiodothyronine (T_3)	Influence metabolism and bone, teeth, and brain growth
	Influence lipid and carbohydrate metabolism
Calcitonin	Stimulates bone development and ossification
Parathyroid Gland	
Parathyroid hormone (PTH)	Influences calcium and phosphorus metabolism
	Regulates phosphorus excretion
	Regulates calcium resorption from bone, blood, intestines
Pancreas	
Insulin (product of the beta cells)	Promotes glucose, protein, lipid metabolism
	Promotes transport of glucose across cell membrane
	Promotes hepatic storage of glucose

Modified from Wong, DL, et al: *Whaley and Wong's nursing care of infants and children,* ed 6, St Louis, 1999, Mosby.

| TABLE 19-1 | Major Endocrine Hormones and their Actions—cont'd |

Gland/Hormone	Actions
Pancreas—cont'd	
Glucagon (product of the alpha cells)	Counters regulatory hormone to insulin with epinephrine, growth hormone, glucocorticoid Increases blood glucose from stimulation of breakdown of glycogen stores in liver Decreases protein synthesis and lipolysis
Adrenal Cortex	
Mineralcorticoid: Aldosterone	Causes sodium resorption by renal tubules and potassium excretion
Sex hormones: Androgens	Influences secondary sex characteristics in boys and girls
Glucocorticoids: Cortisol Cortisone	Facilitates fat, protein, carbohydrate metabolism Acts as antagonist to insulin Causes an anti-inflammatory action Promotes gluconeogenesis Influences protein and fat catabolism, immunologic functions Promotes sodium and water retention with a loss of potassium
Adrenal Medulla	
Calecholamines: Epinephrine	Increases contractility and excitability of heart muscle Increases basal metabolic rate Increases blood flow to muscles, brain, viscera
Norepinephrine	Regulates glycogenolysis, lipolysis Stimulates alpha and beta receptors
Ovaries	
Estrogen	Stimulates development and maintenance of secondary sex characteristics Stimulates protein anabolism Provides protective functions to prevent osteoporosis and atherosclerosis Prepares endometrium for implantation of fertilized ovum
Progesterone	Prepares uterus for pregnancy; helps maintain pregnancy Prepares breasts for lactation Promotes protein catabolism
Testes	
Testosterone	Stimulates development and maintenance of primary and secondary sex characteristics in boys Stimulates sperm production Stimulates protein anabolism for growth

3. Major processes controlled by the endocrine glands include growth, maturation, metabolic function, and reproduction
4. Regulation of hormone levels is controlled by feedback systems
5. Endocrine problems occur from hyperfunction or hypofunction of the endocrine glands

B. **Fetal development of the endocrine system**
 1. The endocrine glands are well developed at birth; however, their functions are immature
 2. The thyroid gland develops during 7 to 14 weeks' gestation
 3. The gross features of the pituitary gland are recognizable by the end of the first trimester
 4. Parathyroid glands form during the fifth week of gestation from the dorsal wings of the third and fourth pharyngeal pouches
 5. Ovaries are distinguishable from testes by 6 weeks' gestation
 6. The pancreas contains the islets of Langerhans, which are endocrine tissues that arise from parenchymatous pancreatic tissues during the third month of fetal life

C. **Assessment of endocrine function**
 1. Health history
    a. General
       (1) Past growth measurements, heights and weights of family members
       (2) Endocrine disorders in relatives
    b. Nutrition
       (1) Timing and content of meals
       (2) Recent changes in appetite or weight
       (3) Plotting of growth patterns on growth chart
    c. Elimination
       (1) Change in usual pattern of elimination
       (2) Characteristics of urine and stool
    d. Activity
       (1) Changes in child's endurance and participation in physical activity
       (2) Frequency of physical activity
 2. Related laboratory and diagnostic studies
    a. Radiographic surveys—bone age and skull series: used as assessment of skeletal growth and maturation, which is controlled by hormones (primarily pituitary growth and thyroid hormones)
    b. Endocrine studies—stimulation tests for growth hormone and thyroid-releasing hormone
 3. Physical examination
    a. Obtain vital signs and compare to norms for age
    b. Obtain accurate physical measurements and plot on growth chart: height, weight, and head circumference

     c. Head and neck

       (1) Inspect for facial anomalies, prominence of the eyes, asymmetry in the neck

       (2) Presence of thyroid masses or enlargement

     d. Chest: breast development is noted in both males and females and compared with *Tanner* stage, a series of 5 phases in the development of secondary sexual characteristics

     e. Pelvic region

       (1) Female genitalia changes: inspect for enlarged clitoris and labial fusion

       (2) Male genitalia: inspect for penis size, location of urethra, testicular development and size, and scrotal development

       (3) Distribution and configuration of pubic hair

     f. Integument

       (1) Hair distribution and texture

       (2) Acne

       (3) Hyperpigmentation or depigmentation

  D. Commonly used medications for endocrine disorders

     1. Thyroid hormone: levothyroxine sodium

     2. Antidiabetic agent: insulin

II. Diabetes mellitus

  A. Description: metabolic disorder characterized by inability of the pancreas to secrete insulin (Table 19-2, p. 562)

     1. Insulin-dependent diabetes mellitus (IDDM): type 1: characterized by pancreatic beta cell destruction, usually resulting in absolute insulin deficiency

     2. Non-insulin-dependent diabetes mellitus (NIDDM): type 2: characterized by improper insulin utilization and some insulin deficiency

  B. Etiology and incidence: type 1 (Table 19-2, p. 562)

     1. Cause unknown; however, affected persons are believed to have a genetic predisposition that results in an autoimmune response

     2. A viral infection may act as the precipitating factor

     3. This most common metabolic disorder has a peak incidence between 5 and 7 years of age and during early adolescence; affects one to two children per thousand

     4. Type 2 diabetes usually is seen in adults over age 45 who are overweight and have a family history of diabetes

     5. Type 1 more often occurs in young children and in adolescents. Type 2 in these age groups is associated with being overweight, and the incidence of type 2 in children is increasing. Children with type 1 are commonly thin, without a weight problem.

  C. Pathophysiology (type 1)

     1. With insulin deficiency, glucose is unable to enter the cell, resulting in hyperglycemia

TABLE 19-2 **Comparison of Characteristics of Types 1 and 2 Diabetes Mellitus**

Characteristic	Type 1	Type 2
Age at onset	Less than 20 yr	Over 30 yr
Type of onset	Abrupt	Gradual
Sex ratio	Males slightly more than females	Females outnumber males
Percentage of diabetic population	5-8%	85-90%
Heredity:		
Family history	Sometimes	Frequently
Human leukocyte antigen	Associations	No associations
Twin concordance	25-50%	90-100%
Ethnic distribution	Primarily whites	Increased incidence in Native Americans, Hispanics
Presenting symptoms	Three Ps common: Polyuria, Polydipsia, Polyphagia	May be related to long-term complications
Nutritional status	Underweight	Overweight
Insulin (natural):		
Pancreatic content	Usually none	Over 50% normal
Serum insulin	Low to absent	High or low
Primary resistance	Minimum	Marked
Islet cell antibodies	80-85%	Less than 5%
Therapy:		
Insulin	Always	20-30% of patients
Oral agents	Ineffective	Often effective
Diet only	Ineffective	Often effective
Chronic complications	>80%	Variable
Ketoacidosis	Common	Infrequent

From Wong DL, et al: *Whaley and Wong's nursing care of infants and children,* ed 6, St. Louis, 1999, Mosby.

2. When glucose is unavailable for cellular metabolism, the body uses other sources of energy such as fats and protein, resulting in diabetic ketoacidosis (DKA)
3. Insulin deficiency also increases the effects of counter-regulatory hormones: epinephrine, glucagon, cortisol, and growth hormone

D. Assessment

1. Assessment findings
   a. Three cardinal symptoms: polydipsia, polyphagia, and polyuria ("3 p's")
   b. Weight loss and fatigue
   c. Hyperglycemia
   d. Yeast infections
   e. Abdominal discomfort
   f. Dehydration
   g. Enuresis—incontinence of urine; when incontinence occurs at night, it is called *nocturnal enuresis*
2. Complications
   a. DKA: dehydration; Kussmaul's respirations, which are deep and rapid; and acetone breath

> ⚠ **Warning!**
>
> DKA is a complete state of insulin deficiency and a life-threatening situation.

   b. Hypoglycemia (insulin shock) and hyperglycemia (Table 19-3, p. 564)
   c. Microvascular changes
      (1) *Neuropathy,* decreased sensation in the hands and feet
      (2) *Retinopathy,* decreased vision to the severest degree of blindness
      (3) *Nephropathy,* renal dysfunction to the severest degree of chronic failure
   d. Limited joint mobility in some cases
3. Laboratory studies
   a. Blood glucose
      (1) Fasting specimen, levels over 120 mg/dl
      (2) Random sample, levels over 200 mg/dl
      (3) In DKA, levels over 300 mg/dl
   b. WBC count—increased with predominantly polymorphonuclear lymphocytes or increased neutrophils
   c. Ketones—increased in blood and urine
   d. Glycosolated hemoglobin test—provides objective measurement of glycemic control; performed every 2 to 3 months; measurement represents average blood glucose levels during the past 3 to 4 months; serum levels indicating glucose control usually range from 6% to 8%. Also called Hemoglobin A_{1C}

TABLE 19-3	Comparison of Manifestations of Hypoglycemia and Hyperglycemia	
Variable	**Hypoglycemia**	**Hyperglycemia**
Onset	Rapid (minutes)	Gradual (days)
Mood	Labile, irritable, nervous, weepy	Lethargic
Mental status	Difficulty concentrating, speaking, focusing, coordinating	Dulled sensorium Confused
Inward feeling	Shaky feeling, hunger Headache Dizziness	Thirst Weakness Nausea, vomiting Abdominal pain
Skin	Pallor Sweating	Flushed Signs of dehydration
Mucous membranes	Normal	Dry, crusty
Respirations	Shallow, rapid	Deep, rapid (Kussmaul)
Pulse	Tachycardia	Less rapid, weak
Breath odor	Normal	Fruity, acetone
Neurologic	Tremors Late: hyperreflexia, dilated pupils, convulsion	Diminished reflexes Paresthesia
Ominous signs	Shock, coma	Acidosis, coma
Blood:		
Glucose	Low: below 60 mg/dl	High: 250 mg/dl or higher
Ketones	Negative, trace	High, large
Osmolarity	Normal	High from hemoconcentration
pH	Normal	Low (≤7.25)
Hematocrit	Normal	High from hemoconcentration
Bicarbonate	Normal	Less than 20 mEq/L
Urine:		
Output	Normal	Polyuria (early) to oliguria (late)
Sugar	Negative	High
Acetone	Negative, trace	High

From Wong DL, et al: *Whaley and Wong's nursing care of infants and children*, ed 6, St Louis, 1999, Mosby.

E. **Therapeutic management**
1. Insulin
   a. Regular (short-acting) and (intermediate-acting) isophane insulin suspension [Neutral Protamine Hagedorn (NPH)] are administered SQ as two or more doses daily, or as continuous SQ infusion with a portable infusion pump; dosage is individualized based on blood glucose monitoring
      (1) Amount of morning regular insulin is determined by the previous day's late morning and lunchtime blood glucose values

(2) Morning intermediate-acting dosage is determined by previous day's late afternoon and dinner blood glucose levels

Insulin Action

Type	Onset (hr)	Peak (hr)	Duration (hr)
Humalog Insulin lispro	Within 15 min	40-60 min	About 2 hr
Short-acting:			
Regular	½-1	2-4	6-8
Semilente			
Intermediate-acting:			
NPH	1-2	6-12	18-26
Lente	1-2	6-12	24-26
Long-Acting:			
Ultralente	4-6	14-24	28-36

    b. Most commonly, 60% to 75% of daily dose is administered before breakfast

       (1) Remainder is taken before the evening meal

       (2) Intensive therapy is required for children with difficult-to-control diabetes and adolescents experiencing a growth spurt. Multiple injections of short- or intermediate-acting insulin are given through the day.

  2. Nutrition—a consistent meal plan is encouraged

    a. Meals and snacks must be eaten based on the peak insulin action

    b. Food intake must be consistent with the needs of a healthy child, except for the elimination of concentrated sugar

    c. The American Diabetes Association (ADA) exchange list facilitates dietary management by individual portion size and is prescribed by the number of each exchange from the four food groups

  3. Exercise—is part of the total diabetic management plan

    a. Because blood glucose levels decrease with exercise, insulin needs will decrease with consistent daily exercise

    b. Daily exercise should be performed at a consistent time to prevent glucose swings

  4. Home blood glucose monitoring aims to maintain serum blood glucose in a range of 80 to 120 mg/dl

F. Nursing management: acute care

  1. Nursing diagnoses

    a. Altered nutrition: less than body requirements

    b. Risk of injury

    2. Expected outcomes

      a. Child maintains nutritional requirements adequate to support growth and development while diabetes is controlled

      b. Child's serum glucose level is maintained within a range of 80 to 120 mg/dl

      c. Child exercises without injury to self and without wide fluctuations in serum glucose levels

    3. Interventions

      a. Assess for signs of hyperglycemia or DKA

      b. Assess blood glucose level three to four times a day if indicated

      c. Administer insulin as ordered

      d. Provide appropriate referrals for diet instruction to ensure calories balance with energy expenditure

      e. Ensure that meals are on time and provide between-meal and nighttime snacks

      f. Reinforce diet instructions

      g. Review meal planning with the family and child as indicated

      h. Provide opportunities for physical exercise

    4. Additional nursing diagnoses

      a. Noncompliance

      b. Risk for impaired skin integrity

      c. Risk for fluid volume deficit

      d. Ineffective family coping

G. Evaluation

    1. Child maintains a daily blood glucose level of over 60 mg/dl and under 120 mg/dl or within physician-prescribed guidelines

    2. Family and child comply with medical regimen for control of diabetes

    3. Child and family demonstrate correct technique of insulin administration and blood glucose monitoring

    4. Child has minimal episodes of extreme glucose levels and wide fluctuations in glucose levels

III. Hypothyroidism

  A. Description: common endocrine disorder that results from inadequate production of thyroid hormone

  B. Etiology and incidence

    1. Classification of causes

      a. Congenital—caused by gene mutation, hypopituitarism, or thyroid dysgenesis

      b. Acquired—examples: thyroidectomy, irradiation, iodine deficiency, thyroiditis, or infection

    2. Hypofunction of the thyroid gland is far more common in childhood than is hyperfunction

3. *Hyperthyroidism,* a condition characterized by a high concentration of thyroid hormone that increases metabolic function, is found mainly in adolescents with Graves' disease
4. Congenital hypothyroidism is the most common cause of primary hypothyroidism; occurs in 1 of 4000 live births
5. Diseases such as TB and mumps may contribute to the development of thyroiditis

C. **Pathophysiology**
1. Development and prognosis of the disease depends on the type of defect, age of onset, and severity of deficiency
2. Thyroid gland secretions
   a. Thyroxine (T_4): regulates metabolic rate; promotes mobilization of fats and gluconeogenesis; plays an important role in bone, teeth, and brain development
   b. Triiodothyronine (T_3): actions are the same as for T_4
   c. Thyrocalcitonin: regulates calcium and phosphorus metabolism; contributes to ossification and bone development; inhibits bone resorption—loss of calcium from the bone
3. Thyroid-stimulating hormone (TSH) is released from the anterior pituitary gland in the brain and stimulates the thyroid to function
4. Complications include retarded skeletal growth, delayed eruption of teeth, mental retardation, ataxia, and strabismus

D. **Assessment**
1. Assessment findings
   a. Infants
      (1) Slow growth
      (2) Facial appearance—small forehead; flattened nasal bridge; and large, protruding tongue
      (3) Hoarse cry
   b. Children
      (1) Dry skin, sparse, and brittle hair
      (2) Constipation
      (3) Mental decline and sleepiness
      (4) Periorbital puffiness
2. Diagnostic procedures
   a. Laboratory studies
      (1) Thyroid hormones by radioimmunoassays—decreased T_3, T_4, and TSH
      (2) Protein-bound iodine—increases after 2 months of age
   b. Diagnostic studies
      (1) Thyroid scan—determines size, location, and shape of gland; radioactive iodine uptake by thyroid is scanned
      (2) Evaluation of T_4 serum level—periodic as follow-up
      (3) Evaluation of bone age—periodic as follow-up
      (4) Ultrasonography—determines the location, size, and type of nodule on the thyroid gland, if it is fluid- or tissue-filled

E. **Therapeutic management: medications**
1. Hormones—levothyroxine sodium (Synthroid) as the replacement for decreased or absent thyroid function
2. Vitamins—calcitrol to ensure adequate calcium levels during periods of growth

F. **Nursing management: acute care**
1. Nursing diagnosis: fatigue related to imbalance in energy production
2. Expected outcome: child maintains optimal activity within disease and developmental limitations
3. Interventions
   a. Assess therapeutic response to thyroid replacement administration, including linear growth and activity level
   b. Monitor for signs of drug toxicity: irritability, nervousness, tachycardia, tremors, diarrhea, insomnia

> ⚠ **Warning!**
>
> Report signs of fatigue, persistent constipation, or the return of the original complaints because these signs indicate the drug dosage needs to be adjusted upward. For findings of irritability, nervousness, tachycardia, tremors, diarrhea, and insomnia, the dosage needs to be adjusted downward.

   c. Schedule follow-up for monitoring of serum levels of T_3 and T_4 at least yearly or if significant changes in weight, energy levels, or other findings are observed

G. **Evaluation**
1. Family complies with daily thyroid replacement regimen
2. Child displays improved function and activity level without signs of hypothyroidism

IV. Hypopituitarism

A. **Description: decreased or inadequate secretion of pituitary hormones**
B. **Etiology and incidence**
1. Hypopituitarism occurs as a result of
   a. Tumors in pituitary or hypothalamic region, which is the most common cause
   b. Irradiation
   c. Infection: tuberculosis and toxoplasmosis
   d. Head trauma: perinatal, child abuse, and skull fracture
2. Most commonly affects boys
C. **Pathophysiology: production or release of growth hormone interference causes these changes**
1. Decreased linear growth associated with decreased production of the hormone that affects bone growth

   2. Increased protein catabolism results in decreased muscle mass, hair thinning, and delayed growth
   3. Decreased fat catabolism causes excess subcutaneous fat and hypoglycemia
D. **Assessment**
   1. Assessment findings
      a. History: normal weight and length at birth; familial pattern of autosomal recessive inheritance
      b. Retarded growth pattern: short stature, below third percentile on the growth chart at 1 year of age
      c. Appears younger than chronologic age; often overweight
      d. Delayed eruption of permanent teeth
      e. Delayed sexual development
      f. Premature aging later in life
   2. Diagnostic procedures
      a. Laboratory study—serum or urine growth hormone level to reveal absent or decreased growth hormone
      b. Diagnostic studies
         (1) Physical examination—review of child's growth in height and weight
         (2) Skeletal survey—reveals delayed skeletal maturation
         (3) X-ray films of wrist and skull—determine bone infection or tumor
         (4) CT scan—identifies lesion site and size
E. **Therapeutic management**
   1. Medications: growth hormone replacement—biosynthetic form
   2. Surgical: removal of tumor, if present
F. **Nursing management: acute care**
   1. Nursing diagnoses
      a. Altered growth and development
      b. Body image disturbance
   2. Expected outcome: child demonstrates positive response to growth hormone therapy
   3. Interventions
      a. Assess child's height and weight with progress monitored on a growth chart
      b. Administer injections of growth hormone
      c. Assess for growth hormone overdose: hypoglycemia followed by hyperglycemia
G. **Evaluation**
   1. Family complies with growth hormone replacement regimen
   2. Child achieves adult height
   3. Child participates in group activities with peers

V. Home care: family education topics and referrals

A. Diabetes

1. Disease process and therapy: pathology, activity and exercise needs, notification of physician if child vomits more than once, if blood glucose remains >240 mg/dl, or if urinary ketones remain high

2. Management: in the event of illness, insulin needs to be maintained or increased; lifelong therapy is required

3. Diet: review or reinforce the prescribed diet plan, and inform parents that food intake depends on activity level and insulin intake; review concept of food exchanges, adequate caloric intake according to age, importance of proper meal times, and when to provide snacks

4. Activity: importance of daily exercise; define hypoglycemia and causes; teach symptoms and actions to treat; eating a snack before exercise and at night before bedtime (see Table 19-3, p. 564)

5. Hygiene: importance of personal hygiene, including regular dental checkups, foot care

6. Medication: proper insulin administration technique; proper insulin handling, mixing, and storage; rotation of injection sites; correct use of pump and injection site care

7. Glucose testing: instruct family on method of testing blood glucose (Chemstrips or glucose monitoring system), maintenance of equipment and care of supplies

8. Follow-up: importance of record-keeping: insulin, test results, responses to diet and exercise; early symptoms of complications: hypoglycemia and hyperglycemia; yearly eye examinations; laboratory tests for renal impairment

9. Safety: wearing medical alert bracelet

10. Referrals: dietician; home health nurse; child and parent support groups

B. Hypothyroidism

1. Disease process: nature of disease; need for life-long replacement therapy

2. Medications: administration of thyroid replacement; assess for increased pulse rate, which indicates excess thyroid hormone; necessity of yearly (at least) monitoring of serum levels

3. Activity: inform parents to expect gradual improvement in activity level; report fatigue or the return of the original findings to the physician for a dose readjustment

4. Referrals: genetic counseling

C. Hypopituitarism

1. Disease process: pathology; discuss probability that the child will eventually reach adult height and that puberty will be delayed by 1 to 2 years

2. Medication: need for frequent injections; growth hormone administration, preparation, storage, and dosing schedule (administer at bedtime); side effects to be tolerated and those to be reported
3. Psychosocial: treat child at appropriate level for age
4. Follow-up: need for continued monitoring for growth and epiphyseal closure
5. Referrals: Human Growth Foundation; Short Stature Foundation

WEB Resources

www.jdf.org/index.html

Website for the Juvenile Diabetes Foundation (JDF) whose mission is to find a cure for diabetes and its complications. Site contains family resources, as well as JDF chapter information, publications, and research updates.

www.ucsc.edu/misc/diabetes

Website sponsored by the Barbara Davis Center for Childhood Diabetes of the University of Colorado School of Medicine, a treatment center for Type I diabetes: nutrition news, recipes, research information, and an "ask the expert" feature.

www.mc.vanderbilt.edu/peds/pidl/indexhtm

The Vanderbilt Pediatric Interactive Digital Library is a learning resource for health care professionals sponsored by the Department of Pediatrics at Vanderbilt University. Topics include endocrinology (growth hormone deficiency, hypothyroidism) with references.

REVIEW QUESTIONS

1. A 7-year-old child complains of shakiness, hunger, and headache. Based on these findings, the school nurse should suspect the student has which of these conditions?
   1. Diabetic ketoacidosis (DKA)
   2. Hyperglycemia
   3. Hypoglycemia
   4. Polyphagia

2. A mother of a child newly diagnosed with diabetes is receiving nutritional counseling. Which of these statements by the mother indicates the need for further instruction?
   1. "Calories and nutrient proportions have to be consistent on a daily basis."
   2. "Chocolate milk with meals is acceptable."
   3. "Meals and snacks must be eaten at the same time each day."
   4. "Cola may be exchanged for fruit juice."

3. A 7-year-old child diagnosed with diabetic ketoacidosis (DKA) is likely to exhibit which of these findings?
   1. Frequent episodes of vomiting
   2. Dilated pupils
   3. Rapid, deep respirations
   4. Warm skin and diaphoresis

4. Which of these laboratory findings of an infant diagnosed with hypothyroidism is useful in determining whether the treatment is effective?
   1. Iodine level
   2. Methimazole (Tapazole) level
   3. CPK, LDH, CK-MB
   4. Serum T_4 and T_3, and TSH

5. The mother of a child newly diagnosed with type 1 diabetes asks why insulin needs to be injected. The nurse responds that the child cannot take oral insulin because it
   1. Is not tolerated well in oral form by children
   2. Is not available in pill form
   3. Is destroyed by the digestive enzymes
   4. Will cause gastric ulcers

ANSWERS, RATIONALES, AND TEST-TAKING TIPS

Rationale	Test-Taking Tips

1. Correct answer: 3

Increased adrenergic activity and increased secretion of catecholamines cause signs of hypoglycemia. These changes produce nervousness, headaches, and hunger. Findings associated with DKA include dehydration from the diuresis; rapid, deep respirations; electrolyte imbalances; and metabolic acidosis. Findings associated with hyperglycemia include lethargy; deep and rapid respirations; and fruity, acetone breath, which is also a finding with DKA. In option 4, this is one of the three cardinal signs of diabetes: the "polys": polyphagia, polydipsia, and polyuria.

Relate the findings in the stem to a personal experience such as working all day without eating. You were probably shaky, hungry, and may have had a headache or become ill-tempered.

2. Correct answer: 2

Low-carbohydrate snacks are emphasized in the diet of the child with diabetes. Nutritional counseling emphasizes a consistent menu with complex carbohydrates and consistent meal times. Substitutions with foods of equal carbohydrate content usually are acceptable without effecting blood glucose control.

The most important approach to use with these types of questions is careful reading. Be sure to note that the question is about "the need for further instruction." Select an incorrect statement, option 2. Before you go to the next question, simply reread this question once more and then read your choice to ensure you have chosen the best option. You increase your ability to select the best answer when you read the question and the chosen option one final time.

3. Correct answer: 3

In this metabolic acidotic state, the respiratory system attempts to return the pH to normal by the elimination of carbon dioxide through an increase in the RR

Recall that DKA is associated with Kussmaul's respirations. Associate the K in DKA with the K in Kussmaul's respirations. Note that in both hyperglycemia and

CHAPTER 19 Nursing Care of Children with Endocrine Disorders

Rationale	Test-Taking Tips

and respiratory depth. These respirations are described as Kussmaul's respirations. Nausea and vomiting are early findings consistent with hyperglycemia before the client is in DKA. The findings in options 2 and 4 are consistent with hypoglycemia.

hypoglycemia the RR is rapid. The difference is that in hyperglycemia, breathing is deep—think deep in sugar level and in hypoglycemia—think shallow or low sugar level in the blood.

4. Correct answer: 4

Effective treatment is determined by a restoration of the state of euthyroid—normal T_3, T_4, and TSH. Iodine is essential for thyroid hormone production. Tapazole is prescribed for hyperthyroidism. The items in option 3 are cardiac enzymes used to detect myocardial damage. These enzymes are elevated when the heart muscle is injured or necrosis occurs.

Remember the three Ts (serum tests for Thyroid function): T_3, T_4, and TSH.

5. Correct answer: 3

Insulin is not effective when taken orally because the GI tract enzymes breaks down the protein molecule before it can be absorbed and reach the blood stream. Type 1 diabetes mellitus, typically found in children, requires exogenous insulin to control the blood glucose level because the pancreas—the beta cells—do not produce insulin. Hypoglycemic agents available in oral form are given to adults and children with type 2 diabetes. Type 2 results when the pancreas does not produce enough insulin or in the event of insulin resistance. Oral hypoglycemic agents stimulate the pancreas to produce more insulin. Option 4 is a false statement.

Eliminate initially that which you know is false, option 4. Eliminate option 1 because it is unlikely that *all* children would not tolerate a medication. Next, make an educated guess that if option 3 had occurred, then option 2 would follow. Thus, select option 3, which best answers the question. Be alert. If the stem had the fact that a child was diagnosed with *type 2 diabetes,* then oral hypoglycemic agents may be appropriate to give these children. In some instances children may have type 2 diabetes from obesity and inactivity. They will need similar interventions as the adults with this diagnosis.

20

Essential Odds and Ends: Nursing Care of Children with Special Needs

FAST FACTS

1. Sensory impairments that lead to visual or auditory deprivation place children at risk for impaired developmental skills: cognitive, perceptive, communication, and socialization.
2. Auditory impairments are classified as conductive, sensorineural, or mixed.
3. Standardized charts are used to estimate the distribution of burns in children.
4. Burns of the face, hands, feet, or perineum place the child at risk and require hospital admission.

CONTENT REVIEW

I. Attention deficit–hyperactivity disorder (AD-HD)
   A. Description: syndrome of varying severity characterized by learning and behavior disabilities; affects children, adolescents, and rarely adults
   B. Etiology and incidence
      1. Frequency is three times more common in males than in females; affects 3% to 5% of school-aged children
      2. Exact cause is unknown; factors involved include genetics, neurotransmitter abnormality, low birth weight (LBW), nicotine and alcohol abuse by mother, and the environment

      3. Seen more often in children with a family member having AD-HD (father, uncle)

C. Assessment

    1. Assessment findings (Box 20-1)

    2. Diagnostic evaluation

      a. Complete medical and developmental history

      b. Observation of home and school behaviors

      c. Physical examination, including detailed neurologic workup and hearing evaluation

      d. Psychological testing to determine intelligence and achievement levels, and visual-perceptual difficulties

      e. Screen for other potential causes: lead poisoning, hearing loss, and seizures

D. Therapeutic management

    1. Behavioral therapy and psychotherapy—behavior modification techniques and family therapy

    2. Appropriate classroom placement—small, orderly, structured setting with minimal distractions and stimuli

    3. Counseling for those children who exhibit symptoms of anxiety and depression

    4. Medications

      a. Psychostimulants: methylphenidate hydrochloride (Ritalin), dextroamphetamine sulfate (Dexedrine), and pemoline (Cylert)

      b. Antidepressants: bupropion (Wellbutrin); selective serotonin reuptake inhibitors (SSRIs): sertraline hydrochloride (Zoloft), paroxetine (Paxil), and fluoxetine hydrochloride (Prozac)

      c. Antihypertensives: clonidine hydrochloride (Catapres)

E. Nursing management: acute

    1. Nursing diagnoses: risk for injury related to hyperactivity, impaired verbal communication related to inattention

    2. Expected outcome: the child safely and effectively participates in a structured school environment

    3. Interventions

      a. Assess the child's environment for safety hazards

      b. Administer medications as ordered; assess for side effects: anorexia, insomnia, and tachycardia

    4. Nursing diagnoses: compromised ineffective family coping; risk for care-giver role strain

    5. Expected outcome: the child and family discuss and implement effective coping strategies

    6. Interventions

      a. Assess coping strategies currently being used by family and child

      b. Review effective parenting techniques, including discipline techniques and rewards for appropriate behavior

      c. Assist the child with social skills through the use of role playing and modeling; point out the positive aspects of the child's behavior

Box 20-1
Diagnostic Criteria for Attention Deficit–Hyperactivity Disorder

A. Either 1 or 2:
  1. Six (or more) of the following symptoms of inattention have persisted for at least 6 months to a degree that is maladaptive and inconsistent with developmental level:
    Inattention
    a. Often fails to give close attention to details or makes careless mistakes in schoolwork, work, or other activities
    b. Often has difficulty sustaining attention in tasks or play activities
    c. Often does not seem to listen when spoken to directly
    d. Often does not follow through on instructions and fails to finish schoolwork, chores, or duties in the workplace (not due to oppositional behavior or failure to understand instructions)
    e. Often has difficulty organizing tasks and activities
    f. Often avoids, dislikes, or is reluctant to engage in tasks that require sustained mental effort (such as schoolwork or homework)
    g. Often loses things necessary for tasks or activities (e.g., toys, school assignments, pencils, books, or tools)
    h. Is often easily distracted by extraneous stimuli
    i. Is often forgetful in daily activities
  2. Six (or more) of the following symptoms of hyperactivity-impulsivity have persisted for at least 6 months to a degree that is maladaptive and inconsistent with developmental level:
    Hyperactivity
    a. Often fidgets with hands or feet or squirms in seat
    b. Often leaves seat in classroom or in other situations in which remaining seated is expected
    c. Often runs about or climbs excessively in situations in which it is inappropriate (in adolescents or adults, may be limited to subjective feelings of restlessness)
    d. Often has difficulty playing or engaging in leisure activities quietly
    e. Is often "on the go" or often acts as if "driven by a motor"
    f. Often talks excessively
    Impulsivity
    g. Often blurts out answers before questions have been completed
    h. Often has difficulty awaiting turn
    i. Often interrupts or intrudes on others (e.g., butts into conversations or games)
B. Some hyperactive-impulsive or inattentive symptoms that caused impairment were present before age 7 years.
C. Some impairment from the symptoms is present in two or more settings (e.g., at school [at work] and at home).
D. There must be clear evidence of clinically significant impairment in social, academic, or occupational functioning.
E. The symptoms do not occur exclusively during the course of a pervasive developmental disorder, schizophrenia, or other psychotic disorder and are not better accounted for by another mental disorder (e.g., mood disorder, anxiety disorder, dissociative disorder, or personality disorder).

From American Psychiatric Association: *Diagnostic and statistical manual of mental disorders,* ed 4, Washington, DC, 1994, American Psychiatric Association.

      7. Additional nursing diagnoses

        a. Self-esteem disturbance

        b. Impaired social interaction

  F. Evaluation

      1. Parents demonstrate correct administration of stimulant

      2. Parents demonstrate effective parenting techniques

      3. Child and family demonstrate effective coping strategies

      4. Child functions within expected limits in the school and home environments

II. Mental retardation

  A. Description: disorder characterized by below average general intellectual function (IQ of 70 or below); classifications include mild, moderate, severe, and profound levels of deficit

  B. Etiology and incidence

      1. Causes

        a. Severe—genetic (Down syndrome), biochemical, infectious (rubella), developmental, and metabolic (phenylketouria [PKU])

        b. Mild—maternal lifestyle factors: cigarette smoking, poor nutrition, and chemical abuse

        c. Acquired—causes include meningitis, lead poisoning, and head and brain injury

      2. Down syndrome accounts for 25% of all cases of MR

  C. Assessment

      1. Most mentally retarded children have a history of normal development for the first 2 years followed by a decline in developmental abilities

      2. Psychometric testing: Stanford-Binet test, Wechsler Intelligence Scale for Children (revised) to determine the level of disability and function

      3. Behaviors

        a. Delayed developmental milestones: language and cognitive skills

        b. Poor eye contact during feeding, slow feeding

        c. Nonresponsiveness; irritability

        d. Decreased spontaneous activity

      4. Family assessment: low family intelligence or environmental deprivation

      5. Diagnostic procedures: chromosome analysis, radiography, tomography, EEG, metabolic disorder testing

  D. Therapeutic management: the goal is early recognition

      1. Infant stimulation and physical therapy programs

      2. Skills: ADL, self-help, verbal, social, and adaptive behaviors

      3. Behavior modification

  E. Nursing management

      1. Nursing diagnosis: altered growth and development related to impaired cognitive functioning

   2. Expected outcomes
      a. Child and family participate in infant stimulation program
      b. Child's maximal potential for development is realized
      c. Child behaves in socially acceptable manner to the degree able
   3. Interventions
      a. Review recent psychological and physical assessment findings; assess child's current level of functioning
      b. Involve family in early intervention programs: infant stimulation
      c. Assess progress at regular intervals
      d. Use positive reinforcement for specific tasks
      e. Encourage learning of self-care skills
   4. Nursing diagnosis: altered family processes
   5. Expected outcome: family demonstrates acceptance of child and the situation
   6. Interventions
      a. Assist the family with the decision to care for the child at home or locate a residential site for placement
      b. Emphasize the child's strengths and potential abilities; encourage the family to include the child in planning
      c. Encourage verbalization of concerns and feelings related to the child and the situation
F. **Evaluation**
   1. Family demonstrates acceptance of the child
   2. Child and family participate in support services

III. Sensory impairment

A. **Description: those impairments leading to visual or auditory deprivation, or both, that place children at risk for impaired development skills: cognitive, perceptive, communication, and socialization**
B. **Etiology and incidence**
   1. Common visual disorders in childhood include refractive disorders (myopia, hyperopia), strabismus, injury from foreign bodies, and conjunctivitis
   2. Auditory disturbances are classified as **conductive, sensorineural,** or mixed type
      a. Damage to inner structures or auditory nerve results in sensorineural hearing loss; causes include excessive exposure to loud noises, ototoxic drugs, and infection
      b. Conductive hearing loss, the most common type of hearing loss, results from interference of transmission of sound to the middle ear
C. **Assessment**
   1. Assessment findings
      a. Visual: symptoms depend on type of visual impairment (Table 20-1, p. 580)

Text continued on p. 582

TABLE 20-1 Types of Visual Impairment from Refractive Errors

Defect, Description, Pathophysiology	Clinical Manifestations	Treatment
Myopia (nearsightedness): ability to see objects clearly at close range but not at a distance; results from the eyeball being too long, causing the image to fall in front of the retina	Behavioral manifestations: Rubs eyes excessively Tilts head or thrusts head forward Has difficulty reading or doing other close work; blinks eyes excessively or is irritable when doing close work Holds book close to the eyes; writes or colors with the head close to the table Clumsy; walks into objects; is unable to see objects clearly Does poorly in school, especially in subjects that require demonstration, such as arithmetic Signs and symptoms: Dizziness Headache Nausea after close work	Corrected with biconcave lenses that focus rays on the retina
Hyperopia (hypermetropia, or farsightedness): ability to see objects clearly at a distance but not at close range; results from the eyeball being too short, causing the image to focus beyond the retina	Because of accommodative ability, the child can usually see objects at all ranges Most children are normally hyperopic until about 7 years of age	If correction is required, use convex lenses to focus rays on the retina
Astigmatism: unequal curvatures in the refractive apparatus; results from unequal curvatures in the cornea or lens that cause light rays to bend in different directions	Depends on the severity of refractive error in each eye May have clinical manifestations of myopia	Corrected with special lenses that compensate for refractive errors

Disorder	Clinical Manifestations	Treatment
Anisometropia: different refractive strengths in each eye; may develop amblyopia as the weaker eye is used less	Depends on the severity of refractive error in each eye May have clinical manifestations of myopia Poor vision in the affected eye	Treated with corrective lenses, preferably contact lenses, to improve vision in each eye so they work as a unit
Strabismus ("squint" or "cross-eye"): mal-alignment of the eyes *Esotropia*: inward deviation of the eye *Exotropia*: outward deviation of the eye May result from muscle imbalance or paralysis, poor vision, or congenital defect; because the visual axes are not parallel, the brain receives two images, and amblyopia can result	Behavioral manifestations: Squints eyelids together or frowns Closes one eye to see; tilts head to one side Has difficulty focusing from one distance to another Inaccurate judgment in picking up objects Unable to see print or moving objects clearly If combined with refractive errors, may see any of the manifestations listed for refractive errors Signs and symptoms: Diplopia Photophobia Dizziness, headache "Crossed" eye	Treatment depends on cause of strabismus May involve occlusion therapy (patching stronger eye) to increase visual stimulation to weaker eye Early diagnosis essential to prevent vision loss
Amblyopia ("lazy eye"): reduced visual acuity in one eye; results when one eye does not receive sufficient stimulation; each retina receives different images, resulting in diplopia (double vision); the brain accommodates by suppressing the less intense image; the visual cortex eventually does not respond to stimulation with loss of vision in that eye	Depends on the primary visual defect, such as anisometropia or strabismus	Preventable if treatment of the primary visual defect begins before 6 years of age.

Modified from Wong DL, et al: *Whaley and Wong's nursing care of infants and children*, ed 6, St. Louis, 1999, Mosby.

    b. Auditory
      (1) Infant
        (a) Lack of startle or blink reflex to loud sounds
        (b) Failure to localize sounds by 6 months of age
        (c) Absence of babble or vocalization by 7 months of age
      (2) Child
        (a) Failure to develop intelligible speech by 2 years of age
        (b) Use of gestures to indicate desires rather than verbalization after 15 months of age
        (c) Vocal play, head banging, or foot stamping for vibratory sensation
  2. Diagnostic studies: early discovery of sensory problems is essential
    a. Vision
      (1) **Snellen chart**—E symbol or letter (for children able to read the alphabet) to determine distant visual acuity
      (2) Cover-uncover test of each eye—determines eye muscle imbalance
      (3) Visual field testing—determines peripheral vision abnormalities
      (4) Fundoscopic examination—reveals absent red reflex, retinal hemorrhages, and retinal detachment
    b. Hearing
      (1) Crib-o-gram—neonatal screening tool that analyzes hearing responses by comparing an infant's motor activity before, during, and after a sound is introduced; determines abnormal infant motor response to sound
      (2) Audiometry—determines the degree of hearing loss; brainstem auditory-evoked potential
      (3) **Rinne** and **Weber** tests—determine conductivity or sensorineural hearing deficits by using a tuning fork
      (4) Tympanometry—reveals middle ear pressure
D. Therapeutic management
  1. Medications
    a. Antibiotics—ophthalmic ointments or drops to treat eye infections; oral antibiotics or eardrops to treat middle ear infection
    b. Anti-inflammatory drugs—ophthalmic or ear drops to decrease eye or ear inflammation
  2. Surgery
    a. Vision: corrective surgery for strabismus and eye trauma
    b. Hearing: cochlear implants for sensorineural loss; insertion of tympanotomy tubes for otitis media
  3. Other treatments
    a. Vision: corrective lens, patching of one eye for strabismus to strengthen eye muscles in the lazy eye
    b. Hearing: hearing aids, speech therapy, sign language, and the use of a telecommunication device

E. **Nursing management for the hospitalized child with a sensory deficit**
   1. Vision
      a. Sensory perceptual alteration: visual
      b. Expected outcome: child demonstrates progression in developmental tasks
      c. Interventions
         (1) Assess visual acuity; perform or facilitate visual tests for acuity, strabismus, and amblyopia as indicated
         (2) Face child when speaking; offer explanation of what is happening in the environment
         (3) Orient child to the room; arrange furniture with child's safety in mind
         (4) State name when entering the room; explain any procedure before starting
         (5) Assist with proper use of corrective devices: glasses or contact lenses
         (6) Administer ophthalamic medications, as ordered
         (7) Teach the family the correct method and concerns about eye and ear medication administration
         (8) Provide information about special programs to learn independent behavior, braille reading and writing, and special computer equipment
         (9) Provide toys that stimulate the senses of hearing and touch
   2. Hearing
      a. Sensory-perceptual alteration: auditory
      b. Expected outcome: child adapts to hearing loss with maintenance of independence in activities and of communication with others
      c. Interventions
         (1) Assess auditory acuity; facilitate auditory testing to determine the degree of hearing loss
         (2) Face the child when speaking; speak slowly and distinctly; do not shout
         (3) Assist with use and care of a hearing aid
         (4) Provide opportunities for socialization; emphasize self-care
   3. Additional nursing diagnoses
      a. Altered growth and development
      b. Risk for injury
      c. Altered family processes
F. **Evaluation**
   1. Child maintains independence with progression in developmental tasks
   2. Child correctly uses assisting devices or aids
   3. Family participates in formal rehabilitation program or support services

IV. Burns

A. **Etiology and incidence**

1. Second leading cause of death from trauma in childhood
2. Children less than 4 years of age are the most likely to require hospitalization because of burns
3. Causes of burns
   a. Thermal agents—flame, direct contact, hot water, and steam
   b. Chemical agents—acids or alkali
   c. Electrical agents—electrical cords
   d. Radioactive agents—X-rays or ultraviolet exposure
4. House fires are the cause of most fire fatalities in children; children playing with matches are responsible for 1 in 10 house fires
5. Most burn injuries are caused by thermal agents

B. **Pathophysiology**

1. The extent of tissue destruction is related to the intensity of the heat source, duration of contact, and speed by which heat energy is dissipated by burned surface
2. There are standardized charts to estimate burn distribution in children less than 5 years of age and older children (Figure 20-1); documentation is expressed as the percentage of total body surface area (BSA).

> ⚠️ **Warning!**
>
> The standard "rule of nines" used for adults is not appropriate for young children. A modified "rule of nines" proposes that for each year of life over 2 years of age, 1% is deducted from the head and 0.5% is added to each leg.

3. Current classification of burn depth of tissue injury
   a. Superficial (first degree)—minimal tissue damage; painful
   b. Partial-thickness burn (second degree)—involves epithelium and portion of corium; very painful
   c. Full-thickness burn (third and fourth degree)—skin of all layers destroyed, as well as underlying tissues or muscles; *not painful*
4. Burns are assessed according to severity
   a. Minor burns: partial-thickness burns of less than 10% of total BSA in children; full-thickness burns of less than 2% of BSA offer no risk of cosmetic or functional impairment or disability
   b. Moderate burns: partial-thickness burns of 10% to 25% of total BSA; full-thickness burns of less than 10% of BSA; offer minimal risk of cosmetic or functional impairment, except in small children or when the burns involve critical areas such as the face, feet, hands, or genitalia in children under 10 years of age
   c. Major or critical burns: partial-thickness burns of 25% of total BSA in children; full-thickness burns of 10% of BSA or more;

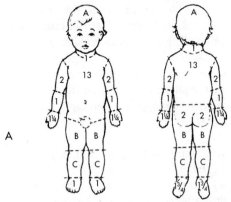

RELATIVE PERCENTAGES OF AREAS AFFECTED BY GROWTH			
AREA	BIRTH	AGE, 1 YR	AGE, 5 YR
A = ½ of head	9½	8½	6½
B = ½ of one thigh	2¾	3¼	4
C = ½ of one leg	2½	2½	2¾

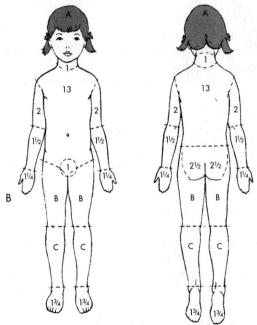

RELATIVE PERCENTAGES OF AREAS AFFECTED BY GROWTH			
AREA	AGE, 10 YR	AGE, 15 YR	ADULT
A = ½ of head	5½	4½	3½
B = ½ of one thigh	4½	4½	4¾
C = ½ of one leg	3	3¼	3½

Figure 20-1 Extent of burn injury. **A,** Children from birth to age 5 years of age. **B,** Older children. (From Wong DL, et al: *Whaley and Wong's nursing care of infants and children,* ed 6, St. Louis, 1999, Mosby.)

burns that involve the face, eyes, ears, hands, feet, and perineum; high-voltage electric burn injury; all burn injuries associated with chemical, inhalation, or major trauma; major burns are likely to result in functional or cosmetic impairment or disability

    d. Burns of the face, hands, feet, or perineum, even though small in area, often require hospitalization from the risk of airway obstruction, severe hypoxia, and rapid fluid shifts

5. Local and systemic responses of the body to an initial burn injury:
    a. Local
        (1) Edema formation—results from altered hydrostatic pressure and capillary permeability
        (2) Fluid and protein loss—results from skin loss
        (3) Reduced blood flow to affected area
        (4) GI system: gastric ileus
        (5) Respiratory system: pulmonary inhalation injury, edema, and bacterial pneumonia
    b. Systemic
        (1) Burn shock—from reduced circulation or vascular volume, which results in decreased cardiac output
        (2) Metabolic acidosis
        (3) Reduced renal perfusion
        (4) Increased metabolic rate and altered growth rate

6. Three phases of burn care
    a. Acute emergent: begins immediately after the injury as the body reacts with an inflammatory response and a large shift of extracellular fluid into the damaged tissues
        (1) First 48 hours from the time of the initial injury
        (2) Priorities
            (a) Assess the ABCs (airway, breathing, and circulation)
            (b) Assess for associated trauma
            (c) Conserve body heat—cover areas that are not burned
            (d) Administer fluids—the priority at this time to prevent shock
            (e) Monitor serum potassium levels, which typically are elevated from the death of cells
    b. Management: occurs during the time the wound is healing until wound closure, that is, from day 3 until about 3 months
        (1) Priorities
            (a) Fluid overload monitoring
            (b) Infection prevention
            (c) Wound care
            (d) Nutritional support
            (e) Pain management
            (f) Physical therapy

    c. Rehabilitation: occurs as the child attempts to return to an optimal level of function, and may last from a few years to a lifetime

      (1) Priorities

        (a) Regaining independence

        (b) Prevention or minimization of deformities and scarring

        (c) Contracture or scar revisions

        (d) Emotional support

        (e) Physical and occupational therapy

7. Burn complications in children

    a. Inhalation injury to upper and lower airways

    b. Acute bronchitis and bronchopneumonia

    c. Wound sepsis

    d. **Curling** or stress ulcer from the increase of hydrochloric acid in the stomach

    e. CNS dysfunction: encephalopathy—symptoms include hallucinations, seizures, and coma

    f. Compartment syndrome due to rapid fluid shift to the interstitial spaces

C. Assessment

1. Wound condition
2. Child's overall condition and behaviors
3. Signs of complications
4. Need for pain management when first or second degree burns are present

D. Therapeutic management

1. Airway maintenance
2. Fluid replacement: Parkland formula-guideline for fluid resuscitation 4 ml/kg per percent of BSA for second and third degree burns; half of the total in the first 8 hours, with the remainder over the next 16 hours

⚠ Warning!

The most reliable indicators of fluid resuscitation are changes in the urinary output, sensorium, and capillary refill.

3. Medications

    a. Analgesics: acetaminophen for minor burns, morphine for major burns; midazolam (Versed) and fentanyl used for procedures to debride the burned areas

    b. Anesthetics: nitrous oxide, ketamine

    c. Tetanus immunization

⚠ Warning!

Tetanus toxoid, or tetanus immune globulin, or both are administered if there is no history of immunization or it has been more that 5 years since the last immunization for tetanus.

4. Management of burn wound
   a. Primary excision used with large full-thickness burns
   b. Debridement in conjunction with hydrotherapy
   c. Methods of burn wound management
      (1) Open wound left uncovered with the application of an antimicrobial cream or ointment
      (2) Modified—cream or ointment applied directly to wound or by means of thin gauze; wound then covered with gauze or net covering
      (3) Occlusive—cream-impregnated gauze placed on wound, layers of bulky gauze applied, secured with stretched gauze or net
      (4) Exposure—wound left open to air; crust forms on partial thickness and eschar forms on full-thickness burns
   d. Topical antimicrobials most commonly used
      (1) 1% silver sulfadiazine (Silvadene): causes a sensation of coldness when applied; effective against many gram-positive and gram-negative organisms; burning, stinging, and swelling indicate an allergic reaction
      (2) 10% mafenide acetate (Sulfamylon): causes discomfort when applied; effective against many gram-positive and gram-negative organisms; effective in deep flame and electrically-caused wounds
      (3) 0.5% silver nitrate solution: stains skin, linens, and clothes; effective against *Pseudomonas* and *Staphylococcus* organisms; does not interfere with wound healing; difficult to apply
      (4) Bacitracin-bacteriocidal and bacteriostatic agents against gram-positive organisms
   e. Skin coverings
      (1) Temporary grafts include allograft (homograft) and xenograft (heterograft); porcine (pig skin) commonly used in children
      (2) Permanent grafts include *autograft* (from child's own body) and *isograft* (tissue from genetically identical individual)
      (3) Synthetic skin substitutes: BCG matrix, Biobrane, and calcium alginate
      (4) Artificial skin: Integra prepares the wound to accept an autograft
      (5) Cultured epithelium: child's skin is cultured to form a thin epithelial layer that is applied to the burn wound

E. **Nursing management**
   1. Nursing diagnoses
      a. Acute emergent phase
         (1) Nursing diagnoses: risk for an ineffective breathing pattern related to smoke inhalation; impaired gas exchange

(2) Expected outcome: child demonstrates unlabored breathing pattern and respirations between a rate of 16 and 24
(3) Interventions
   (a) Assess for signs of respiratory distress: restlessness, confusion, labored breathing, diminished or adventitious breath sounds, and sternal retractions
   (b) Monitor airway, breathing, and circulation (ABCs), as ordered
   (c) Continuously monitor oxygen saturation levels to maintain at over 90%
   (d) Administer oxygen and corticosteroids, as ordered
   (e) Elevate head of bed; keep intubation tray at bedside
(4) Nursing diagnosis: risk for fluid volume deficit related to fluid loss through burns
(5) Expected outcome: fluid volume is restored with appropriate potassium levels and with an adequate urine output of 1 ml/kg/hr
(6) Interventions
   (a) Assess for signs of fluid volume deficit
   (b) Monitor vital signs, mental state, and peripheral perfusion
   (c) Monitor serum potassium levels and the urine for specific gravity changes to be increased with dehydration
   (d) Monitor input and output and hourly urine output; maintain Foley catheter, if present
   (e) Assess daily weights: compare to the severity of the fluid lost versus the fluid given
   (f) Monitor H&H for decreases from blood loss or overhydration
   (g) Administer IV fluids and electrolytes, as ordered
   (h) Administer diuretics and albumin, as ordered
b. Acute and management phase
  (1) Nursing diagnoses: impaired skin integrity; risk for infection; pain
  (2) Expected outcomes
   (a) Child maintains skin integrity without infection
   (b) Child verbalized relief from or minimal pain
  (3) Interventions
   (a) Assess the percentage of BSA burned with the use of a burn chart appropriate for the child's age
   (b) Assess the condition and location of the burn; assess pain level using pediatric pain rating scale; administer analgesics before onset of severe pain and at regular intervals
   (c) Elevate the burned extremities above the level of the heart

(d) Assess the child for signs of infection: drainage, odor, and delayed healing of the burn; change in vital signs; increased WBCs; and increased temperature

(e) Maintain infection control techniques

(f) Enforce strict hand washing technique

(g) Use hydrotherapy tub, as ordered, to cleanse and debride the burns

(h) Apply a bacteriostatic agent and give an analgesic agent before painful procedures, as ordered

(i) Maintain extremities in alignment to prevent contractures

(j) Dress wounds with the use of sterile technique, as ordered

(k) Observe for signs of curling ulcer or hemorrhage: bloody or coffee-brown emesis, melena, epigastric pain, or abdominal distention

(l) Administer antacids or Histamine H_2 receptor antagonists to decrease the risk of gastric ulcer development or bleeding

(4) Nursing diagnosis: altered nutrition—less than body requirements

(5) Expected outcome: child has adequate nutrition with the maintenance of 90% of child's weight before injury

(6) Interventions

(a) Obtain child's weight before injury; assess eating habits, preferred foods, and food allergies

(b) Administer oral fluids or nasogastric feedings

(c) Administer TPN, as ordered

(d) Monitor daily weights for significant changes

(e) Provide a high-calorie, high-protein diet

(f) Supplement the diet with high doses of vitamins B and C, iron, and zinc

(g) Gradually advance the liquid diet to a regular diet and provide nutritious snacks

(h) Encourage the family to bring the child's favorite foods from home

(i) Provide positive reinforcement for eating

c. Rehabilitative phase

(1) Nursing diagnosis: body image disturbance

(2) Expected outcome: child exhibits behaviors that indicate body image has been restored or maintained

(3) Interventions

(a) Assess child for feelings about the change in appearance, difficulty with school and social situations, behaviors of withdrawal or depression

(b) Encourage child to express feelings and concerns about the restrictions in lifestyle and altered appearance

        (c) Support child in decision-making, with encouragement for independence as appropriate

        (d) Discuss with family the impact of the burns on the child's body systems and the psychosocial development needs

        (e) Stress the importance of family support and of child participation in peer activities

        (f) Suggest follow-up counseling with child-life worker or counselor

2. Other nursing diagnoses
   a. Acute emergent phase
      (1) Ineffective airway clearance
      (2) Impaired physical mobility
   b. Management
      (1) Risk for fluid overload
      (2) Risk for altered tissue perfusion
      (3) Anxiety and fear
   c. Rehabilitative phase
      (1) Ineffective family processes
      (2) Self-care deficit

F. Evaluation
1. Child exhibits an absence of fluid and electrolyte imbalance
2. Child exhibits an absence of skin impairment and infection
3. Child verbalizes improved body image and makes social contacts outside of the family
4. Family and child participates in psychological counseling as necessary

V. Child maltreatment

A. Description: the physical or psychological assault or the neglect of a child; there are four types of child of child maltreatment (Box 20-2, p. 592)

B. Etiology and incidence
1. More than 2 million children receive protective services each year
2. Three factors predispose a child to physical injury by parents or other caregivers
   a. Parental characteristics—parents have been victims themselves; isolated
   b. Child characteristics—temperament, physical or cognitive disability, illegitimacy, or hyperactivity
   c. Environmental characteristics—divorce, marital problems, financial strain, alcoholism, drug addiction, and poor housing
   d. See also Munchhausen by proxy syndrome in the glossary

C. Assessment (see Box 20-2, p. 592)

Text continued on p. 594

Box 20-2
Clinical Manifestations of Potential Child Maltreatment

PHYSICAL NEGLECT
Suggestive Physical Findings

Failure to thrive

Signs of malnutrition, such as thin extremities, abdominal distention, lack of subcutaneous fat

Poor personal hygiene, especially of teeth

Unclean and/or inappropriate dress

Evidence of poor health care, such as nonimmunized status, untreated infections, frequent colds

Frequent injuries from lack of supervision

Suggestive Behaviors

Dull and inactive; excessively passive or sleepy

Self-stimulatory behaviors, such as finger-sucking or rocking

Begging or stealing food ⎫
Absenteeism from school ⎪
Drug or alcohol addiction ⎬ in older child
Vandalism or shoplifting ⎭

EMOTIONAL ABUSE AND NEGLECT
Suggestive Physical Findings

Failure to thrive

Feeding disorders, such as rumination

Enuresis

Sleep disorders

Suggestive Behaviors

Self-stimulatory behaviors such as biting, rocking, sucking

During infancy, lack of social smile and stranger anxiety

Withdrawal

Unusual fearfulness

Antisocial behavior, such as destructiveness, stealing, cruelty

Extremes of behavior, such as overcompliant and passive or aggressive and demanding

Lags in emotional and intellectual development, especially language

Suicide attempts

PHYSICAL ABUSE
Suggestive Physical Findings

Bruises and welts

  On face, lips, mouth, back, buttocks, thighs, or areas of torso

  Regular patterns descriptive of object used, such as belt buckle, hand, wire hanger, chain, wooden spoon, squeeze or pinch marks

  May be present in various stages of healing

From Wong DL, et al: *Whaley and Wong's nursing care of infants and children*, ed 6, St. Louis, 1999, Mosby.)

Box 20-2
Clinical Manifestations of Potential Child Maltreatment—cont'd

PHYSICAL ABUSE—cont'd
Suggestive Physical Findings—cont'd

Burns
  On soles of feet, palms of hands, back, or buttocks
  Patterns descriptive of object used, such as round cigar or cigarette burns, "glovelike" sharply demarcated areas from immersion in scalding water, rope burns on wrists or ankles from being bound, burns in the shape of an iron, radiator, or electric stove burner
  Absence of "splash" marks and presence of symmetric burns
  Stun gun injury—lesions circular, fairly uniform (up to 0.5 cm), and paired approximately 5 cm apart
Fractures and dislocations
  Skull, nose, or facial structures
  Injury may denote type of abuse, such as spiral fracture or dislocation from twisting of an extremity or whiplash from shaking the child
  Multiple new or old fractures in various stages of healing
Lacerations and abrasions
  On backs of arms, legs, torso, face, or external genitalia
  Unusual symptoms, such as abdominal swelling, pain, and vomiting from punching
  Descriptive marks such as from human bites or pulling out of hair
Chemical
  Unexplained repeated poisoning, especially drug overdose
  Unexplained sudden illness, such as hypoglycemia from insulin administration

Suggestive Behaviors

Wariness of physical contact with adults
Apparent fear of parents or of going home
Lying very still while surveying environment
Inappropriate reaction to injury, such as failure to cry from pain
Lack of reaction to frightening events
Apprehensiveness when hearing other children cry
Indiscriminate friendliness and displays of affection
Superficial relationships
Acting-out behavior, such as aggression, to seek attention
Withdrawal behavior

SEXUAL ABUSE
Suggestive Physical Findings

Bruises, bleeding, lacerations or irritation of external genitalia, anus, mouth, or throat
Torn, stained, or bloody underclothing
Pain on urination or pain, swelling, and itching of genital area
Penile discharge
Sexually transmitted disease, nonspecific vaginitis, or venereal warts
Difficulty in walking or sitting
Unusual odor in the genital area

Continued

Box 20-2
Clinical Manifestations of Potential Child Maltreatment—cont'd

SEXUAL ABUSE—cont'd
Suggestive Physical Findings—cont'd
Recurrent urinary tract infections
Presence of sperm
Pregnancy in young adolescent

Suggestive Behaviors

Sudden emergence of sexually related problems, including excessive or public masturbation, age-inappropriate sexual play, promiscuity, or overtly seductive behavior
Withdrawn behavior, excessive daydreaming
Preoccupation with fantasies, especially in play
Poor relationships with peers
Sudden changes, such as anxiety, loss or gain of weight, clinging behavior
In incestuous relationships, excessive anger at mother for not protecting daughter
Regressive behavior, such as bed-wetting or thumb-sucking
Sudden onset of phobias or fears, particularly fears of the dark, men, strangers, or particular settings or situations (e.g., undue fear of leaving the house or staying at the daycare center or the baby-sitter's house)
Running away from home
Substance abuse, particularly of alcohol or mood-elevating drugs
Profound and rapid personality changes, especially extreme depression, hostility, and aggression (often accompanied by social withdrawal)
Rapidly declining school performance
Suicidal attempts or ideation

From Wong DL, et al: *Whaley and Wong's nursing care of infants and children,* ed 6, St. Louis, 1999, Mosby.)

⚠ Warning!

Inconsistencies between the history and the injury are important criteria on which to base a decision to report child maltreatment.

D. **Nursing management**
  1. Nursing diagnosis: risk for injury
  2. Expected outcome: child is free of additional maltreatment
  3. Interventions
     a. Assess child for injury, fractures, and burns
     b. Assess interpersonal relationship behaviors between the child and family
     c. Assess the child's reaction to health care personnel
     d. Assess the history or the present evidence of injury
     e. Complete a thorough history in a nonthreatening manner
     f. Provide a safe environment for the child
     g. Provide treatment for the current injury

     h. Document thoroughly: the child's physical condition, the child's interaction or behaviors with parents, the results from the interview with family members

     i. Report findings to the proper authorities; make referrals for alternate placement

     j. Establish a therapeutic relationship with the family and child

   4. Additional nursing diagnoses

     a. Fear; anxiety

     b. Altered parenting

   5. Expected outcomes

     a. Child exhibits positive interactions with family members

     b. Family members demonstrate appropriate parenting behaviors

   6. Interventions

     a. Assess current support systems; convey an attitude of concern

     b. Provide a consistent care-giver to enhance trust and consistency for the collection of information

     c. Provide care for the child until the parent is ready to participate

     d. Provide the parents with opportunities to verbalize their emotions

     e. Participate in a multidisciplinary approach to refer the family to home care or an appropriate government agency

     f. Introduce the parents to effective child rearing techniques and expected child growth and development behaviors and milestones

   7. Additional nursing diagnoses

     a. Knowledge deficit

     b. Self-concept disturbance

E. Evaluation

   1. Child is free of additional injury in the home or alternative placement environment

   2. Parents demonstrate appropriate parenting activities

   3. Parents participate in counseling, support services, and legal system requirements

VI. Home care: family education topics and referrals

A. AD-HD

   1. Safety: advise parents to assess the environment for safety hazards

   2. Medications: teach parents the correct administration of stimulants or other medications; explain the side effects

   3. Psychosocial: assist family to use effective coping strategies; review parenting techniques, include discipline and rewards for appropriate behavior; emphasize importance of a stable environment

   4. Referrals: special education services; individual psychotherapy in addition to family therapy; support groups for child and parents

B. Mental retardation

   1. Development: involve the family in early intervention programs: infant stimulation; assist family to set realistic goals for the child;

encourage family to have the child learn self-care skills; assist family to use special day-care programs and educational classes that include vocational training

2. Psychosocial: emphasize the need for setting limits, discipline, social interaction, and preparation for sexual maturation

3. Referrals: provide information about support services, community agencies, and opportunities for child socialization

C. **Sensory impairment**

1. Development: provide toys that stimulate the senses of hearing and touch or that promote social interaction and an increase in the potential for hearing; encourage the learning of sign language by the child and parents

2. Assistive devices: teach proper use and care of a hearing device; provide information on amplification devices for phone, teletypewriters, signaling devices for the doorbell and phone, and closed-captioned television

3. Safety: teach the importance of environmental safety to promote maximum mobility

4. Referrals: provide information about the following: special programs to learn independent behavior, braille reading and writing, and rehabilitation programs that teach independence

D. **Burns**

1. Wound care: assist family to obtain needed equipment and supplies; teach the proper method of cleaning the wound, changing the dressing, and using sterile technique

2. Nutrition: encourage high-calorie, high-protein meals and snacks

3. Activity: perform range-of-motion exercises and activities to prevent contractures

4. Socialization: collaborate with the school nurse to ease the child's return to school

5. Referrals: occupational and physical therapists, support groups for parents and children

E. **Child maltreatment**

1. Psychosocial: effective child rearing techniques, child growth and development, normal attachment and bonding

2. Referrals: special support groups and counseling; appropriate community organizations such as Alcoholics Anonymous; and legal organizations

WEB Resources

www.americanschdeaf.org/asd/

The American School for the Deaf provides a comprehensive program for the development of the intellect and enhancement of the quality of life for the deaf. This website furnishes information about education and vocational programs for deaf children and their families. Other resources include information on sign language and video games.

www.nih.gov/nidcd
    National Institute on Deafness and other communication disorders provides information for research funding and updates and for news and events, including a report on informed consent for deaf persons.

www.asha.org/
    This website is sponsored by the American Speech, Language and Hearing Association for audiologists, speech and language pathologists and other professionals; students; and consumers. It provides information on legislation, research issues and activities, and professional activities. Parents may access information to find a speech pathologist, a self-help group, summer programs for children, and on topics such as infant hearing.

www.afb.org
    Website of the American Foundation for Blindness provides a guide to toys for blind children.

www.kempcenter.org/
    Kemp Prevention Research Center for Family and Child Health directed by the University of Colorado provides child abuse information, including frequently asked questions by parents.

www.child.cornell.edu/
    This site is sponsored by the Child Abuse Prevention Network for professionals in the field of child abuse and neglect. It provides resources to support the identification, investigation, treatment, and follow-up for child abuse, maltreatment, and neglect.

www.cdc.gov/ncip/duip
    This site is sponsored by the Division of Unintentional Injury of the National Center for Injury Prevention and Control. It provides resources for prevention, statistics, and references on unintentional injuries such as burns.

www.vch.org/
    The University of Iowa sponsors this site, which provides client education materials for children with burn injuries.

www.aamr.org
    Website for the American Association on Mental Retardation that provides a bookstore, conference news, and abstracts.

REVIEW QUESTIONS

1. The nurse overheard these statements by the mother during emergency room treatment of an 18-month-old child suspected of being abused. Which comment by the mother should be reported?
    1. "I blame myself for this injury."
    2. "I want to know what is going to be done for my child."
    3. "I wish my child were potty trained."
    4. "My sister helps care for my child."

2. A 7-year-old is diagnosed with attention deficit-hyperactivity disorder (AD–HD). To promote optimal functioning, which of these approaches should be used?
    1. Encourage the use of a delayed reward system
    2. Encourage a diet that emphasizes processed foods
    3. Obtain placement for the child in a small, structured classroom
    4. Obtain a prescription for antidepressant medications

3. The parents of a severely burned child have received information about the importance of nutritional support. Which of these diet selections made by the parents indicates an understanding of what they have been taught?
    1. Beef and cheese taco, yogurt, and skim milk
    2. Cheeseburger, celery and carrot sticks, cola
    3. Chicken nuggets, milkshake, and pudding
    4. Tossed salad, cheese sticks, a banana, and tea

4. When a child is admitted to the hospital because of suspected maltreatment, the nurse is aware that legal proceedings may be necessary. Because of this possibility, which of these actions should receive priority?
    1. Assessment of the child's developmental level
    2. Determination of the extent of the child's injuries
    3. Documentation of the physical findings and interactions during admission
    4. Notification of the parents about diagnostic tests

5. A preschool child who has been burned exhibits a decreased interest in eating. Which of these actions should the nurse take to increase the child's intake?
    1. Ask the mother to feed the child
    2. Eliminate snacks
    3. Offer smaller and more frequent feedings
    4. Withhold dessert until the meal is eaten

ANSWERS, RATIONALES, AND TEST-TAKING TIPS

Rationale	Test-Taking Tips

1. Correct answer: 3

A characteristic of some abusive families is inadequate knowledge of normal developmental expectations. A child does not demonstrate physiologic and psychological readiness for toilet training until 18 to 24 months of age. Guilt and anger are expected reactions of parents who blame themselves for their child's illness. Option 2 illustrates a parental method of dealing with the frustrations related to a lack of information about the procedures and treatments for their child. Abusive parents may have fewer support systems and supportive relationships than do parents who are not abusive.

Reread each of the options and note that options 1, 2, and 4 are based in reality. Option 3 is different. The statement is a "wish" or "want." Ask if this is a realistic wish. It is not, and therefore it indicates a need for knowledge about normal child development.

2. Correct answer: 3

Children with attention deficit–hyperactivity disorder (AD-HD) benefit from a stable and predictable environment with regular routines and minimal stimuli. The provision of rewards for desired behaviors should be an immediate action. Although controversial, some children with AD-HD demonstrate improved behavior when certain processed food additives and artificial colorings are eliminated from their daily diets. The most frequently prescribed medications are sympathomimetic amines, for example, methylphenidate (Ritalin). Antidepressants are used sparingly because of the cardiac side effects such as tachycardia.

Approach your choice with an educated guess. Eliminate option 1 because of the key term "use delayed reward." Eliminate option 2 because "processed foods" are commonly inappropriate foods to use in most given diseases or problems. Eliminate option 4 because antidepressant medication is not recommended for AD-HD. Select option 3.

3. Correct answer: 3

The diet for a severely burned child must provide sufficient protein and calories to prevent negative nitrogen balance and weight loss. Extra calories should be derived from carbohydrates because fat sources, although higher in total calories, will not spare protein.

The key term in the stem is "severely burned." Think of a need for high calories. Eliminate options 2 and 4 because fresh vegetables have minimal calories. Select option 3 over 1 because skim milk, in option 1, has fewer calories.

4. Correct answer: 3

Besides observable physical evidence of abuse, the type of history revealed by family members or caregivers and their interactions with the child are significant factors in legal proceedings. Therefore, documentation of these observations is essential. The other actions, verbal and mental, are appropriate for the plan of care. However, the priority is written actions. Documentation can best be used in court proceedings.

Note the key term "legal proceedings" and associate it with the need for written communication. Cluster the other options under the category of unwritten communication. Select option 3.

5. Correct answer: 3

Serving small, frequent meals at least six times daily facilitates the habit of eating by self. The preschool child will typically eat small amounts frequently and prefers finger foods. Many children, especially of preschool age, eat better when they feed themselves. Nourishing snacks should be encouraged to boost caloric intake. Children with burns usually need 5000 to 7000 kcal/day. Meals, including desserts, should provide sufficient protein to prevent negative nitrogen balance.

Small, frequent meals usually are a good choice for diet questions. Options with the word "eliminate" usually are not a correct answer. The word eliminate falls under the category of an absolute word such as never.

Appendix A
Growth and Development

Age & General Stages	Play Type and Age-Appropriate Developmental Activities/Toys	Significant Other	Erikson Stage
0 to 1 year INFANCY	SOLITARY PLAY—mobiles, rattles, musical boxes, squeeze or soft toys, large wooden beads, spools, balls, pots and pans	mother	trust vs. mistrust

1 to 3 years
TODDLER
  favorite word
  "NO"
	PARALLEL PLAY—push-pull toys, pounding pegs, cars, trucks, blocks, telephone, dolls, clay, stuffed toys, large crayons, coloring books, play dress-up in Mom and Dad's clothes	mother and father
		negative stage
			autonomy vs. shame and doubt

Age & General Stages	Play Type and Age-Appropriate Developmental Activities/Toys	Significant Other	Erikson Stage
3 to 6 years PRESCHOOL favorite word "WHY"	COOPERATIVE PLAY WITH OTHER CHILDREN— housekeeping toys, ground equipment, wagons, tricycles, big wheel cycles, water colors, finger paints, clay, material for cutting and pasting, coloring books, simple jigsaw puzzles, dolls, TV, play dress-up in costumes: Snow White, cowboys	basic family play age	initiative vs. guilt
6 to 12 years SCHOOL AGE Rules are important	TEAM PLAY—dolls, trains, model kits, games, jigsaw puzzles, magic tricks, books (jokes, comic, adventure, mystery), TV, video games, audio equipment (tapes or discs w/headphones), bicycles, go-carts, initial individual interest such as hobbies, Scouts, and collections	peers	industry vs. inferiority
12 to 18 years ADOLESCENCE	TEAM/INDIVIDUAL—pagers, telephone conversations, movies, sports, games, reading, hobbies, crossword puzzles	peers	identity vs. identity diffusion
ADULTS 18 years to 30's young adult	INDEPENDENCE EDUCATION CAREER CHOICES	chosen significant other	intimacy vs. isolation
30's to mid 40's adult	CAREER CHOICES FAMILY	significant other/basic family	generativity vs. stagnation
mid 40's to 60 years older adult	CAREER CHANGE SELF—how many years are left FAMILY	significant other/basic family	generativity vs. stagnation
over 60's senescence	SELF/FAMILY FRIENDS LEFT	basic family self	integrity vs. despair

MILESTONES IN THE FIRST YEAR

1 Month
Holds head up briefly when prone. Head is one-inch larger than chest circumference at birth. Head circumference increases by ½ inch per month for the first 6 months. Eyes follow light or bright moving objects. Sleeps about 18 hours/day.

2 Months
When prone, can lift head to 45 degrees off the table. Posterior fontanel closed. Demonstrates "social smile." Vocalizes, which is distinct from crying. Turns head to side when sound is made at the level of the ear.

3 Months
Is able to raise head and shoulders with forearm. Sleeps about 15 hours/day. Babbles, chuckles, and coos. Sits with support. Reflexes begin to go away—grasp, startle. Night sleep pattern begins. Briefly holds toy.

4 Months
Raises head and shoulders to 90-degree angle. The Moro, tonic neck, rooting, and extrusion reflexes have disappeared. Begins to drool; feeds well from a spoon. Laughs out loud. Reaches for objects and toys; grasps objects with both hands. Eye–hand coordination begins. Digestive enzymes start being produced in the mouth; is able to swallow pureed food from spoon. Start first with formula mixed with cereal, then progress to pureed: fruits (to be given first), then vegetables, and then meats. Give foods one at a time to be able to detect food allergies. Note that a controversy exists of when and what to feed; recommended that parents consult their health care provider.

5 Months
Holds head erect when sitting; sits for short periods with support; rolls over. Grasps objects voluntarily. Teething begins with the lower central incisors coming in first—drooling, fretful, crying, slight temperature elevation and mild diarrhea may occur—bites; chews. Makes vowel and consonant sounds. Differentiates family from strangers.

6 Months
Sits alone for short periods; sits in high chair; plays peek-a-boo and pat-a-cake; raises arms to be picked up. Birth weight doubles. Holds bottle; feeds self finger foods. Recognizes name; utters one syllable; turns head and eyes towards sound. Recognizes and fears strangers.

7 to 9 Months
Sits alone; crawling begins about 7 months; holds spoon—hand preference is evident. Transfers objects from one hand to the other. Cup feeding can begin between 8 and 9 months in preparation for weaning. Amuses self with self-centered play; eye to eye contact with others occurs. May exhibit fear of being left alone by 9 months.

9 to 11 Months

Creeping or walking on hands and feet begins. Uses thumb and index finger to grasp objects, which is the pincer grasp. Pulls self to standing position by 9 months.

12 Months

Starts to walk or tries to. The head and chest circumferences are equal. Birth weight triples. Understands simple verbal commands; speaks several words. May develop attachment to favorite toy or security blanket; engages in repetitive play. Uses spoon; holds own bottle or cup; can be weaned from breast or bottle.

MILESTONES AFTER THE FIRST YEAR

18 Months

Walks alone; climbs stairs with help; begins to use spoon properly; holds, lifts and drinks from a cup. Babinski reflex goes away; chest grows larger than head. Distinguishes self from others; plays alone but likes to be near others; enjoys books with pictures. Bladder sphincter control begins to develop; indicates when wet; start potty training for voiding during the day. Has a vocabulary of about 20 words. Anxious around strangers.

24 Months (2 years)

Goes up and down stairs one at a time; climbs on furniture; runs; rides tricycle; likes push-pull toys and stuffed animals. Develops fine motor coordination; uses a spoon well; builds a tower of 6 blocks; scribbles with crayons or pencils. Understands up to 500 words; has a vocabulary of about 250 words; uses 2 and 3 word sentences. Bowel sphincter control begins to develop; starts daytime bowel training. Fears parents leaving; begins peer friendships.

36 Months (3 years)

Goes up and down stairs with alternating feet; is able to copy a cross and circle and feed and dress self. Has complete set of deciduous teeth. Uses 3 and 4 word sentences; has a vocabulary of about 900 words; identifies some colors. States the need to go to the toilet and goes alone. Knows own sex. Starts to interact and share with others; begins make-believe play and cooperative or group play. Able to separate from parents for short periods. Asks many questions; recalls visual images.

48 Months (4 years)

Skips and hops on one foot; has good motor coordination; throws ball overhead; catches ball reliably; bathes self with direction; laces shoes & buttons clothes; brushes teeth. Is completely potty trained. Has a vocabulary of about 1500 words; asks many questions; counts but has no concept of numbers. Begins to understand time; draws with form and meaning but not with detail; reading readiness is present. Is more socially aware; seeks out peer relationships and enjoys cooperative play.

Glossary

Abortion   Termination of pregnancy before fetal viability.

Abruptio placenta   Premature separation of a normally implanted placenta (fundal implantation).

Acrocyanosis   Bluish tinge to hands and feet of newborns especially when exposed to the environment. The cyanosis diminishes during the first 24 hours after birth, but slight cyanosis may reappear for as long as 7 to 10 days after birth if the newborn is chilled or exposed to the cold. It should disappear quickly once the newborn is warm.

Afterload   Resistance against which the left or right ventricle must eject its volume of blood during contraction; resistance is produced by the volume of blood already in the vascular system, the degree of blood viscosity, and the vessel walls: for the right ventricle the pulmonary vascular system (called pulmonary vascular resistance, PVR; however, sometimes this abbreviation is used to mean "peripheral vascular resistance") and for the left ventricle the systemic vascular system (called systemic vascular resistance, SVR).

Albumin   Water-soluble, heat-coagulable protein; can be given IV as a plasma-volume expander.

Allis sign   Shortening of leg on affected side in infant with congenital dysplasia of the hip.

Ambiguous genitalia   External genitalia that are not normal and morphologically typical of either sex, as occurs in pseudohermaphroditism.

Amblyopia   Reduced vision in an eye that appears to be structurally normal when examined by an ophthalmoscope; such condition may lead to strabismus.

Amniocentesis   Insertion of a needle transabdominally into the uterus to obtain a sample of amniotic fluid for the purpose of genetic screening and determination of fetal well-being and maturity.

Amniotic fluid   Clear, slightly yellow, alkaline fluid that surrounds the fetus; usually is 1 L.

Amniotic membranes   Amnion (inner) and chorion (outer) membranes that enclose the fetus in amniotic fluid and protect it from infectious microorganisms that may ascend up through the maternal vagina.

Amniotomy   Artificial rupture of the membranes.

Anaphylactic hypersensitivity Immmunoglobulin E- or G-dependent, immediate-acting humoral hypersensitivity response to an exogenous antigen.

Antepartal (prenatal, gestational) period Time of fetal development and maternal adaptation to pregnancy that begins with conception and ends with the onset of labor.

Apgar score Method used to determine the newborn's immediate adaptation to extrauterine life by assessing heart rate, respiratory effort, muscle tone, reflex irritability, and color.

Appropriate for gestational age (AGA) Designation given to a newborn whose birth weight meets the growth expectations for gestational age; weight falls between the 10th and 90th percentiles or within two standard deviations of the mean for gestational age.

Arterial oxygen (PaO$_2$) Force with which oxygen molecules, physically dissolved in blood, are constantly trying to escape; expressed as partial pressure, PaO$_2$; normal = 80-100.

Ascites Abnormal intraperitoneal accumulation of a fluid containing large amounts of protein and electrolytes; may be detectable when more than 500 ml of fluid has accumulated.

Attachment A process whereby an enduring bond is established between the infant and its parents and family.

Augmentation of labor Methods used to enhance existing uterine contractions to facilitate the progress of labor.

Aura Sensation of light or warmth experienced just before the onset of a seizure or migraine headache.

Automatism A mechanical, repetitive, and undirected behavior that is not consciously controlled, as seen in psychomotor epilepsy, hysterical states, and such acts as sleepwalking.

Azotorrhea Excessive protein in the stool.

Bearing down effort Effective use of abdominal muscle contractions with uterine contractions to facilitate descent and birth of the fetus during the second stage of labor.

Biophysical Profile Test using external fetal monitoring and ultrasound scan to assess fetal status by evaluating the fetal heart rate after movement (Non-Stress Test), fetal breathing movements, fetal body movements, fetal muscle tone, and amniotic fluid volume.

Brudzinski's sign Involuntary flexion of the arm, hip, and knee when the neck is passively flexed, as seen with irritated meninges such as in meningitis or cerebral bleeding.

Bruit Abnormal sound or murmur heard while auscultating a carotid artery, organ, or gland.

Bryant traction Skin traction device used for hip dislocation in children under 2 years of age and weighing less than 12 to 14 kg. Hips are flexed at a 90 degree angle, with knees extended.

Cardinal movements of labor Mechanism of labor whereby the powers of labor combined with resistance from the passage force the fetus to change the position of its head as it moves downward.

Cell-mediated immunity Delayed type IV hypersensitivity reaction, mediated primarily by sensitized T cell lymphocytes as opposed to antibodies; responsible for defense against certain bacterial, fungal and viral pathogens, malignant cells, and other foreign protein or tissue.

Cervical ripening Softening and thinning of the cervix in preparation for labor.

Cesarean birth Transabdominal delivery of the fetus through an incision, usually horizontal, into the lower abdomen and uterus.

Chorionic villus sampling Removal of a tissue sample from the fetal portion of the developing placenta, chorionic villi, for the purpose of genetic testing.

Chromosome Threadlike strands composed of the hereditary material known as deoxyribonucleic acid (DNA); many genes, which are small segments of DNA, comprise each chromosome.

Cold stress Hypothermic state that increases the newborn's risk for respiratory distress, hypoxia, metabolic acidosis, and hypoglycemia.

Compartment Group of muscles, surrounded by tough, inelastic tissue or burn.

Compartment syndrome Complication after a crush injury, fracture reduction, or burn in an extremity. Swelling reduces blood flow to the affected area and compresses the nerves. It is characterized by deep pain unrelieved by analgesia and complaints of numbness with a loss of ability for movement of the distal portion of the extremity.

Conception The process whereby a sperm fertilizes (unites with) an ovum to create a zygote, the first cell of a new human being.

Conductive Form of hearing loss in which sound is inadequately conducted through the external or middle ear to the sensorineural apparatus of the inner ear; sensitivity to sound is diminished but clarity (interpretation of sound) is not changed.

Congenital disorders Disorders present at birth related to interferences in the process of fetal growth and development; causes can be a combination of abnormal chromosomes or genes and environmental factors.

Contraction stress test (CST) Test performed to assess the response of the fetal heart rate to uterine contractions to determine fetal risk for hypoxia during labor as a result of uteroplacental insufficiency during contractions.

Corium Also called the dermis. A layer of skin, just below the epidermis, consisting of papillary and reticular layers and containing blood and lymphatic vessels, nerves, nerve endings, glands, and hair follicles.

Couvade Culturally determined paternal behaviors during pregnancy and birthing.

Curling ulcer Also called Curling's stress ulcer. A duodenal ulcer that develops in persons who have severe burns on the surface of the body.

Diaphysis Shaft of a long bone; consists of a tube of compact bone enclosing the medullary cavity.

Dilation Widening of the cervical os to 10 cm.

Dystocia Labor that is abnormal, dysfunctional, or difficult as a result of ineffective uterine contractions, fetal problems, or pelvic inadequacy.

Dysuria Painful urination, usually the result of a bacterial infection or obstructive condition in the urinary tract.

Ectopic pregnancy   Implantation of the fertilized ovum occurs at a site other than the body of the uterus, most often in the fallopian tube.

Effacement   Thinning and shortening of the cervical canal.

Embryo   Term used to refer to the fertilized ovum from day 15 until 8 weeks' gestation.

Encephalitis   Inflammatory process of the central nervous system, producing altered functioning of the brain and spinal cord; caused by a number of organisms including bacteria and viruses.

Endometritis   Uterine infection usually at the placental site that can spread to the fallopian tubes and peritoneum creating a major threat to fertility and life.

Enuresis   Incontinence of urine, especially while sleeping (nocturnal enuresis).

Epiphyseal plate   Thin layer of cartilage between the epiphysis (the head of the long bone), which is a secondary bone-forming center, and the shaft of the bone; the new bone forms along the plate.

Epidural hemorrhage   Arterial intracranial bleeding with findings evident within 24 to 48 hours.

Episiotomy   Perineal incision performed to enlarge the vaginal outlet.

Epithelium   Covering of the internal and external organs of the body, lining of vessels, body cavities, glands, and organs; the cells are bound together by connective tissue.

Erythema toxicum   Newborn rash characterized by round, erythematous areas with small, raised, yellowish centers; often a response to the environment.

Erythrocyte   Also called red blood cell (RBC). Major cellular element of the circulating blood containing hemoglobin confined within a lipoid membrane; principal function is to transport oxygen; normally lives 110 to 120 days after which it is removed from the blood stream and broken down by the reticuloendothelial system in the liver.

Erythropoietin   Glycoprotein hormone synthesized mainly in the kidneys and released into the blood stream in response to anoxia for stimulation, regulation, and production of erythrocytes.

External fetal monitoring   Noninvasive method of continuously or intermittently monitoring uterine contractions and fetal heart rate patterns using a tocotransducer and an ultrasound transducer.

Fetal position   Location of a set point on the fetal presenting part in a section or quadrant of the maternal pelvis. This changes as the fetus uses the cardinal movements of labor to pass through the pelvis.

Fetal presentation (presenting part)   The part of the fetus that enters the pelvic inlet first: head (cephalic), buttocks or feet (breech), or shoulder.

Fetus   Term used to refer to the embryo from 8 weeks' gestation until the pregnancy ends.

Fourth trimester   The 3-month period of adjustment the postpartum woman and her family undergo as a result of the process of pregnancy and birth, and the impact of newborn care responsibilities.

Gametes   Sperm and ova.

Gavage feeding   Feeding by way of a gastric tube inserted through the mouth (preferred site in newborns) or nose. This type of feeding is required when a newborn is unable to obtain sufficient nutrients and fluids orally.

Gene   Small segment of DNA found on chromosomes.

Gestational diabetes   Diabetic state that develops in some nondiabetic women during the second half of their pregnancies, usually the third trimester.

Gland   Any one of many organs in the body, comprised of specialized cells that secrete or excrete materials not related to their ordinary metabolism; some lubricate, others produce hormones, and others such as the spleen and lymph take part in the production of blood components.

Glasgow coma scale (GCS)   Quick, practical, and standard system for assessing the degree of conscious impairment in critically ill clients and predicting the duration and ultimate outcome of coma. Primarily used in head-injured clients. The GCS involves three determinants: eye opening, verbal responses, and motor responses.

Gravida   Refers to the total number of times the woman has been pregnant, regardless of the outcome.

Hemarthrosis   Also called hemoarthros. The extravasation of blood into a joint.

Hematoma   Accumulation of blood within the connective tissue of the pelvis or genitalia (labia, vagina, vulva, perineum) as a result of bleeding from a blood vessel damaged during the childbirth process.

Hernia   Protrusion of an organ through an abnormal opening in the muscle wall of the cavity that surrounds it.

High-risk pregnancy   Pregnancy in which the life and health of the maternal-fetal unit is in jeopardy.

Hormone   Complex chemical substance produced in one part of the body or a gland that initiates or regulates the activity of an organ or group of cells in another part of the body. Secretion of hormones by the endocrine glands is regulated by other hormones, neurotransmitters, and a negative feedback system.

Humidification   Process of increasing the relative humidity of the atmosphere around a client through the use of aerosol generators or steam inhalers that exert an antitussive, cough-inhibiting effect. It acts by decreasing the viscosity of bronchial secretions.

Humoral immunity   One of two forms of immunity that responds to antigens; results from the development and continuing presence of circulating antibodies, produced by the plasma or B-cell lymphocytes. Antibodies are carried in immunoglobulins IgA, IgG, and IgM.

Hydrotherapy   Use of water to treat various physical or mental disorders.

Hyperemesis gravidarum   Excessive, intractable vomiting during pregnancy, most often during the first 16 weeks. It results in weight loss and in fluid, electrolyte, metabolic, and nutritional imbalances.

Hyperglycemia   Greater than normal amount of glucose in the blood. In diabetes mellitus it is best diagnosed by the glucose tolerance test of which the normal test results are: (fasting) 70 to 115 mg/dl; (30 min and 1 hour) less than 200 mg/dl; (2 hour) less than 140 mg/dl; (3 and 4 hours) 70 to 115 mg/dl.

Hyperopia   Also called hypermetropia, hypermetropy. Farsightedness, a condition resulting from an error of refraction in which rays of light entering the eye are brought into focus behind the retina.

Hypoglycemia   Less than the normal level of glucose in the blood; best tested by a random serum glucose; glucose level less than 50 mg/dl.

Hypoxemia   Abnormal deficiency of oxygen in the arterial system; chronic hypoxemia stimulates erythrocyte production, leading to secondary polycythemia; if caused by decreased alveolar oxygen tension or underventilation, improvement occurs with oxygen administration; if caused by shunting of blood from the right to left heart without exchange of gases in the lungs, improvement is achieved by bronchial hygiene and positive end expiratory pressure therapy.

Hypoxia   Inadequate oxygen at the cellular level; tissues most sensitive to hypoxia are the brain, heart, lungs, and kidneys.

Hypoxic drive   Low arterial oxygen pressure stimulus to respiration that is mediated through the carotid and aortic bodies, also called chemoreceptors for partial arterial pressure of carbon dioxide.

Induction of labor   Stimulation of the onset and progress of labor.

Infant mortality rate   Number of deaths in the first year of life per 1000 live births.

Influenza   Highly contagious infection of the respiratory tract caused by a myxovirus and transmitted by airborne droplet infection; incubation period is 1 to 3 days followed by sudden onset of fever, chills, and malaise; complete recovery in 3 to 10 days after symptomatic treatment; fever and constitutional symptoms distinguish it from the common cold.

Insulin   Naturally occurring hormone secreted by the beta cells in the pancreas in response to increased levels of glucose in the blood.

Internal fetal monitoring   Invasive method of continuously monitoring uterine contractions and fetal heart rate patterns using an intrauterine pressure catheter and a spiral electrode.

Involution   Process whereby the reproductive organs, including the uterus, return to their approximate pre-pregnant state.

Kernig's sign   Inability to completely extend the leg when the thigh is flexed on the abdomen; indicates meningeal irritation from meningitis or cerebral bleeding.

Lanugo   Fine downy hair found on the shoulders, back, pinna of ears, and forehead of the newborn.

Large for gestational age (LGA)   Designation given to a newborn whose birth weight exceeds the growth expectations for gestational age; weight is above the 90th percentile or two standard deviations above the mean for gestational age; often referred to as macrosomia.

Letting-go/interdependence stage   Last stage of the maternal psychosocial recovery process characterized by the giving up of the role as a pregnant woman for the role of mother and re-establishment of other roles such as that of partner and spouse.

Leukocyte   White blood cell that functions as a phagocyte of bacteria, fungi, and viruses; five types of leukocytes are classified by the presence or absence of granules in the cytoplasm of the cell—agranulocytes: (1) lymphocytes, (2) monocytes and granulocytes, (3) neutrophils, (4) basophils, and (5) eosinophils.

Low birth weight   Weight at birth is less than 2500 g as a result of intrauterine growth retardation, preterm birth, or both.

Macewen's sign   The "cracked pot" sound that is produced as a result of increased intracranial pressure in hydrocephalus. The increased volumes causes bones to thin and sutures to become separated and palpable.

Malabsorption   Impaired absorption of nutrients from the gastrointestinal tract.

Mastitis   Infection of breast tissue; may be unilateral or bilateral.

Maternal mortality rate   Number of maternal deaths related to the complications of pregnancy, birth, and the puerperium per 100,000 live births.

McBurney's point   Site of extreme sensitivity, localized rebound tenderness, in acute appendicitis; situated about one third the distance between the right anterior superior iliac spine and the umbilicus.

Meconium   Thick, dark-green fecal substance found in fetal intestines; may be passed into the amniotic fluid when the fetus experiences hypoxia.

Meninges   Three membranes enclosing the brain and spinal cord, composed of the dura, arachnoid, and pia mater (listed external to internal); the arachnoid and pia mater become inflamed in bacterial meningitis.

Menstrual cycle   Recurring, hormone-regulated process of follicle maturation and endometrial development that results in ovulation and preparation of the uterus for implantation of a fertilized ovum.

Milia   Plugged sebaceous glands that look like pimples on newborns; found on the face, especially the chin and nose; require no intervention since they occur naturally and resolve spontaneously.

Moro reflex   Immediate extension and abduction of newborn's arms with fingers fanning out as the thumb and forefinger form a C as a result of a sudden, intense stimulus; adduction and flexion of the arms into an embrace-type position follows the initial response.

Multifactorial inheritance   Pattern of inheritance that reflects the interaction of several genetic and environmental factors that create mild to severe defects, depending on the number of factors present.

Munchausen syndrome by proxy (MSBP)   Fictitious illness involving the infliction of physical harm on a child, usually by the mother, in an effort to gain attention of the medical staff. Methods used to cause symptoms in the child include chronic poisoning and suffocation. Warning signs are when an illness does not respond to treatment, history of the complaint is inconsistent with the presenting clinical findings, or the parents desire to interact with the health care team and to stay with child. Priorities are to protect child and siblings, and to consult the child protection team when MSBP is suspected.

Myopia   Also called shortsightedness and nearsightedness. Condition caused by the elongation of the eyeball or by an error in refraction so that parallel rays are focused in front of the retina.

Negative feedback   To decrease the function in response to a stimulus; for example, the follicle-stimulating hormone decreases as the amount of circulating estrogen decreases.

Neonatal period   First 28 days of life.

Non-stress test   Screening test performed to assess the response of the fetal heart rate to periods of fetal movement.

Nonreassuring FHR pattern   Fetal heart rate changes that reflect the warning signs of mild hypoxia.

Oligohydramnios Diminished volume of amniotic fluid; hydramnios or polyhydramnios refers to excessive amniotic fluid.

Opisthotonos Prolonged severe spasm of the muscles causing the back to arch acutely, the head to bend back on the neck, the heels to bend back on the legs, and the arms and hands to flex rigidly at the joints; more common in children with meningitis or hydrocephalus. They are best positioned on their side when this occurs.

Ortolani's sign Also called Ortolani's click. A click or popping sensation felt by examiner when a selected technique is used to evaluate range of motion for the hips of infants.

Oxytocics Medications that stimulate the uterus to contract.

Para The number of pregnancies delivered after the age of fetal viability.

Partial pressure of CO_2 ($PaCO_2$) Portion of total arterial blood gas pressure exerted by carbon dioxide; normal, 35 to 45.

Passage Maternal bony pelvis and soft tissues of the lower uterine segment, cervix, vagina, introitus, and pelvic floor muscles.

Passenger The fetus.

Pavlik harness Device used for congenital dislocated hip for infants less than 6 months of age.

PEFR Peak expiratory floor rate.

Periods of reactivity Periods comprising the transition to extrauterine life; the transition lasts approximately the first 6 to 8 hours of life and is characterized by instability of the newborn's behavioral states and physiologic function.

Phototherapy Treatment for hyperbilirubinemia that uses a light source such as a fluorescent light bulb panel or fiber-optic panel or blanket to facilitate bilirubin breakdown for excretion.

Pica Craving to eat substances that are nonnutrients or nonfood substances, such as clay, starch, ice, paint chips, crayons, glue, chalk, dirt, and hair.

Placenta Organ specific to pregnancy that is formed as the chorionic villi are imbedded into the decidua.

Placenta previa Placenta is implanted in the lower uterine segment rather than in the fundus.

Platelet Smallest cell in the blood that contains no hemoglobin and is essential for the coagulation of blood and to maintain hemostasis.

Porcine xenograft Also called heterograft. A temporary biologic graft from the skin of a pig used to cover a burn during the first few days, reducing the amount of fluid loss from the open wound; this type of graft is rejected quickly.

Post-term gestation Birth occurs after the 42nd week of gestation.

Postmaturity/dysmaturity syndrome Newborn exhibits the detrimental effects of placental insufficiency from a prolonged pregnancy.

Postpartum (postnatal) period/puerperium The 6- to 8-week period of maternal recovery after giving birth.

Postpartum blues/baby blues Mild, transient let down feeling or depression that occurs approximately 3 days after birth and again 1 month later; typically lasts from 3 days to 1 week.

Postpartum check   Systematic approach used for the assessment of essential factors (breasts, fundus, lochia, perineum, and so on) indicative of maternal physical recovery after birth.

Postpartum depression with or without psychotic features   Severe mood disorder that is prolonged in nature and requires professional intervention.

Postpartum hemorrhage   Blood loss of over 500 ml after a vaginal birth, over 1000 ml after a cesarean birth, a 10% change in hematocrit from the time of admission for childbirth, or a need for erythrocyte transfusion.

Post-term gestation   Birth occurs after 42 weeks' gestation.

Powers of labor   Forces that facilitate fetal descent and birth, namely, uterine contractions (primary power) and abdominal muscle contractions (secondary power).

Preconception care   Health assessment and guidance within the year before becoming pregnant to ensure optimal physical and psychosocial condition for pregnancy.

Pregnancy-induced hypertension (PIH)   Syndrome associated with pregnancy that begins after the 20th week of pregnancy through the early postpartum period; it is characterized by hypertension alone (transient hypertension) or in combination with varying degrees of edema and proteinuria (preeclampsia, eclampsia).

Preload   Stretch of the myocardial fiber at end diastole, which is reflected by the ventricular end diastolic pressure and volume.

Premonitory signs of labor   Signs that signal the approach of the onset of labor.

Prenatal care   Early, comprehensive health care during pregnancy.

Prepared childbirth techniques   Use of relaxation exercises, breathing techniques, and effleurage during labor and childbirth to reduce pain, stress, and tension; enhance rest; and conserve energy.

Preterm gestation   Birth occurs before 38 weeks' gestation but after the age of fetal viability has been reached at approximately 20 to 24 weeks' gestation.

Preterm labor   Labor that begins after 20 to 24 weeks' gestation but before the end of 37 weeks' gestation.

Prolonged/post-term pregnancy   Pregnancy that lasts 42 weeks or more.

Proprioception   Sensation pertaining to stimuli originating within the body regarding position and muscular activity.

Reassuring FHR pattern   Fetal heart rate reflective of fetal well-being, adequate oxygenation, and expected responses to the stress of labor.

Rebound tenderness   Sign of inflammation of the peritoneum in which pain is elicited by the sudden release of a hand pressing on the abdomen; common finding in peritonitis and appendicitis.

Respiratory distress syndrome (RDS)   Ineffective function of the newborn's respiratory system as a result of immaturity of the lungs and respiratory center and limited production of surfactant.

Reye syndrome (RS)   Combination of encephalopathy and fatty infiltration of the internal organs that may follow acute viral infections and has an association with the administration of aspirin, especially in persons under 18 years of age.

Rinne test   Also called rinne tuning fork test. A method of distinguishing conductive from sensorineural hearing loss; sensorineural loss—sound heard longer by air conduction; conductive loss—sound heard longer by bone conduction.

Romberg test   Also called Romberg's sign. Sign of loss of position in which an individual loses balance when standing erect with feet together and eyes closed.

Rooting reflex   Newborn turns head and opens mouth when side of cheek, lips, or mouth are stimulated with a finger or nipple.

Sensorineural hearing loss   Sound normally is conducted through the external and middle ear but a defect in the inner ear or acoustic nerve results in hearing loss; sound discrimination may or may not be affected.

Small for gestational age (SGI)   Designation given to a newborn whose birth weight is less than the growth expectations for gestational age; weight is below the 10th percentile or two standard deviations below the mean for gestational age.

Snellen chart   Chart used in testing visual acuity by letters, numbers or symbols arranged on the chart in decreasing size from top to bottom; the test is done from a distance of 20 feet.

Status asthmaticus   Acute, severe, and prolonged asthma attack.

Steatorrhea   Fat in stools; bulky, foul odor to stools

Stevens-Johnson syndrome   Severe form of erythema multiforme characterized by severe lesions of the skin and mucous membranes, fever, and multiple systemic manifestations; presumed to be a hypersensitivity to a drug or may follow an upper respiratory tract infection. Treatment includes bed rest, antibiotics for pneumonia, steroids, analgesics, mouthwashes, and sedatives.

Strabismus   Abnormal ocular condition in which the eyes are crossed.

Stricture   Abnormal temporary or permanent narrowing of the lumen of a hollow organ such as the esophagus, pylorus of the stomach, ureter, or urethra caused by inflammation, external pressure, or scarring.

Stridor   Abnormal, high-pitched, musical sound caused by an obstruction of the trachea or larynx; usually heard during inspiration.

Subdural hemorrhage   Venous bleeding; common in infancy from falls or violent shaking; findings may not be evident for weeks or months.

Sunset eyes   Finding in a child with hydrocephalus in which the eyes deviate downward.

Surfactant   Substance that coats the lining of alveoli facilitating their expansion and contraction during respiration; prevents alveolar collapse or atelectasis.

Taking-hold   Stage of maternal psychosocial recovery beginning about 3 days after birth, which is characterized by vacillation between the need for nurturing and the need to take charge of self and the newborn.

Taking-in   Stage of maternal psychosocial recovery during the first 1 to 2 days after giving birth when maternal dependency needs predominate.

Talipes   Refers to deformities that involve the foot and ankle; usually congenital.

Tension of O$_2$ (PaO$_2$)   Gases dissolved in blood are constantly trying to escape; expressed as partial pressure; normal oxygen tension is 80 to 100; for clients with chronic obstructive pulmonary disease, 60 to 80.

Teratogen   Environmental substances or exposures known to be harmful to humans and that may adversely effect fetal and newborn growth and development.

Term gestation   Birth occurs after 37 weeks' but before end of 42 weeks' gestation.

"Tet" spells   Also known as "blue spells," acute episodes of anoxia that are preceded by crying or feeding, which increase oxygen requirements. Prompt treatment includes morphine and oxygen administration, IV fluid replacement, and possible blood transfusions.

Thermoneutral environment   An environment that assists the newborn to maintain a stable body temperature between 97.7° F and 99.5° F, with minimal expenditure of oxygen and nutrients; radiant warmers, incubators, close wrapping and bundling, with coverings on the head, hands and feet, can be used to create this environment.

Tocolytic   Medications that suppress labor.

Tocotransducer   Device placed on the abdomen over the uterine fundus to assess the duration and frequency of uterine contractions.

Trimester   One of three divisions of pregnancy, with the first trimester lasting from week 1 to 13, the second trimester from week 14 to 26, and the third trimester from week 27 until birth.

Ultrasound scan   Diagnostic test that uses sound waves to reflect off of tissue; allows visualization of the contents of the uterine cavity, including the fetus, placenta, and amniotic fluid.

Ultrasound transducer   Device placed on the abdomen over the point of maximum intensity to assess the fetal heart rate pattern.

Umbilical cord   Cord that connects the fetus to the placenta; composed of two arteries and one vein.

Unifactorial (single gene) inheritance   A particular trait, health problem, or defect controlled by one gene as a result of a variety of transmission patterns.

Upper respiratory infection (URI)   Infection located from the trachea upward in the respiratory tract; usually includes the common cold, laryngitis, pharyngitis, rhinitis, sinusitis, and tonsillitis.

Urgency   Feeling of a need to void urine immediately.

Uterine atony   Uterine hypotonia noted as a boggy or flaccid fundus.

Vernix caseosa   White, odorless, cheesy substance that covers the newborn's integument at birth.

Volkmann's (ischemic) contracture   A serious, persistent flexion contracture of the forearm and hand caused by ischemia.

Weber test   Method of assessment in auditory acuity, especially useful in determining whether defective hearing in an ear is a conductive loss caused by middle ear problems or a sensorineural loss; a vibrating tuning fork is placed in the center of the person's forehead, the midline vertex, or the maxillary incisor; if there is sensorineural loss in one ear, the unaffected ear perceives the sound as louder; if conductive hearing loss is present, the sound is louder in the affected ear because sound is received only by bone conduction.

Wheeze   Sound characterized by a high-pitched musical quality; caused by a high-velocity flow of air through narrowed bronchi; may be heard with a stethoscope, during breathing as a lower airway sound on both inspiration and expiration or may be audible without a stethoscope.

Bibliography

Aderhold K, Roberts J: Phases of the second stage of labor. *J Nurse Midwifery* 1991, 36(5):267.

American Academy of Pediatrics, Committee on Genetics: Folic acid for the prevention of neural tube defects. *Pediatrics* 1993, 92(3):493-494.

American Academy of Pediatrics: Report of the Committee on Infectious Diseases, ed 22, Elk Grove, 1991, American Academy of Pediatrics.

American College of Obstetricians and Gynecologists (ACOG): Postpartum hemorrhage. ACOG Technical Bulletin 243. Washington, DC, 1998, ACOG.

American Psychiatric Association: *Diagnostic and Statistical Manual of Mental Disorders* (DSM-IV), ed 4. Washington, DC, 1994, American Psychiatric Association.

Andrews H, Roy C: *The Roy Adaptation Model.* Norwalk, CT, 1991, Appleton & Lang.

Apgar V: The newborn (Apgar) scoring system: reflections and advice. *Pediatr Clin North Am* 1966, 13(8):695.

Bajo K, Hager J, Smith J: Keeping moms and babies together. *AWHONN Lifelines* 1998 2(2):44-48.

Ballard J, Khoury J, Wedig K, et al: New Ballard Score, expanded to include extremely premature infants. *J Pediatr* 1991, 119:417-423.

Barkauskas V, Baumann L, Stoltenberg-Allen K, Darling-Fisher C: *Health and Physical Assessment,* ed 2. St. Louis, 1998, Mosby.

Beck C: Postpartum depression: stopping the thief that steals motherhood. *AWHONN Lifelines* 1999, 3(4):41-44.

Biancuzzo M: Six myths of maternal posture during labor. *Am J Maternal Child Nurs* 1993, 8(5), 264-269.

Biancuzzo M: *Breastfeeding the Newborn.* St. Louis, 1999, Mosby.

Bishop EH: Pelvic scoring for elective induction. *Obstet Gynecol* 1964, 24(2):266-268.

Brown ML: Dilemmas facing nurses who care for Munchausen syndrome by proxy. *Pediatr Nurs* 1997, 23:416-418.

Chess S, Thomas A: Temperamental differences: a critical concept in child health care. *Pediatr Nurs* 1985, 11:167-171.

Cook A, Wilcox G: Pressuring pain: alternative therapies for labor pain management. *AWHONN Lifelines* 1997, 1(2):36-41.

Corrarino J: Perinatal hepatitis B: update and recommendations. *Am J Maternal Child Nurs* 1998, 23(5):246-252.

Cosner K, de Jong E: Physiologic second-stage labor. *Am J Maternal Child Nurs* 1993, 18(1):38-43.

Cowan M: Home care of the pregnant woman using terbutaline. *Am J Maternal Child Nurs* 1993, 18(2):99-105.

Crawford N, Pruss A: Preventing neonatal hepatitis B infection during the perinatal period. *J Obstet Gynecol Neonatal Nurs* 1993, 22(6):491-497.

Enkin M, Keirse M, Renfrew M, Neilson J: Effective care in pregnancy and childbirth: a synopsis. *Birth* 1995, 22(2):101-110.

Erikson E: *Childhood and Society.* New York, 1963, WW Norton.

Erikson E: *Identity: Youth and Crisis.* New York, 1968, WW Norton.

Fishbein E, Burggraf E: Early postpartum discharge: how are mothers managing? *J Obstet Gynecol Neonatal Nurs* 1998, 27(2):142-148.

Fleming B, Munton M, Clarke B, Strauss S: Assessing and promoting positive parenting in adolescent mothers. *Am J Maternal Child Nurs* 1993, 18(1):32-37.

Fortier J, Carson V, Well S, Shubkagel B: Adjustment to newborn: sibling preparation makes a difference. *J Obstet Gynecol Neonatal Nurs* 1991, 20(1):73-79.

Freda M, Mikhail E, Polizzotto R, et al: Fetal movement counting: which method? *Am J Maternal Child Nurs* 1993, 18(6):314-321.

Gebauer C, Lowe N: The biophysical profile: antepartal assessment of fetal well-being. *J Obstet Gynecol Neonatal Nurs* 1993, 22(2):115-124.

Gilbert E, Harmon J: *Manual of High Risk Pregnancy and Delivery,* ed 2. St. Louis, 1998, Mosby.

Gordon S: Lyme disease in children. *Pediatr Nurs* 1994, 20(4):415-418.

Gupton A, Heaman M, Ashcroft T: Bed rest from the perspective of the high-risk pregnant woman. *J Obstet Gynecol Neonatal Nurs* 1997, 26(4):423-430.

Hanson L: Second stage positioning in nurse-midwifery practices. Part 1: position use and preferences. *J Nurse Midwifery* 1998, 43(5):320-325.

Hanson L: Second stage positioning in nurse-midwifery practices. Part 2: factors affecting use. *J Nurse Midwifery* 1998, 43(5):326-330.

Hazinski M: Cardiovascular disorders. In *Nursing Care of the Critically Ill Child,* ed 2. Edited by Hazinski M: St. Louis, 1992, Mosby.

Jones Criteria Update: *JAMA* 1992, 268(15):2070.

Kenner C, Amlung S, Flandermeyer A: *Protocols in Neonatal Nursing.* Philadelphia, 1998, WB Saunders.

Koniak-Griffin D: Maternal role attainment. *Image J Nurs Sch* 1993, 25(3), 257-261.

Lawrence R: *Breastfeeding,* ed 5. St. Louis, 1999, Mosby.

Lerner H: Sleep position of infants: applying research to practice. *Am J Maternal Child Nurs,* 1993, 18(5):275-277.

Lowdermilk D, Perry S, Bobak I: *Maternity and Women's Health Care,* ed 7. St. Louis, 2000, Mosby.

MacDorman M, Atkinson J: Infant mortality statistics from the 1997 period: linked birth/infant death data set. *National Vital Statistics Reports* 1999, 47(23):1-24.

Maloni J, Ponder M: Father's experience of their partner's antepartum bed rest. *Image J Nurs Sch* 1997, 29(2):183-188.

Mandeville L, Troiano N: *High-Risk Intrapartum Nursing,* ed 2. Philadelphia, 1999, JB Lippincott.

Mattson S, Smith J: *Core Curriculum for Maternal-Newborn Nursing,* ed 2. Philadelphia, 2000, WB Saunders.

McGregor L: Short, shorter, shortest: improving the hospital stay for mothers and newborns. *Am J Maternal Child Nurs* 1994, 19(2):91-96.

McKay S, Barrows T: Reliving birth: maternal responses to viewing videotape of their second stage labors. *Image J Nurs Sch* 1992, 24(1):27-31.

McKerny LM, Salerno E: *Pharmacology in Nursing,* ed 20. St. Louis, 1998, Mosby.

Mitchell A, Steffenson N, Hogan H, Brooks S: Group B *Streptococcus* and pregnancy: update and recommendations. *Am J Maternal Child Nurs* 1997, 22(5):242-248.

Moore M: Biochemical markers for preterm labor and birth. *Am J Maternal Child Nurs* 1999, 24(2):80-86.

Moore M, Freda, M: Reducing preterm and low birth weight births: still a nursing challenge. *Am J Maternal Child Nurs* 1998, 23(4):200-208.

Mosby's Medical, Nursing and Allied Health Dictionary, ed 5. St. Louis, 1999, Mosby.

Owen CL: New directions in asthma management. *AJN* 1999, 99(3):26-33.

Patrick T, Roberts J: Current concepts in preeclampsia. *Am J Maternal Child Nurs* 1999, 24(4):193-200.

Peterson L, Besuner P: Pushing techniques during labor: issues and controversies. *J Obstet Gynecol Neonatal Nurs* 1997, 26(6):719-726.

Piaget J: *The Theory of Stages of Cognitive Development.* New York, 1969, McGraw-Hill.

Proctor S: What determines quality in maternity care? Comparing the perceptions of childbearing women and midwives. *Birth* 1998, 25(2):85-93.

Radabaugh S, Everhart A: Cesarean births: reducing the incidence while improving outcomes. *AWHONN Lifelines* 1999, 3(1):28-34.

Rollant P: Acing multiple choice tests, *AJN Career Guide,* Vol. 36, January 18-21, 1994.

Rollant P: *Soar to Success Do Your Best on Nursing Tests.* St. Louis, 1999, Mosby.

Rubin R: *Maternal Identity and the Maternal Experience.* New York, 1984, Springer.

Seidel HM, Ball JW, Dains JE: *Mosby's Guide to Physical Examination.* St. Louis, 1995, Mosby.

Shermer R, Raines D: Positioning during the second stage of labor: moving back to basics. *J Obstet Gynecol Neonatal Nurs* 1997, 26(6):727-734.

Simkin P: Reducing pain and enhancing progress in labor: a guide to nonpharmacologic methods for maternity caregivers. *Birth* 1995, 22(3):161-171.

Simpson K, Poole J: *Cervical Ripening and Induction and Augmentation of Labor.* Washington, DC, 1998, Association of Women's Health, Obstetric, and Neonatal Nurses (AWHONN).

Sleutel M, Golden S: Fasting in labor: relic or requirement. *J Obstet Gynecol Neonatal Nurs* 1999, 28(5):507-512.

Smith K, Cook F: Current treatment options for ectopic pregnancy. *Am J Maternal Child Nurs* 1997, 22(1):21-25.

Soeffner M, Hart M: Back to class: helping high-risk moms cope with hospitalization. *AWHONN Lifelines* 1998, 2(3):47-51.

Speer KM: *Pediatric Care Planning.* Springhouse, 1999, Springhouse.

Tanner J: Issues and advances in adolescent growth and development. *J Adolescent Health Care* 1987, 8:470-478.

Thureen P, Deacon J, O'Neill P, Hernandez J: *Assessment and Care of the Well Newborn.* Philadelphia, 1999, WB Saunders.

Tinkle M, Sterling B: Neural tube defects: a primary prevention role for nurses. *J Obstet Gynecol Neonatal Nurs* 1997, 26(5):503-512.

Tucker S: *Pocket Guide to Fetal Monitoring,* ed 3. St. Louis, 1996, Mosby.

Van de Vusse L: The essential forces of labor revisited: 13 Ps reported in women's stories. *Am J Maternal Child Nurs* 1999, 24(4):176-184.

Ventura S, Martin J, Curtin S, Mathews T: Births: final data for 1997. *National Vital Statistics Reports* 1999, 47(18):1-96.

Wong DL: *Essentials of Pediatric Nursing,* ed 5. St. Louis, 1997, Mosby.

Wong DL: *Whaley and Wong's Nursing Care of Infants and Children,* ed 6. St. Louis, 1999, Mosby.

Wong DL: *Wong and Whaley's Clinical Manual of Pediatric Nursing,* ed 4. St. Louis, 1996, Mosby.

Index

A

Abdominal muscle contractions and labor, 123

ABO blood type incompatibility, 324

Abortion
  causes of, 90
  manifestations and management of, 92t-93t

Abruptio placenta and bleeding, 94, 139

Acquired heart disease; *see* Rheumatic fever

Acquired immune deficiency syndrome
  assessment of, 418-419
  common conditions related to, *418*
  description of, 417-418
  etiology of, 418
  evaluation of, 420
  home care of children with, 421-422
  management of, 419-420
  pathophysiology of, 418

Acrocyanosis, defined, 273t

Actinomycin-D, 415t

Active range-of-motion exercises and hemophilia, 411

Acute gastroenteritis, 474, 475t-476t

Acute poststreptococcal glomerulonephritis
  assessment of, 511
  description of, 510
  etiology of, 511
  evaluation of, 512
  home care of children with, 520
  management of, 512
  pathophysiology of, 511

AD-HD; *see* Attention deficit-hyperactivity disorder

Adolescent mothers
  grandparents as caregiver for newborn with, 220-221
  and pregnancy, 35
  support for, 217

Adrenal cortex, actions of, 559t

Adrenal medulla, actions of, 559t

Afterload, defined, 373

AIDS; *see* Acquired immune deficiency syndrome

Alcohol's effects on fetal growth and development, 14

Alleles, defined, 2

Amblyopia, 581t

Amniocentesis
  defined, 5
  in high-risk pregnancy, 74-76

Amniotic fluid
  assessment of features of, 137
  defined, 8

Amniotic membranes
  assessment of, 137-139
  defined, 8
  rupture before onset of labor, 194-195

Anemias
  aplastic, 408-409
  iron-deficiency, 401
  sickle cell, 404-408

Anesthesia
  administered during labor, 143t
  effect on blood pressure, 167
  general, 146t

L

Labor; *see also* Preterm labor and birth
 assessment of, 132-135
 augmentation of, 196
 childbirth techniques in, 133-134
 fetal descent during, 128-132
 interventions to facilitate, 131-132
 managing pain in, 139-140, 142t-146t
 maternal positions during, *148*
 and maternal stress, 183
 mechanism of, 130-131, *131-132*
 nursing diagnosis for complications of,
  201
 nursing implications of inducing,
  198t-199t
 passage of, 123, 128
 powers of
  primary, 120-123
  secondary, 123
 psychosocial reactions to, 147, 149
 rupture of membranes before onset of,
  194-195
 signs of, 119
 stages and phases of
  active, 124t, 126t, 147
  first, 124t-125t
  fourth, 127t, 157, 159-160
  latent, 124t, 125t, 147
  second, 125t-126t, 147
  third, 127t, 149
  transition, 125t, 126t, 147
 stimulation of process of, 196-197
 stressors of, 167
Laboratory tests of newborn, 294-297
Lactation, nutritional requirements during,
 64t-66t
Lanugo, defined, 291t
Large for gestational age, defined, 294
Laryngeal spasm, 436
Laryngotracheobronchitis
 acute, 439t
 assessment of, 438
 description of, 438
 etiology of, 438
 home care of children with, 455
 management of, 438
 pathophysiology of, 438
 progression of symptoms in, *440*
 treatment of, 438, 440
Latex allergy and spina bifida, 350

Leopold maneuvers
 defined, 55
 determining fetal heart sounds using,
  168, *169*
Leukemia
 assessment of, 412-414
 classification of, 412
 description of, 412
 etiology of, 412
 evaluation of, 417
 home care of children with, 421
 management of, 414, 417
 pathophysiology of, 412
 tissue involvement in, *413*
Levels of consciousness and neurologic
 status, *334*
Lightening
 defined, 119
 maternal discomforts caused by, 35
Lochia, 157, 159, 227t
Low birth weight
 AD-HD in children with, 575
 ineffective adaptation of neonate due
  to, 274t
 and infant mortality, 268
 and intrauterine stressors, 315
Low-risk pregnancy
 defined, 48
 fetal health assessment in, 50, 54-56
 laboratory tests for, 61t-63t
LTB; *see* Laryngotracheobronchitis
Lumbar puncture for diagnosing
 neurologic disorders, 338t

M

Macewen sign, 343
Magnesium sulfate, administration of,
 192t-193t
Magnetic imaging resonance for diagnosing
 neurologic disorders, 338t
Magnet reflex, 282t
Major burns, 584
Mast cell stabilizer, 433t
Mastitis, defined, 259
Maternal age
 and chromosomal abnormalities, 3
 parental attachment related to, 213
 recovery from birth related to, 216
Maternal health habits before and during
 pregnancy, 13-14